Contemporary Endoscopic Spine Surgery

(Volume 3)

Advanced Technologies

Edited by

Kai-Uwe Lewandrowski
Center For Advanced Spine Care
Tucson
Arizona
USA

Jorge Felipe Ramírez León
Fundación Universitaria Sanitas
Clínica Reina Sofía – Clínica Colsanitas
Centro de Columna – Cirugía Mínima Invasiva
Bogotá, D.C.
Colombia

Anthony Yeung
University of New Mexico
School of Medicine
Albuquerque
New Mexico, USA

Assistant Editors

Hyeun-Sung Kim
Department of Neurosurgery
Nanoori Gangnam Hospital
Seoul
Republic of Korea

Xifeng Zhang
Department of Orthopedics
First Medical Center
PLA General Hospital
Beijing 100853
China

Gun Choi
Neurosurgeon and Minimally Invasive Spine Surgeon
President Pohang Wooridul Hospital
South Korea

Stefan Hellinger
Department of Orthopedic Surgery
Arabellaklinik
Munich
Germany

Álvaro Dowling
Endoscopic Spine Clinic
Santiago
Chile

Contemporary Endoscopic Spine Surgery

(Volume 3)

Advanced Technologies

Editors: Kai-Uwe Lewandrowski, Jorge Felipe Ramírez León and Anthony Yeung

Assistant Editors: Hyeun-Sung Kim, Xifeng Zhang, Gun Choi, Stefan Hellinger and Álvaro Dowling

ISSN (Online): 2810-952X

ISSN (Print): 2810-9538

ISBN (Online): 978-981-5051-54-4

ISBN (Print): 978-981-5051-55-1

ISBN (Paperback): 978-981-5051-56-8

need for a court order if at any point you breach any terms of this License Agreement. In no event will any delay or failure by Bentham Science Publishers in enforcing your compliance with this License Agreement constitute a waiver of any of its rights.

3. You acknowledge that you have read this License Agreement, and agree to be bound by its terms and conditions. To the extent that any other terms and conditions presented on any website of Bentham Science Publishers conflict with, or are inconsistent with, the terms and conditions set out in this License Agreement, you acknowledge that the terms and conditions set out in this License Agreement shall prevail.

Bentham Science Publishers Pte. Ltd.
80 Robinson Road #02-00
Singapore 068898
Singapore
Email: subscriptions@benthamscience.net

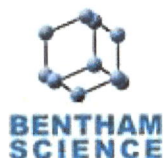

ENDORSEMENTS

ISASS

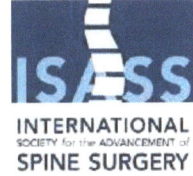

The International Society for the Advancement of Spine Surgery (ISASS; formerly The Spine Arthroplasty Society) has its roots in motion preservation as an alternative to fusion. Since then, it has worked to achieve its mission of acting as a global, scientific and educational society with a surgeon-centered focus. ISASS was organized to provide an independent venue to discuss and address the issues involved with all aspects of basic and clinical science of motion preservation, stabilization, innovative technologies, MIS procedures, biologics, and other fundamental topics to restore and improve motion and function of the spine. ISASS has a robust international membership of orthopedic and neurosurgery spine surgeons and scientists. ISASS is dedicated to advancing evolutionary and innovative spinal techniques and procedures such as endoscopic spine surgery. Every editor of Contemporary Endoscopic Spine Surgery represents ISASS as a member, author, reviewer, or editor of its quarterly circulation – The International Journal of Spine Surgery (IJSS). The contributors of *Contemporary Endoscopic Spinal Surgery* have succeeded in compiling an exhaustive and up-to-date reference text. It is an example of our society's mission pursuit of surgeon education and scientific study. It is my pleasure to endorse this comprehensive text on behalf of ISASS.

Domagoj Coric
President
International Society for the Advancement of Spine Surgery (ISASS)
Illinois
USA

SBC

SBC
Sociedade Brasileira
de Coluna

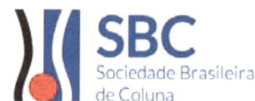

Founded on October 12, 1994, the Brazilian Spine Society (Sociedade Brasileira de Coluna - SBC) is a scientific, non-profit organization whose primary objective is the advancement of spine surgery through basic research and clinical study in orthopedics and neurosurgery. SBC is actively engaged in the accreditation and continued education of spine surgeons in Brazil. It prides itself on bringing the latest high-grade scientific evidence on novel technological advances and therapies to its professional members. SBC pursues this mission with its quarterly circulation Coluna/ Columna and its online courses, including Introduction to Endoscopy. The authors and editors of Contemporary Endoscopic Spine Surgery have put forward a comprehensive reference text essential to SBC's core curriculum of teaching spinal endoscopy to the next generation of surgeons. The presented clinical protocols for the endoscopic treatment of cervical and lumbar spine conditions are vetted and validated by peer-reviewed articles published by its contributors. It is my pleasure to endorse Contemporary Endoscopic Spine Surgery on behalf of the Brazilian Spine Society.

Cristiano Magalhães Menezes
President of the Brazilian Spine Society (Sociedade Brasileira de Coluna - SBC)
São Paulo
Brazil

MISS OF COA

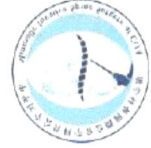

The Minimally Invasive Spine Surgery (MISS) of Chinese Orthopaedic Association (COA) was founded in 2003, which is one of the most special subsidiary societies of Chinese Medical Association, aiming to promote and develop minimally invasive orthopedics especially spine surgeries in China.

The MISS society organizes global discussions and encourages our members to participate international efforts and cooperation to improve surgeon education. With this mission in mind, it is my pleasure to endorse Contemporary Endoscopic Spine Surgery on behalf of the MISS of COA. Many international editors and contributors are from China, who have made great efforts, contributions and dedications to this book. They share with and update readers all over the world about the latest endoscopic spinal surgery techniques. I am confident that *Contemporary Endoscopic Spinal Surgery* can be a textbook for spine surgeons. It should be used as medical school advanced lessons materials for continuing education courses. In sum, it is my pleasure and honor to support it on behalf of the MISS of COA.

Huilin Yang
Chairman of MISS of COA
Professor & Chairman of Orthopedic Department
The First Affiliated Hospital of Soochow University
Suzhou
China

SICCMI

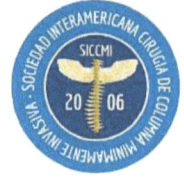

SICCMI (Sociedad Interamericana De Cirugia De Columna Minimamente Invasive) was founded in 2006 with similar objectives pursued by the editors of Contemporary Endoscopic Spine Surgery: the advancement and mainstreaming of minimally invasive spine surgery (MIS). SICMII members joined to implement MIS in all countries of South America, the Caribbean, Central America, and North America. Endoscopic surgery is performed by many of its key opinion leaders at the highest level, some of which have contributed to this multi-volume text. Four of the editors are active SICCMI members in leadership positions. The book contents are exhaustive and comprehensive, encompassing topics of the cervical and lumbar spine and advanced technology applications. Contemporary Endoscopic Spine Surgery will serve as SICCMI's core curriculum and course material for endoscopic surgery of the spine. It is my pleasure to endorse it on behalf of SICCMI.

President of SICCMI
Manuel Rodriguez
President-Elect of SICCMI, Department of Neurosurgery
ABC Medical Center
Ciudad de México, Mexico

SBMT

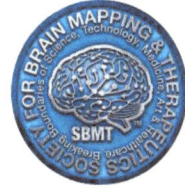

As a nonprofit organization, the Society for Brain Mapping and Therapeutics (SBMT) focuses on improving patient care by translating new technologies into life-saving diagnostic and therapeutic procedures. Contemporary Endoscopic Spine Surgery is a prime example of achieving excellence in education and scientific discovery. Authors and editors from around the globe came together to present the reader with the most up-to-date endoscopic spine surgery protocols and their supporting clinical evidence. SBMT has an active spine section led by productive innovator surgeons – some of which have demonstrated their leadership with their editorial contributions to *Contemporary Endoscopic Spinal Surgery*. The editors have embraced multidisciplinary collaborations across many cultural and geographic barriers. Their effort represents one of the core principles of SBMT's mission: to identify and bridge gaps in modern patient care with technological advances. It is my pleasure to endorse *Contemporary Endoscopic Spinal Surgery* on behalf of SBMT.

Babak Kateb
Founding Chairman of the Board of Directors
CEO and Scientific Director of SBMT
Californias
USA

SILACO

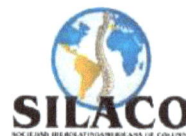

SILICO (Sociedad Ibero Latinoamericana de Columna) had its beginnings in the meetings of the Scoliosis Research Society with the first Hispano-American Congress held in 1991 in Buenos Aires Argentina. Since then, it has morphed into an organization that promotes the study of treatments and prevention of spinal conditions by bringing together spine care professionals from all subspecialties. The scientific activities of our biannual Ibero-Latin American Congress are focused on the promotion of surgeon education to the highest academic standards via international relationships between members from the Americas, Spain and Portugal.

Contemporary Endoscopic Spine Surgery resembles such a collaborative effort where authors worldwide have come together to update the reader on the latest endoscopic spinal surgery techniques.

SILACO has incorporated Contemporary Endoscopic Spine Surgery into its core curriculum and plans on using it as course material for its continuing education courses. It is my pleasure to endorse it on behalf of SILACO.

Jaime Moyano
President of SILACO
Editor Revista De Sociedad Ecuatoriana De Ortopedia y Traumatología
de la Sociedad Ecuatoriana De Ortopedia Y Traumatología
Quito, Ecuador

SOMEEC

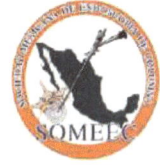

SOMEEC- Sociedad Mexicana de Endoscopia de Columna- is Mexico's prime organization uniting spine surgeons with a diverse training background having a fundamental interest in endoscopic surgery. SOMEEC organizes annual meetings where member surgeons and international faculty update each other on their latest clinical research to promote spine care *via* endoscopic spinal surgery technique. Two of the senior lead editors of *Contemporary Endoscopic Spinal Surgery* have been active international supporters of SOMEEC. I am pleased to endorse their latest three-volume reference text, which will become an integral centerpiece of SOMEEC's continuing medical educational programs.

Cecilio Quinones
Past President of the Sociedad Mexicana de Endoscopia de Columnas

KOSESS

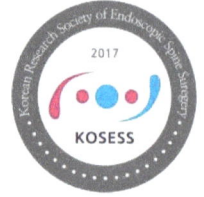

The Korean Research Society of Endoscopic Spine Surgery (KOSESS) was established in 2017. KOSESS was founded to bring endoscopic spine surgeons in the Republic of Korea together to advance the subspecialty of endoscopic spine surgery with high-quality clinical research. It is reflected in *Contemporary Endoscopic Spine Surgery* by the numerous contributions of Korean authors. It is *Contemporary Endoscopic Spine Surgery*. It is my pleasure to endorse it on behalf of KOSESS.

Hyeun-Sung Kim (Harrison Kim)
President of the Korean Research Society of the Endoscopic Spine Society
(KOSESS)
Seoul
Republic of Korea

KOMISS

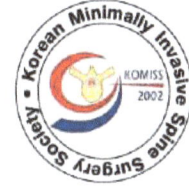

Since its establishment in 2002, the *Korean Minimally Invasive Spinal Surgery Society* (KOMISS) has had a leading role in developing new clinically applicable technologies to advance patient care with less invasive yet more effective therapies. The superiority of minimally invasive spine surgery in Korea is demonstrated by its competitiveness on the world stage at the highest academic level. It is reflected in *Contemporary Endoscopic Spine Surgery* by the numerous Korean authors who have contributed to this timely reference text with their groundbreaking clinical research on endoscopic spine surgery. I am proud of their accomplishments and want to congratulate them on acting as KOMISS ambassadors by carrying the message of Korean excellence in minimally invasive spinal surgery the world over within *Contemporary Endoscopic Spine Surgery*. It is my pleasure to endorse it on behalf of KOMISS.

Dae Hyun Kim
President of KOMISS
Seoul
Republic of Korea

NATIONAL ACADEMY OF MEDICINE OF COLOMBIA

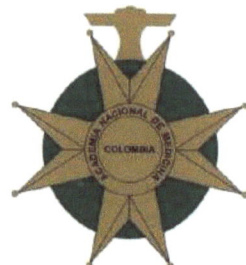

After reviewing the table of content and some representative chapters, I am happy to inform you that the Board of Directors of the National Academy of Medicine of Colombia grants academic endorsement of your book series entitled Contemporary Endoscopy Spine Surgery. Kai-Uwe Lewandrowski, Jorge Felipe Ramírez, and Anthony Yeung produced a text of great interest and scientific impact.

On behalf of the National Academy of Medicine, I would like to express my admiration and respect for your dedication to scientific research that led to this great work's culmination. It meets the high standards required by our National Academy to support such a production spearheaded by one of our most esteemed members - Dr. Jorge Felipe Ramírez.

Gustavo Landazabal Bernal
General Secretary
National Academy of Medicine of Colombia
Bogota, Colombia

IITS

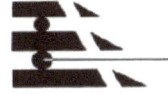

International Intradiscal Therapy Society

The International Intradiscal Therapy Society (IITS) was founded in 1987, initially headquartered in Belgium, Wisconsin, and led by Dr. Eugene Nordby, the first Executive Director of IITS. Members were primarily orthopaedic surgeons, anesthesiologists, radiologists, and rheumatologists dedicated to the treatment, research, and education involving The FDA-approved and validated level I studies that supported intradiscal spinal therapies.

From 2013-2017, the society began operating under International Intradiscal and Transforaminal Therapy Society (IITTSS) to reflect the advancements in endoscopic spine surgery augmenting Intradiscal therapy. The organization wanted to include and reflect the state-of-the-art evolution in intradiscal therapy with advances by intradiscal visualization of pain generators through the endoscope. However, the society reverted to IITS.

IITS now sponsors workshops on intradiscal therapy in conjunction with other International societies when it lost its original pharma support. IITS disseminates a newsletter to provide its membership, other healthcare professionals, and the general public information on the safest and cost-effective techniques to treat conditions such as herniated nucleus pulposus and other intradiscal spinal disorders.

IITS is a 501C3 non-profit organization whose focus is on intradiscal therapy aided by the endoscope as the least invasive, visually-guided treatment for discogenic pain, including extra-discal and complex foraminal decompression and stabilization procedures. The disc has been validated as the primary initial source of common back pain.

Two of the senior lead editors of Contemporary Endoscopic Spinal Surgery have been in active leadership roles in International Spine Organizations as consultants, full and associate professors, and directors. I am pleased to endorse their latest three-volume reference text, which will become integral to IITS' ongoing course programs.

Anthony Yeung
Executive Director of IITS
Desert Institute for Spine Care
Phoenix, Arizona
USA

SLAOT

SLAOT

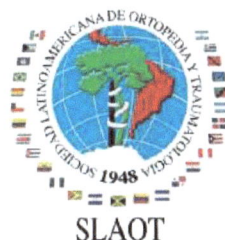

The Sociedad Latinoamericana de Ortopedia y Traumatologia (SLAOT)/ Latin American Society of Orthopaedics and Traumatology is a non-profit, autonomous, scientific organization of orthopaedic surgeons and orthopaedic care professionals. SLAOT has an organization structure that brings together professionals with a diverse scientific interest. It promotes continuous professional development and education at the highest level. *Contemporary Endoscopic Spine Surgery* is of interest to SLAOT because of its illustrative use of cutting-edge technology and discussion of validated clinical endoscopic spinal surgery protocols. It is my pleasure to endorse *Contemporary Endoscopic Spine Surgery* on behalf of SLAOT.

Horacio Caviglia
President of SLAOT FEDERACION
USA

CONTENTS

PREFACE

Spinal endoscopy is a technology-driven subspecialty of spinal surgery. The increased clinical traction and acceptance of minimally invasive endoscopic spinal surgery techniques result in successful technology transfers from other industries. Image quality in endoscopy is perceived by magnification, depth of field, resolution, color truth, and high image contrast, as well as low distortion and homogeneous illumination up to the edge of the image. The introduction of HD technology in 2005 to the general consumer market forced endoscope manufacturers to develop endoscopes that provided optimized image quality for the HD Video chain. Some of these technological advancements in 2000 coincided with the introduction of the endoscope into transforaminal spinal surgery. Newer clinical indications for endoscopic spine surgery are aimed to replace traditional translaminar surgeries. This expansion of the endoscopic spinal surgery platform is fueled by technology transfers from the space-, military- or consumer sector developments in the area of illumination, image quality, and high-definition video quality. It also hinges on the development of more durable and stress-resistant spinal endoscopes requiring continued expert surgeon input. Illustrating the application of these technological advancements in endoscopic spine surgery is at the heart of the third volume of the Bentham Series entitled *"Contemporary Endoscopic Spine Surgery."*

The editors have come together to develop a multi-authored and clinically focused medical monograph entitled *Contemporary Endoscopic Spine Surgery: Advanced Technologies* to give the reader a most up-to-date snapshot of the current and future technology advances in spinal endoscopy. The publication is intended for Orthopedic Spine & Neurosurgeons interested in treating common painful conditions of the spine with minimally invasive endoscopic techniques. A wide array of highly timely and clinically relevant topics have been assembled for this purpose. They range from the historical review of intradiscal therapies and foraminoplasty techniques, the discussion of the disruptive approach to personalized pain generator-oriented spine care *versus* population-based evidenced-based treatment strategies in context with modern clinical classification systems, the application of lasers, radiofrequency, and regenerative medicine strategies, the use of artificial intelligence and decision algorithms employed in the interpretation of advanced imaging studies to more accurately identify pain generators and their management with denervation and surgical strategies, the management of postoperative sequelae and complications, the indications for efficacious use of interspinous implants and fusion techniques, to the cost of implementing and maintaining a clinical endoscopic spine care program and advanced endoscopic technique for the most challenging clinical problems.

Future advances in clinical protocols will likely be driven by higher image quality standards that may provide the basis for artificial intelligence applications in image recognition, robotics, integration and automatization of surgical processes. *Contemporary Endoscopic Spine Surgery: Adavanced Technologies* was written with these trends in mind. The editors hope that the readers will find it an informative knowledge resource they will continue to revert to when implementing a lumbar endoscopic spinal surgery program in their practice setting.

Kai-Uwe Lewandrowski
Center for Advanced Spine Care of Southern Arizona
and
Surgical Institute of Tucson
Tucson, AZ
USA

Departmemt of Orthopaedics
Fundación Universitaria Sanitas
Bogotá, D.C.
Colombia

Department of Orthopedics at Hospital Universitário Gaffree
Guinle Universidade Federal do Estado do Rio de Janeiro
Rio de Janeiro
Brazil

Jorge Felipe Ramírez León
Fundación Universitaria Sanitas
Clínica Reina Sofía – Clínica Colsanitas
Centro de Columna – Cirugía Mínima Invasiva
Bogotá, D.C.
Colombia

Anthony Yeung
University of New Mexico
School of Medicine
Albuquerque
New Mexico
USA

List of Contributors

Álvaro Dowling	Department of Orthopaedic Surgery, USP, Ribeirão Preto, Brazil
André Luiz Calderaro	Centro Ortopedico Valqueire, Departamento de Full Endoscopia da Coluna Vertebral, Rio de Janeiro, Brazil
Anthony Yeung	University of New Mexico School of Medicine, Albuquerque, New Mexico Desert Institute for Spine Care, Phoenix, AZ, USA
Bu Rongqiang	Department of Orthopedics, Beijing Yuho Rehabilitation Hospital, Beijing, 100853, China
Byapak Paudel	Department of Neurosurgery, Nanoori Gangnam Hospital, Seoul, Republic of Korea Department of Orthopaedics & Traumatology, Grande International Hospital, Kathmandu, Nepal
Du Jianwei	Department of Orthopedics, Affiliated Hospital of Yangzhou University, Yangzhou, 225001, China
Friedrich Tieber	Medical Technologies Consulting, Augsburg, Germany
Hyeun-Sung Kim	Nonhyeon-dong, Gangnam-gu, Nanoori Hospital, Seoul, South Korea
Ibrahim Hussain	Department of Neurological Surgery, University of Miami, Miami, FL 33136, USA
Il-Tae Jang	Department of Neurosurgery, Nanoori Gangnam Hospital, Seoul, Republic of Korea
Jiang Letao	Department of Orthopedics, Affiliated Hospital of Yangzhou University, Yangzhou, 225001, China
Jorge Felipe Ramírez León	Orthopedic and Minimally Invasive Spine Surgeon; Reina Sofía Clinic and Center of Minimally Invasive Spine Surgery, Bogotá Colombia. Chairman, Spine Surgery Program, Universidad Sanitas, Bogotá, D.C., Colombia, USA
Juan Carlos Vera	Molecular Biotechnology Engineer-Universidad de Chile Business Development Manager-VidaCel, Chile
Kai-Uwe Lewandrowski	Center for Advanced Spine Care of Southern Arizona and Surgical Institute of Tucson, Tucson, AZ, USA Departmemt of Orthopaedics, Fundación Universitaria Sanitas, Bogotá, D.C., Colombia, USA Department of Neurosurgery in the Video-Endoscopic Postgraduate Program at the Universidade Federal do Estado do Rio de Janeiro, UNIRIO, Rio de Janeiro, Brazil
Lei-Ming Zhang	Department of Orthopedics, Beijing Yuho Rehabilitation Hospital, Beijing, 100853, China
Max Rogério Freitas Ramos	Federal University of the Rio de Janeiro State UNIRIO, Associate Professor of Orthopedics and Traumatology, Rio de Janeiro - RJ, Brazil Head of Orthopedic Clinics at Gaffrée Guinle University Hospital HUGG, Rio de Janeiro - RJ, Brazil

Michael Y. Wang Professor of Neuosurgery Department of Neurological Surgery, University of Miami, Miami, FL 33136, USA

Narendran Muraleedharan Basme Aptus Engineering, Inc, Scottsdale, Arizona, and Multus Medical, LLC, Phoenix, Arizona, USA

Nicholas A Ransom Director of Endoscopic Spine Clinic, Orthopaedic Spine Surgeon, Santiago, Chile

Nitin Maruti Adsul Department of Neurosurgery, Nanoori Gangnam Hospital, Seoul, Republic of Korea
Sir Ganga Ram Hospital, Ortho-Spine Surgery, New Delhi, India

Paulo Sérgio Teixeira de Carvalho Department of Neurosurgery, Universidade Federal do Estado do Rio de Janeiro, Rio de Janeiro, Brazil

R. Cantú-Leal Department of Spine Surgery, Hospital Christus Muguerza Alta Especialidad in Monterrey, Mexico

R. Cantu-Longoria Orthopaedic Spine Surgeon, Hospital Christus Muguerza Alta Especialidad, Villa Alegre C.P. 64130 Monterrey. N.L, Mexico

Sandeep Shah Multus Medical, LLC, Phoenix, Arizona, USA

Stefan Hellinger Department of Orthopedic Surgery, Arabellaklinik, Munich, Germany

Vikram Sobti Innovative Radiology, PC, River Forest, Illinois, USA

Vincent Hagel Asklepios Hospital Lindau, Spine Center, Lindau, Germany

Xifeng Zhang Department of Orthopedics, First Medical Center, PLA General Hospital, Beijing 100853, China
Department of Orthopedics, Beijing Yuho Rehabilitation Hospital, Beijing, 100853, China

The History and Future Value of Endoscopic Intradiscal Therapy and Foraminoplasty

Anthony Yeung[1] and **Kai-Uwe Lewandrowski**[2,3,4]

[1] *Clinical Professor, University of New Mexico School of Medicine, Albuquerque, New Mexico, Desert Institute for Spine Care, Phoenix, AZ, USA*

[2] *Center for Advanced Spine Care of Southern Arizona and Surgical Institute of Tucson, Tucson AZ, USA*

[3] *Departmemt of Orthopaedics, Fundación Universitaria Sanitas, Bogotá, D.C., Colombia, USA*

[4] *Department of Neurosurgery in the Video-Endoscopic Postgraduate Program at the Universidade Federal do Estado do Rio de Janeiro — UNIRIO, Rio de Janeiro, Brazil*

Abstract: The utilization of spinal endoscopic surgery techniques is on the rise in routine clinical practice and treating painful annular tears, herniated disc, and spinal stenosis. Over the past ten years, we have witnessed an increasing number of surgeons recognizing spinal endoscopy's value. Many of them had difficulty finding access to adequate training while facing reimbursement and acceptance problems. In this chapter, the authors describe the implementation issues at play that they perceive as relevant in the discussion between the healthcare equation's stakeholders. Included in this chapter on the forward-looking perspective of spinal endoscopy is the first author's involvement in the role and value of laser and electrothermal therapy, which is still pertinent but has evolved with advancements in technology and endoscopes and instrumentation.

Keywords: Endoscopic surgery, Foraminoplasty, History & Future, Intradiscal therapy.

INTRODUCTION

Surgeons and surgically trained non-surgeons will advance the future success of endoscopic spinal surgery. The number of endoscopic and minimally invasive spinal surgeries has been predicted to increase the spine surgery market at a compound annual growth rate of 7.57 percent between 2016 and 2020 in North America and Europe alone [1]. The explosion of endoscopic spine surgeries in

---

* **Corresponding author Anthony Yeung**: Clinical Professor, University of New Mexico School of Medicine, Albuquerque, New Mexico, Desert Institute for Spine Care, Phoenix, AZ, USA and ; E-mail: ayeung@sciatica.com

Asia has been recently illustrated by analyzing the country of residence of the authors of scholarly articles published in peer-reviewed SCI(E) journals within the last five years [2]. Authors from China, South Korea, the USA, Germany, and Japan have published the vast majority of papers. The most prolific authors came from a few number of well-recognized institutions, including the Wooridul Spine Hospital in Seoul, South Korea, The Tongji University and the Third Military Medical University in China, the University of Witten/Herdecke in Germany, Brown University, The Center For Advanced Spine Care of Southern Arizona, and from the Desert Institute of Spine Care, Phoenix, in the USA. Endoscopic spinal surgery is expected to become more mainstream globally by increasingly augmenting or replacing traditional open spinal surgeries with less aggressive procedures that are less invasive but equally, if not more beneficial to the patient.

The expanding number of indications that surgeons now identify as appropriate for endoscopic treatment of the spine's common degenerative conditions suggest that there is more to it than merely miniaturizing incisions and performing surgery under local anesthesia sedation. The direct visualization of the intradiscal pathology, pathology in the epidural space, and neural elements in the axilla allow for the diagnosis of pain generators that previously have not been visualized and recognized as treatable conditions. Even more relevant is the ability to correlate the pathophysiology of pain with visualized pathoanatomy with the endoscope. Examples include toxic and painful annular tears, epidural adhesions, scar tissue, and inflammatory granulomas. Other pain inducing patho-anatomy include superior foraminal ligament and facet impingement, facet joint cysts and impaction, tethering of the nerve roots to the pars interarticularis, the pedicles or the intertransverse membrane. Inflammatory irritation of the annulus, posterior longitudinal ligament, lateral and shoulder osteophytes (Tables **1** and **2**), and a myriad of endoscopically visualized intradiscal conditions ranging from fissuring, delamination of the endplates, to gaseous degeneration of the intervertebral disc leaving it hollow, and void of any functional tissues round out the myriad of patho-anatomy documented with the endoscope (Fig. **1**) [3].

With current diagnostic tools, including radiographs, computed tomography (CT), and magnetic resonance imaging (MRI), these conditions are difficult to establish before surgery. These pain generators may be insufficiently imaged with routine preoperative studies or just not included in imaging reporting by the radiologist, hence, leaving a large portion of patients that by new measures are considered either "too young," or "too old" or having too much surgical morbidity without surgical treatment of their painful conditions. However, it will be in this grey area where highly qualified and experienced providers will use the endoscope to correlate the pathophysiology of the patients' symptoms with intraoperatively visualized pathoanatomy that can be decompressed, ablated, thermally modulated, and irrigated to provide pain relief from chemical as well as mechanical irritation and structural defects.

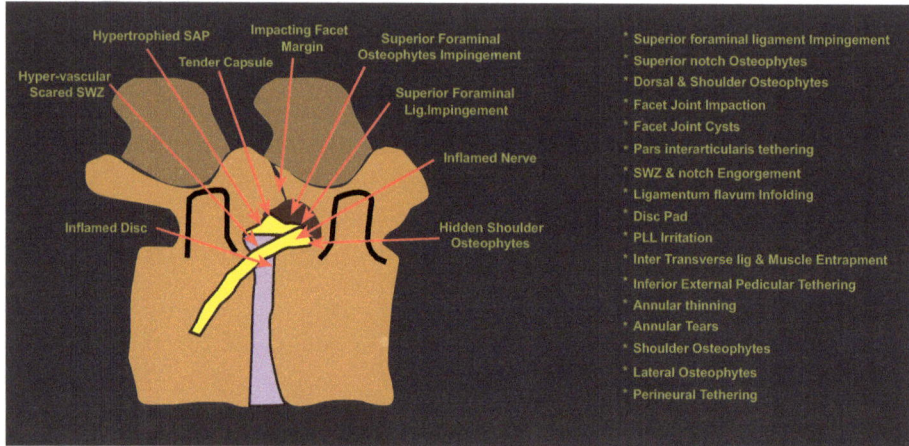

Fig. (1). Illustration of 9 common, and 19 endoscopically documented painful conditions and their anatomic locations in the foramen.

Table 1. Nine common endoscopically lumbar conditions visualized during foraminoplasty.

- Inflammed disc
- Inflammed nerve
- Hypervascular scar
- Hypertrophies superior articular process (SAP), ligamentum flavum impingement
- Tender capsule
- Impacting facet margin
- Superior foraminal facet osteophyte
- Superior foraminal ligament impingement
- Hidden shoulder osteophyte

Table 2. Additional conditions visualized during routine lumbar endoscopy.

- Symptomatic foraminal scar tissue
- Facet joint impingement
- Facet joint cysts
- Parts defect tethering
- PLL irritation
- Annular thinning and tears
- Perineural tethering by scar
- Various foraminal osteophytosis locations
- Endplate tethering and impingement

This endoscopic surgical platform's success depends on the practitioner's cumulative clinical and intraoperative experiences, validated by the direct correlation of a responsive patient under modern monitored anesthesia care (MAC), and recorded response to the endoscopic surgery [4]. Rather than relying on a surgical plan that is deducted mainly from preoperative imaging studies, which by definition limit the list of plausible pain generators virtually only to instability and neural impingement, the clinical approach to employing spinal endoscopy relies on the personalized and individualized diagnostic workup of each patient with much greater attention to detail of the relevant patho-anatomy and its pathophysiological role in the patient's pain syndrome.

Invariably, this not only leads to less aggressive but also to earlier, staged, interventions. Rather than waiting for the advanced clinical end-stage of the degenerative condition to develop, treating pain generators in the early stages of the degeneration of the lumbar motion segment, in the authors' opinion, will be the largest area of expansion of endoscopic spinal surgery. The senior author with 29 years of experience, and early clinical involvement in chymopapain and laser clinical research, has demonstrated his approach to identifying pain generators intraoperatively by interactive feedback with the patient along with surgical case examples with recorded audio and video feedback available for viewing on youtube.com and his website (www.sciatica.com). The viewer will follow the authors' editorialized opinions on performing endoscopic surgery on the sedated yet awake patient's relevant pain generators in these videos. In this chapter, a historical review on the evolution and value of the various intradiscal therapies, including laser and electrothermal technologies and foraminoplasty, is provided as experienced first-hand by the first author.

THE POLITICS, BUSINESS, AND REIMBURSEMENT FOR ENDOSCOPIC SPINE SURGERY

Internationally, spinal endoscopy is already accepted and practiced extensively in Asia. However, its recognition as a mainstream method to treat common degenerative conditions of the spine lags in North America and Europe. A recent opinion survey amongst 430 spine surgeons the world over corroborated this statement [5 - 7]. Surgeons in Asia reported fewer hurdles to implementation, less concern with the cost of capital equipment and disposables, fewer problems with health insurance authorization, and fewer problems with rejection by the medical establishment in their respective countries [8]. Surgeons in North America, and Europe on the other hand, were not only by far fewer, but they were also chiefly concerned with low reimbursement and fear of being called out for operating outside the norms established by the coverage and treatment guidelines of their national professional societies, the health insurance industry, and local governing bodies [5, 7, 8]. Some of these concerns were also echoed by surgeons from Latin America who reported better overall acceptance of endoscopic spinal surgery into the mainstream than surgeons from North America and Europe [5]. These responding surgeons from the Americas and Europe were keenly aware of their advanced endoscopic spinal surgery program colliding with established treatment guidelines by challenging the necessity of aggressive and extensive open spinal surgeries which they are seeking to replace with small targeted endoscopic interventions. This dynamic creates a conflict of opinions and conflict between the stakeholders of this ongoing debate. They represent various economic and political agendas in the healthcare industry as a whole. It is the makeup of the politics of medicine. The high responsiveness of surgeons to the surveys cited herein clearly shows how keenly aware spine surgeons seeking to innovate their clinical practice are of this debate [5 - 8].

The three elephants in the room silently partaking in this ongoing discussion whether spinal endoscopy is "too experimental, too costly, and unproven" on the one hand, or "cutting edge, cost saver, and advanced medicine" on the other hand are the stakeholders in the health insurance, hospital, and medical device industry. All three may have a competing economic interest in the revenue cycle of medicine, which ultimately impacts the surgeon innovator's ability to justify the cost of implementation. The burden of proof of its economic viability is typically placed on the practitioner in the context of clinical superiority. While it is easy to understand that medical device companies are looking to grow sales with innovative products and directly or indirectly contribute to the rise in healthcare costs, even if the individual products and services may help outcomes and make accepted procedures achieve better outcomes, health insurance companies are held to a higher moral standard as they are expected to operate as a real business but should do it to benefit their insured in an economically viable manner. Therefore, most health insurance companies have formulated extensive medical coverage guidelines and implemented a vigorous preauthorization of service bureaucracy to facilitate appropriate utilization without abuse. These coverage guidelines are typically based on a comprehensive review of the evidence-based literature, which is often graded by its quality as level I – high-quality randomized trial or prospective study (RCT), level II - lesser quality RCT; prospective comparative study; retrospective study; untreated controls from an RCT; lesser quality prospective study; development of diagnostic criteria on consecutive patients; sensible costs and alternatives and meta-analysis, level III - case-control study (therapeutic and prognostic studies); retrospective comparative study, level IV - Case series; case-control study (diagnostic studies); poor reference standard; analyses with no sensitivity analyses, and level V – personal opinion. By definition, evidence-based medicine analyzes the effectiveness of various protocols in managing disease in a population as a whole. Simultaneously, such an approach to determine the medical necessity of an intervention or surgery of the spine is at odds with the personalized approach to spine care with endoscopy. All accepted levels of evidence begin with level 5 expertise. Therefore, the evidence-based medicine approach, which may be appropriate for determining drug-based therapies' effectiveness, seems rather ill-fitted for modern personalized spine care that does not fit the double-blind level 1 and 2 trials criteria. Furthermore, contrary to its intent, it may increase the cost by mandating rigid sequential care protocols with ineffective services before definitive care with endoscopic surgery is deemed indicated. To this author's surprise, this dilemma was even recognized by the SPORT trial authors who recently accepted the need for more patient-specific, individualized tools for presenting clinical evidence on treatment outcomes [9] after their initial studies suffered from a high percentage of patient crossover [10, 11].

It is evident that the current debate suffers from intersectional barriers between the stakeholders with business illiteracy on the surgeons' side, and a lag of medical accolades on the commercial and regulatory side where the parties involved simply do not have sufficient knowledge of each other's expertise to the extent that innovation could be vetted more expeditiously and implemented if proven safe, efficacious, and cost-effective regardless of the health care market dynamics in an individual country. This dynamic has played out in Asia, where private reimbursement is not as critical, and there is government-provided health care. Acceptance of spinal endoscopy into the mainstream in North America and Europe will depend on how this debate will be steered by payer systems and by the traditional open surgery-oriented spine surgeons skeptical of percutaneous and endoscopic procedures that they are not trained to perform and are competing with their successful traditional techniques [12].

It is clear though that the U.S. Department of Health and Human Services via its Centers for Medicare & Medicaid Services (CMS) is incentivizing institutions and surgeons alike to move simple spinal decompressions from being performed as an inpatient to an outpatient ambulatory surgery center (ASC) to provide more cost-effective, high-value spine care. New current procedural terminology (CPT) codes have been allowed to perform many spinal surgeries in ASC [13]. In 2017, The American Medical Association (AMA) for the first time included a new spinal endoscopy CPT code (62380) [14]. The new code covers endoscopic decompression of the spinal cord, nerve root, including laminotomy, partial facetectomy, foraminotomy, discectomy, and excision of a herniated intervertebral disc, one lumbar interspace [15]. However, CMS did not assign a final value to CPT 62380 in its final 2017 ruling instead of assigning contractor pricing. Effectively, this means that each Medicare Administrative Contractor (MAC) will set reimbursement determination [16]. As a result, it remains to be seen how this endoscopic CPT role plays out in each healthcare market with sufficient reimbursement for the facility- and professional fee being of concern for ASCs and surgeons. Ultimately, spinal endoscopy is intended to replace more costly open inpatient spinal surgeries. However, financial disincentives may come to bear mainly if the actual reimbursement of endoscopic procedures is lower than the procedures it replaces, and if capital equipment and disposable cost are insufficiently covered. The authors expect that this transition from open to endoscopic procedures will not be swift. Slow embracement of spinal endoscopy by mainstream spinal surgeons in North America and Europe coupled with low reimbursement and lack of formal inclusion into coverage and treatment guidelines will leave the field by default to a smaller group of endoscopic surgeons and multidisciplinary pain management and rehabilitation physicians who do not have nor accept the need for additional surgery training. The latter is simply needed and required for the procedure to be mainstream. Endoscopic spinal surgeons must demonstrate that the procedures they adopt remain safe, efficient, and practical or more effective than the current contemporary techniques they are trying to replace [17].

THE REASON WHY ENDOSCOPIC SPINE SURGERY SHOULD REQUIRE HIGH STANDARDS

U.S. regulatory approval is not needed for physicians to perform endoscopic spinal surgery since physicians are licensed and are overseen by their medical boards, and not the Food and Drug Administration (FDA) who does not regulate the practice of medicine. Credentialing of core privileges at hospitals and surgery centers typically requires that the surgeon presents evidence of having had training in the surgeries she or he is intending to perform. Examples of this include kyphoplasty and fusion surgeries. Kyphoplasty became popular in the United States 20 years ago and gained significant traction 15 years ago. Fusion surgeries have seen a similar rise in utilization within the same time frame. While it is understandable that hospitals require training in more complex and riskier fusion surgeries, having to show evidence of training in kyphoplasty as a by far less aggressive procedure may not seem evident to surgeons. Spinal endoscopy may fall in a similar category where surgery through a small incision may be considered as a smaller, less risky surgery that can be carried out by nearly anyone who had some postgraduate residency or fellowship training in neuro- or orthopedic spinal surgery. This is not the case in endoscopic spine surgery. The casual approach to training future expert surgeons capable of executing endoscopic spinal surgeries in a highly reliable and consistent manner is inappropriate. Many KOLs have published results of their clinical series after many years of trial and error practice to hone in their skills in mastering this demanding procedure that by many is recognized to have a steep learning curve and may not be for everyone [17]. Integration of formal spinal endoscopy training into the core curriculum of neurosurgical and orthopedic residency program should be not just considered but required, and will most likely remain part of the debate.

Besides the complex technical aspects of spinal endoscopy, there is the issue of understanding its indications and surgical principles of best clinical practice. There is no doubt that spinal endoscopy is not merely replacing existing surgeries and their standard clinical indications to the authors. The intradiscal and epiduroscopic visualization during spinal endoscopy has and will continue to recognize pain generators either hitherto unknown or ignored because of the lack of adequate diagnostic and treatment protocols (Fig. **2**) [17]. In other words, it is a new world distinctly different from traditional spine surgery that is simply focused on relieving neural element compression in consideration of instability and deformity; a new world that requires any practitioner embarking on the spinal endoscopy voyage to think differently, and to become familiar with the in's and out's of a successful endoscopic spine practice. At its core, a successful endoscopic spine practice requires close investigative interaction with the patient to treat the pain generator causing the disability [17].

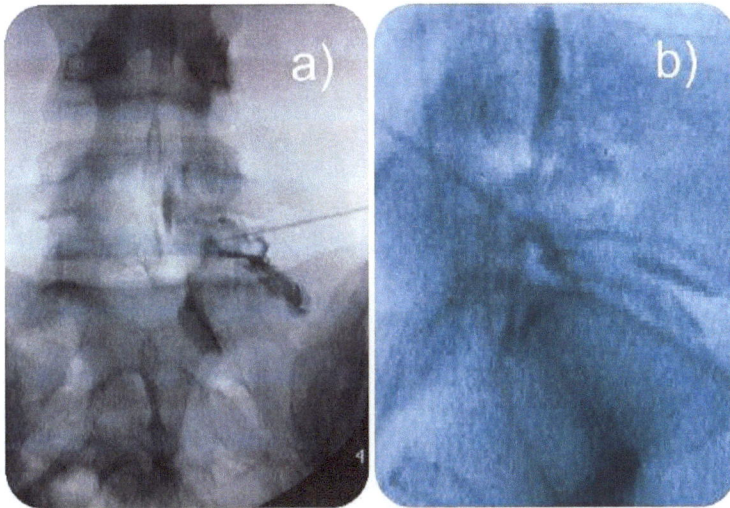

Fig. (2). a) Epidurogram of paracentral HNP demonstrating blockage of the traversing nerve **b)** epidural gram and incidental discogram. The leakage of contrast identifies and extruded HNP. A therapeutic injection providing good relief provides a good prognosis for endoscopic decompression.

In that sense, the endoscopic spine technology's successful application employs new concepts that are "*disruptive*" to traditional degenerative spine surgery concepts. In the authors' opinion, open surgery for many of the degenerative conditions of the spine are appropriate, but has the propensity to be more surgically aggressive than required and may be associated with greater collateral damage from associated muscle de-innervation and the destabilizing effects of the decompression. Ultimately, postoperative adjacent segment disease and epidural fibrosis may add to additional disability and more follow-up surgeries, which in the patients' minds seems outdated and creates apprehensions before spine surgery [18]. The patients demand us to do better by modernizing the approach to managing their sciatica-type low back- and leg pain or their cervical and thoracic pain syndromes. Patient demand, coupled with a push by government and payers to develop more reliable, less complicated, and "less costly" ways to manage the socioeconomic impact of spine-related pain syndrome. Pain management, however, is NOT a minimally invasive subspecialty of surgical pain care.

In current practice, authorization for health insurance coverage of surgical indications is primarily dependent on interpreting the CT and MRI imaging by the reading radiologist [19]. When the radiologist's report "on paper" does not support the treatment requested by the surgeon, denial for a preauthorization insurance company for surgery is often the consequence. This disconnect between these traditional protocols run by payers and governmental review boards and protocols used by the "disruptive" spine surgeon has the potential to lead to significant undertreatment. This has recently been corroborated in a study that found that up to 30% of patients who underwent successful endoscopic decompression for a lumbar herniated disc and spinal stenosis were classified as MRI false negative [19]. These MRI false-negative patients underwent successful surgery with a resolution of symptoms despite the MRI report suggesting that stenosis was not present at the surgical level. Therefore, the Interventional Pain Management Surgery approach will require the definition and validation of more useful clinical prognosticators of a successful outcome after endoscopic spinal surgery [19].

THE ROLE OF INJECTIONS AS PROGNOSTICATORS OF OUTCOME

The interpretation of preoperative advanced imaging studies may be further validated and documented by discography, transforaminal epidurography, and transforaminal therapeutic epidural steroid injections (TESI) containing a local anesthetic, or transforaminal foraminal nerve root blocks by injecting just a local anesthetic to identify the pain generator (Fig. 2). Diagnostic transforaminal injections containing a local anesthetic are an excellent prognosticator of favorable outcomes after a lumbar transforaminal decompression procedure. The concepts of developing new prognosticators of successful surgical outcomes lie in the pathophysiology's correlation with the intraoperative endoscopic visualization of the patho-anatomy responsible for the patient's pain. Correlation between the patient's response to a preoperative interventional work with lidocaine containing TESI has been conclusively demonstrated in a recent study carried out over nine years [20]. Of the 1839 patients, 1750 had intraoperatively visualized stenosis in the lateral recess at the surgical level, and 89 patients did not. The analysis showed true positive (1578); false negative (172), as compared with TESI responses in patients without visualized compressive pathology: false positive (26); and true negative (63). The sensitivity (90.17%), specificity (70.79%), and the positive predictive value (98.38%) of preoperative lidocaine containing TESI concerning the successful clinical outcome of the subsequent endoscopic decompression surgery were calculated. This study demonstrated that diagnostic lidocaine containing transforaminal epidural steroid injection – if it produces more than fifty percent VAS pain score reduction – is a valuable diagnostic tool in predicting improved clinical outcomes after lumbar endoscopic transforaminal decompression.

The only person able to validate this correlation intraoperatively in close interaction with the sedate yet awake patient is the surgeon. The surgeon's evaluation and validation of the preoperative prognosticators, whether imaging studies or diagnostic injections, during surgery cannot be replaced by any other technological prognosticator. Since pain relief relies on the correlation between the pathophysiology and the intraoperatively visualized patho-anatomy for each patient's specific condition, a successful outcome depends on this critical patient surgeon interaction. It cannot be replaced by a rule book of medical necessity criteria or by rigid adherence to advanced imaging reporting discounting the importance of the interaction between the patient and the surgeon [21, 22].

THE ROLE OF IMPROVED ENDOSCOPES AND INSTRUMENTATION

Historically, companies marketing spinal endoscopes, endoscopic- devices, and instruments had to budget significant money for training to stimulate their sales. Advances in endoscopes and surgical equipment will also help the development and adoption of endoscopic surgery [23, 24]. The development of endoscopic implants for the spine may further galvanize the push towards endoscopic spine surgery, particularly if viable reimbursement is associated with these procedures. The feasibility of a stand-alone lumbar interbody fusion cage being placed entirely using an endoscope and instruments adopted for the percutaneous endoscopic transforaminal placement of the cage into the spine has recently been demonstrated [25]. It is evident that creating sustainable revenue cycles for physicians and facilities is needed to retool clinical practices from traditional open to minimally invasive endoscopic spinal surgeries.

THE ROLE OF PHYSICIAN AND CERTIFICATION

For a surgeon to achieve success in the future subspeciality of Endoscopic Surgical Pain Care employing the "disruptive" techniques of correlating patho-anatomy and pathophysiology of pain generators, providers who embrace these spinal endoscopy principles should have surgical training. They should also:

1. Continue research and development of the endoscopic platform. Examples of future impactful developments include intraoperative robotic mechanical and image recognition guidance.

2. Continue to develop endoscopic designs and instrumentation to improve surgeon effectiveness and competence.

3. Support commercially viable manufacturing, marketing, distribution, and training operations to facilitate the expansion of spinal endoscopy to be incorporated into mainstream postgraduate training at a contemporary level.

All physicians who employ spinal endoscopy must be adequately and formally trained. Ideally, surgeon training moves away from weekend cadaver courses run by vendors. It should be included in the core curriculum of neurosurgical and orthopedic residency programs and, at a minimum, be taught in MIS spine fellowship programs. The most effective way to formalize training in spinal endoscopy is to establish standards for certification. The formalization of such minimum required standards for certification and skill level in spinal endoscopy may be challenging to define. It will most likely continue to be at the center of the debate. Despite this perceived difficulty, it is essential and will be demanded by licensing and neurosurgical and orthopedic governing boards for them to be able to endorse it.

THE PATIENT'S POINT OF VIEW & PLACEMENT OF SPINAL ENDOSCOPY

Patients who can seek the best surgeons and are often willing to pay cash and supplement what is not covered by insurance, for not just the best endoscopic surgeons, but surgeons with a known track record for safety and excellent clinical results [26]. Such surgeons will be sought out, similar to recruiting the best professional athletes. Cultural biases may also influence patients in their quest to search out the most appropriate way to treat spine pain. Asians, for example, have accepted specific methods of non-traditional medicine for thousands of years. One can only speculate whether the higher acceptance of alternative medicine in Asia has made it easier for spinal endoscopy in Asian countries to be adopted widely. Every culture has its own biases toward ethnic methods such as Asian alternative medicine methods, including acupuncture, exercise, massage, stretching techniques, reflexology, and naturopathic medicine [27]. Hence, other ethnic groups may have their level of acceptance and methodologies.

In the authors' opinion, the verdict is straightforward: Innovation in medicine in general, besides many other factors, requires money. Therefore, acceptance of endoscopic procedures and technologies as a "surgical" procedure or minimally invasive spinal surgical technique rather than interventional pain management is the most appropriate way to place a fair monetary value on its application, implementation, and expansion into day-to-day clinical practice. Adoption by the majority of surgeons and their respective professional governing boards and specialty societies will depend upon its continued safety, low complication rates, and effectiveness with ongoing innovation. These three factors will always heavily depend on each physician's skills [27, 28].

CONCLUSION

Spinal endoscopy will likely become more mainstream in the years to come. Formalized postgraduate training programs are expected to improve training, helping surgeons to master the learning curve. The substantiation of clinical guidelines should follow to formalize payment schedules that provide adequate reimbursement to build viable endoscopic spinal surgery programs capable of replacing traditional open spinal surgery protocols.

CONSENT FOR PUBLICATION

Not applicable.

CONFLICT OF INTEREST

The authors declare no conflict of interest, financial or otherwise.

ACKNOWLEDGEMENT

Declared none.

REFERENCES

[1]   Adam Schrag. 20 things to know about minimally invasive spine surgery. 2017. https://www.beckersspine.com/mis/item/35569-20-things-to-know-about-minimally-invasive- spine-surgery.html

[2]   Kim JS. A bibliometric study in the field of percutaneous full-endoscopic spine surgery since 1997. Annual NASS Meeting 2018, Los Angeles After Hours: Endoscopic Spine Surgery: Current Trends & Evidence of Spinal Endoscopic Procedures. 2018.

[3]   Pan F, Shen B, Chy SK, *et al.* Transforaminal endoscopic system technique for discogenic low back pain: A prospective Cohort study. Int J Surg 2016; 35: 134-8.
[http://dx.doi.org/10.1016/j.ijsu.2016.09.091] [PMID: 27693825]

[4]   Yeung AT. Lessons learned from 27 years' experience and focus operating on symptomatic conditions of the spine under local anesthesia: the role and future of endoscopic spine surgery as a "disruptive technique" for evidenced based medicine. J Spine 2018; 7: 413.

[http://dx.doi.org/10.4172/2165-7939.1000413]

[5]   Lewandrowski KU, Soriano-Sánchez JA, Xifeng Z, *et al.* Regional variations in acceptance, and utilization of minimally invasive spinal surgery techniques among spine surgeons: results of A global survey. J Spine Surg 2018; 6(Suppl 1): S260-74.

[6]   Lewandrowski KU, Soriano-Sánchez JA, Xifeng Z, *et al.* Surgeon motivation, and obstacles to the implementation of minimally invasive spinal surgery techniques: results of a global survey. J Spine Surg 2018; 6(Suppl 1): S249-59.

[7]   Lewandrowski KU, Soriano-Sánchez JA, Xifeng Z, *et al.* Surgeon training and clinical implementation of spinal endoscopy in routine practice: results of a global survey. J Spine Surg 2018; 6(Suppl 1): S237-48.

[8]   Lewandrowski KU. Kim-JS, Yeung AT. Is Asia truly a hotspot of contemporary minimally invasive and endoscopic spinal surgery? Results of a global survey. J Spine Surg 2018; 6(Suppl 1): S224-36.

[9]   Moulton H, Tosteson TD, Zhao W, *et al.* Considering Spine Surgery: A Web-Based Calculator for Communicating Estimates of Personalized Treatment Outcomes. Spine 2018; 43(24): 1731-8.
        [http://dx.doi.org/10.1097/BRS.0000000000002723] [PMID: 29877995]

[10]   Weinstein JN, Lurie JD, Tosteson TD, *et al.* Surgical vs nonoperative treatment for lumbar disk herniation: the Spine Patient Outcomes Research Trial (SPORT) observational cohort. JAMA 2006; 296(20): 2451-9.
        [http://dx.doi.org/10.1001/jama.296.20.2451] [PMID: 17119141]

[11]   Weinstein JN, Tosteson TD, Lurie JD, *et al.* Surgical vs nonoperative treatment for lumbar disk herniation: the Spine Patient Outcomes Research Trial (SPORT): a randomized trial. JAMA 2006; 296(20): 2441-50.
        [http://dx.doi.org/10.1001/jama.296.20.2441] [PMID: 17119140]

[12]   Yeung AT, Roberts A, Shin P, Rivers E, Paterson A. Suggestions for a Practical and Progressive Approach to Endoscopic Spine Surgery Training and Privileges. J Spine 2018; 7: 414.
        [http://dx.doi.org/10.4172/2165-7939.1000414]

[13]   Yeung AT. The Yeung Percutaneous Endoscopic Lumbar Decompressive Technique (YESSTM). J Spine 2018; 7: 408.
        [http://dx.doi.org/10.4172/2165-7939.1000408]

[14]   Hignite J. Understanding the Impact of the CMS 2017 ASC Payment Rule on Spine Procedures. 2016. https://www.beckersspine.com/spine/item/34156-understanding-the-impact-of-the-cms--017-asc-payment-rule-on-spine-procedures.html

[15]   AMA includes 1st endoscopic spine surgery code in 2017 codebook: 6 things to know. 2017. https://www.beckersspine.com/orthopedic-a-spine-device-a-implant-news/item/33-03-ama-includes-1st-endoscopic-spine-surgery-code-in-2017-codebook-6-things-to-know.html

[16]   Issues CMS. Final physician fee schedule: what spine surgeons should know. 2017. https://www.isass.org/awp/wp-content/uploads/2016/11/Final-2017-PFS-Rule-Summary.pdf

[17]   Wang B, Lü G, Patel AA, Ren P, Cheng I. An evaluation of the learning curve for a complex surgical technique: the full endoscopic interlaminar approach for lumbar disc herniations. Spine J 2011; 11(2): 122-30.
        [http://dx.doi.org/10.1016/j.spinee.2010.12.006] [PMID: 21296295]

[18]   Hersht M, Massicotte EM, Bernstein M. Patient satisfaction with outpatient lumbar microsurgical discectomy: a qualitative study. Can J Surg 2007; 50(6): 445-9.
        [PMID: 18053372]

[19]   Lewandrowski KU. Retrospective analysis of accuracy and positive predictive value of preoperative lumbar MRI grading after successful outcome following outpatient endoscopic decompression for lumbar foraminal and lateral recess stenosis. Clin Neurol Neurosurg 2019; 179: 74-80.
        [http://dx.doi.org/10.1016/j.clineuro.2019.02.019] [PMID: 30870712]

[20] Lewandrowski KU. Successful outcome after outpatient transforaminal decompression for lumbar foraminal and lateral recess stenosis: The positive predictive value of diagnostic epidural steroid injection. Clin Neurol Neurosurg 2018; 173: 38-45.
[http://dx.doi.org/10.1016/j.clineuro.2018.07.015] [PMID: 30075346]

[21] Yeung AT, Yeung CA, Salari N, Field J, Navratil J, *et al.* Lessons Learned Using Local Anesthesia for Minimally Invasive Endoscopic Spine Surgery. J Spine 2017; 6: 377.
[http://dx.doi.org/10.4172/2165-7939.1000377]

[22] Yeung AT. *In-vivo* Endoscopic Visualization of Pain Generators in the Lumbar Spine. J Spine 2017; 6: 385.
[http://dx.doi.org/10.4172/2165-7939.1000385]

[23] Yeung A, Yeung CA. Endoscopic identification and treating the pain generators in the lumbar spine that escape detection by traditional imaging studies. J Spine 2017; 6: 369.

[24] Yeung AT. Transforaminal endoscopic decompression for painful degenerative conditions of the lumbar spine: a review of one surgeon's experience with over 10,000 cases since 1991. J Spine Neurosurg 2017; 6: 2.

[25] Lewandrowski KU. Surgical technique of endoscopic transforaminal decompression and fusion with a threaded expandable interbody fusion cage and a report of 24 cases. J Spine 2018; 7: 2.
[http://dx.doi.org/10.4172/2165-7939.1000409]

[26] Yeung AT. Delivery of spine care under health care reform in the united states. J Spine 2017; 6: 372.
[http://dx.doi.org/10.4172/2165-7939.1000372]

[27] Yeung AT. Intradiscal therapy and transforaminal endoscopic decompression: opportunities and challenges for the future. J Neurol Disord 2016; 4: 303.
[http://dx.doi.org/10.4172/2329-6895.1000303]

[28] Yeung AT. Enhancement of KTP/532 laser disc decompression and arthroscopic microdiscectonmy with a vital dye. Proc SPIE 1880, Lasers in Orthopedic, /dental and /veterinary. Medicine (Baltimore) 1993.
[http://dx.doi.org/10.111/12.148334]

CHAPTER 2

Evidence Based Medicine *versus* Personalized Treatment of Symptomatic Conditions of the Spine Under Local Anesthesia: the Role of Endoscopic *versus* Spinal Fusion Surgery as a "Disruptive" Technique

Anthony Yeung[1] and **Kai-Uwe Lewandrowski**[2,3,4]

[1] *Clinical Professor, University of New Mexico School of Medicine, Albuquerque, New Mexico, Desert Institute for Spine Care, Phoenix, AZ, USA*

[2] *Center for Advanced Spine Care of Southern Arizona and Surgical Institute of Tucson, Tucson AZ, USA*

[3] *Departmemt of Orthopaedics, Fundación Universitaria Sanitas, Bogotá, D.C., Colombia, USA*

[4] *Department of Neurosurgery in the Video-Endoscopic Postgraduate Program at the Universidade Federal do Estado do Rio de Janeiro — UNIRIO, Rio de Janeiro, Brazil*

Abstract: Runaway cost for surgical spine care has led to increased scrutiny on its medical necessity. Consequently, the beaurocracy involved in determining coverage for these services has grown. The call for high-grade clinical evidence dominates the debate on whether endoscopic surgery has a place in treating painful conditions of the aging spine. The cost-effectiveness and durability of the endoscopic treatment benefit are questioned every time technology advances prompt an expansion of its clinical indications. The authors of this chapter introduce the concept of early-staged management of spine pain and make the case for personalized spine care focused on predominant pain generators rather than image-based necessity criteria for surgery often applied in population-based management strategies. The authors stipulate that future endoscopic spine care will likely bridge the gap between interventional pain management and open spine surgery. This emerging field of interventional endoscopic pain surgery aims to meet the unanswered patient demand for less burdensome treatments under local anesthesia and sedation. The very young and old patients often are ignored because their conditions are either not bad enough or too advanced for a successful outcome with traditional spine care. In this watershed area of spine care, the authors predict endoscopic spine surgery will thrive and carve out accepted surgical

* **Corresponding author Kai-Uwe Lewandrowski:** Center for Advanced Spine Care of Southern Arizona and Surgical Institute of Tucson, Tucson, AZ, USA, Department of Orthopaedic Surgery, UNIRIO, Rio de Janeiro, Brazil and Department of Orthoapedic Surgery, Fundación Universitaria Sanitas, Bogotá, D.C., Colombia, USA; Tel: +1 520 204-1495; Fax: +1 623 218-1215; E-mail: business@tucsonspine.com

indications in direct competition with pain management and traditional open spine fusion protocols.

Keywords: Endoscopy future, Pain generators, Personalized spine care, Staged endoscopic pain management.

INTRODUCTION

Clinical treatment guidelines are reflected in the health insurance industry's medical necessity and coverage rules. Many organizations and their "key opinion" leaders (KOLs) structure their medical and surgical treatments' narrative based on consensus finding and peer-reviewed articles. Health care, in general, is becoming more and more regulated and reliant on subsidies by the government or payers, making payments dependent on compliance with their treatments- and coverage guidelines and thereby increasing the bureaucracy in the delivery of healthcare on the backend to the individual patient. Bureaucratic hurdles have created more significant headwinds on the front end of the medical innovation cycle that effectively hamper the dissemination and publication of original and pioneering literature, which by definition starts with low-level V research and expert opinions. This low- level evidence is often unable to survive the rigorous review process of a medical publishing system geared towards publishing higher-level studies. Surgeon innovators often lack resources, institutional, and funding support to conduct prospective randomized single or multicenter trials. Even if able to orchestrate those trials, researchers in academic institutions are dependent on NIH or institutional support to get their clinical research published. Publication fees associated with many open-access Journals and the bureaucracy associated with traditional journals often requiring institutional review board (IRB) approval before submitting even low-level retrospective studies. This dynamic may pose additional unintended hurdles to disseminating novel and disruptive information, which is often created under the premise of reining in runaway healthcare cost.

In spine surgery, introducing new evidence in support of novel treatments can be particularly challenging since it is always compared to evidence relying on fusion as the ultimate solution. Combining these factors may hinder the entry of innovative clinical information into the mainstream peer-reviewed literature because spine surgeons, especially in a private practice setting, are too busy dealing with the increasing non-clinical and managerial workload while trying to pay clinical practice overhead. Academic surgeons may have institutional support, but the new challenges in endoscopic spine surgery can be daunting, whether in an academic or private setting. Endoscopic spine surgery is innovative but lacks traditional evidence-based criteria of conventional spine surgery for several reasons. First, the number of surgeons performing endoscopic spine surgery is still significantly less than surgeons performing traditional and other forms of translaminar minimally invasive spinal surgeries. The objectives of endoscopic spine surgery are different from other forms of spine surgery since it focuses on the patient's individual needs for their painful patho-anatomy of the spinal motion segment rather than treating pain syndromes from overt instability or severe spinal stenosis, which lends itself better for the study of outcomes and cost-effectiveness of lumbar spine surgery in a large population of patients. Third, by definition, endoscopic spine surgery is "disruptive" to the evidence-based medicine (EBM) study approach since there are many more study variables due to a large number of concurrent pain generators that are not considered for treatment with other forms of lumbar spine surgery. Taking all this into consideration, it comes as no surprise that true level I and II studies investigating the merits of endoscopic spine surgery are rare. In awake patients, randomization is not possible. Even level I and II studies are subject to different interpretations by academicians and payors. Most patients cannot receive meaningful treatment until their symptoms are out of control and all non-operative measures have failed. The many patients that cannot find help by institutionalized surgeons turn to alternative medicine and pain management to control their symptoms. Surgery is usually reserved for more severe conditions supported by traditionally accepted imaging studies.

TREATMENT NECESSITY RATIONALES

Radiologic imaging is alone often unable to explain the pain that does not meet medical necessity criteria for surgery. A lumbar MRI scan has been demonstrated not to correlate with the severity and low back pain duration [1]. In the treating physician's and surgeon's judgment, the disability may not be severe enough for consideration by traditional surgeons, especially when the risk and benefits of established spinal treatments and surgeries are factored in. Pain management treatments with narcotics, helpful or not, as well as a multitude of alternative medicine remedies, and durable medical equipment (DME) are often overutilized. For example, braces and home traction devices such as inversion tables are sold without prescription and are typically not covered by insurance. Some payors allow for chiropractic care. The concepts employed in endoscopy spine surgery are disruptive and will likely continue to be disruptive to our current established scientific validation system on large patient populations. If performed expertly and adequately, superior outcomes with endoscopic spine care can be provided in a more cost- effective and less burdensome manner both to the patient and the health care system as a whole.

INSURANCE AUTHORIZATION

Rigid adherence to established protocols may impact reimbursement for endoscopic spine surgery [2]. Payers and insurance companies deny reimbursement for experimental procedures or those which lack level I or II evidence and do not recognize expert opinion [3]. Insurance companies also employ many means to deny reimbursement and fail to honor contracts using arbitrary criteria of post-preauthorization denial of payment for services rendered to patients – many of whom benefited and were rendered pain-free because of the "out-of-the-box" approach with targeted endoscopic procedures. The rigid EBM approach to spine care could delay implementing more cost-effective, innovative technologies – all of which start with level V expert opinions. On the other hand, having high-grade clinical evidence is not a guarantee that a procedure is implemented. One such example is chymopapain. The supporting evidence is high-grade, but was largely ignored. It fell out of favor [4]

THE PERSONALIZED MEDICINE APPROACH

Symptomatic conditions of the spine can be endoscopically evaluated. At the same time, most patients may eventually be taken seriously, mainly if they continue to complain of debilitating pain or are realistic about the anticipated surgical results [5]. Contrary to traditional spine care, where the patient's disability is attempted to be treated in one intervention, the personalized approach to endoscopic spine care takes into account that multiple pain generators may exist with varying degrees of pain and disability. At times it can be confusing as surgeon and patient are trying to prioritize spine care to attend to the most painful condition. Other pain generators may exist and become clinically relevant at a later time in a different functional context. Personalized spine care revolves around these staged management concepts and is embraced by endoscopic visualization and therapy. It has been the first author's focus for 28 years [6].

THE SOCIETAL BURDEN

The cumulative effect of aging in the spine may lead to pain [7]. Validating pain generators early on can be accomplished with diagnostic injections. Ineffective and expensive spine care can be avoided by incorporating endoscopically visualized procedures earlier in the disease process rather than waiting until the underlying degenerative condition progresses to its end-stage, where aggressive and costly fusion surgeries are considered the only option [8, 9]. Directly visualizing and treating the pain generator is the key element of endoscopic spine surgery than any other form of spine surgery cannot replicate [10]. When done under local anesthesia, verbal feedback from the patient during surgery can be incorporated into intraoperative decision-making as to the goal of the operation has been completed. This approach truly represents a personalized patient-centered approach to modern spine care. It is disruptive to the classic evidenced-based approach, whose many concepts were derived from data mining across a sizeable patient population under strict inclusion and exclusion criteria, discounting the detailed intraoperative endoscopic visualization of the painful pathology for each patient. While the EBM insurance coverage guidelines put many patients on a path to under-treatment because the treatments of their painful conditions are deemed a "non-covered" service or their condition is not bad enough by the standards established by the insurance industry, many patients nowadays opt-out of the EBM discussion by seeking out recognized experts and paying them cash. In the opinion of these authors, cash payments will become more acceptable to patients as the cost for insurance coverage and out-of-pocket expenses go up, making outpatient spine care in an ambulatory surgery center (ASC) more competitive, and in some cases, the only option for patients who face increasing hurdles set up in the bureaucracy of traditional inpatient spine care [11, 12]. The implementation of InterQual medical necessity criteria [13] with yearly updates is one example of cost containment measures limiting patients' access to spine care unless there is acute and severe deterioration of neurological function due to overt trauma, instability and spinal cord or cauda equina compression. Elective surgical treatment for a herniated disc and spinal stenosis is preceded by complex pathways and decision trees that have to be satisfied before surgical treatment is granted as medically necessary – a process that weeds out a large number of symptomatic patients as non-surgical candidates committing them to medical pain management which also has become under fire in the context of the opioid crisis in the United States [14 - 17]. Endoscopic visualization of the painful spinal motion segment affords the ability to simplify and breakdown the patient's sciatica low back and leg pain syndrome and to correlate the symptoms to specific structural problems including annular tears, foraminal and lateral recess stenosis due to ligament hypertrophy, facet cysts, tethering of the nerve roots the posterior longitudinal ligament, foraminal ligaments, and intradiscal disc degeneration causing fissuring of the nucleus or delamination from the endplates to name a few. Other clinically relevant information from history and physical examination, imaging studies, preoperative diagnostic injections, and intraoperative epidurogram is used to determine the best course of action. A context-driven spine care model should be applied to determine the need for endoscopic spinal surgery for each patient realizing this decision is more about what not to treat rather than what to treat in the aging spine with multi-level degenerative disease. Prioritizing this type of care by identifying the most predominant pain generator with the described protocol is one of the most challenging aspects of personalizing and tailoring the endoscopic spine surgery approach to the needs of each patient. Functional context is just as important as advanced imaging and diagnostic injection. Relying only on imaged based criteria for endoscopic decompression of the spine is likely the single most inaccurate prognosticator of beneficial intervention and would reintroduce many patients into the cycle of pain management, thus, avoiding definitive early treatment, further contributing to the opioid crisis focusing on managing pain rather than treating the underlying structural problem [8, 18 - 25]. Successful clinical outcomes from the endoscopic visualized spine pain treatment hinge on locating the pain generator correctly because of the small size of the endoscopically treated area. Identifying and directing endoscopy to validated pain generators requires good judgment and experience [26].

Endoscopic visualization of the painful spinal motion segment affords the ability to simplify and breakdown the patient's sciatica low back and leg pain syndrome and to correlate the symptoms to specific structural problems including annular tears, foraminal and lateral recess stenosis due to ligament hypertrophy, facet cysts, tethering of the nerve roots the posterior longitudinal ligament, foraminal ligaments, and intradiscal disc degeneration causing fissuring of the nucleus or delamination from the endplates to name a few. Other clinically relevant information from history and physical examination, imaging studies, preoperative diagnostic injections, and intraoperative epidurogram is used to evaluate and validate the patient's complaint. However, imaging by itself is inadequate to explain complaints of symptoms that may or may not be debilitating in the physician's judgment, and the patient may be dismissed merely or prescribed a drug to mitigate the complaint [26]. This reintroduces the patient into the cycle of pain management by avoiding definitive treatment, thus, contributing to the opioid crisis focusing on pain rather than treating the underlying structural problem.

SPINAL PAIN GENERATORS

Symptoms may sometimes be distorted by other underlying conditions and therefore be misinterpreted by the treating physician. Opioids are often employed to mitigate pain. A spinal work-up is often prompted if the patient presents with weakness and other nerve-mediated symptoms in addition to pain [27]. Pain is typically related to inflammation and weakness to compression of neural elements. The latter requires decompression and the former treatment of the conditions that causes inflammation. Autoimmune diseases may be involved [28]. Patients with peripheral neuropathy may also present with nerve root compression symptoms. Hence, they may benefit from the endoscopic treatment protocols described above. Hyperactivity conditions of the peripheral nerves stemming from the dorsal and ventral ramus may also be excruciating [29]. Patients may represent multiple concurrent painful conditions. Therefore, diagnostic and therapeutic injections are the most reliable way to determine whether image evidence of neural element compression would respond favorably to endoscopic decompression [29, 30].

DISCUSSION

Operating on validated pain generators is key to making endoscopic spine surgery work. Developing protocols focusing on correlating preoperative imaging studies with intraoperatively visualized pathology is key to creating plausible evidence to substantiate the role of endoscopic surgery. In the elderly, these protocols often ignore other pathologies demonstrated on MRI scans. The break with image-based criteria has to be substantiated with other predictors of a successful outcome with the endoscopic surgery compared to open surgery. The use of local anesthesia and sedation may be a key element in determining intraoperatively which of the visualized pathology needs treatment of what kind. The current literature has barely scratched the surface of this complex dynamic. Future research needs to focus on developing more reliable predictors of good surgical outcomes with intervention as image-based criteria have a low predictive value of a positive result.

Most patients should not require a primary fusion surgery at the index level. In the future, endoscopic spine surgery will likely see an expansion of its validated clinical indications. Its safety, efficacy, and cost-effectiveness have been demonstrated. This minimally invasive technique has the potential to bridge the enormous gap between aggressive surgical and all other forms of interventional and non-operative spine care. Patients may elect to pay out of pocket if their health insurance plans do not cover these services. Unfortunately, many spine surgeons are reluctant to provide care to the very old and very young patients. Painful conditions may lack structural correlates fitting their traditional medical necessity criteria for surgery or may be so advanced that only ultra-aggressive spinal fusion surgeries would be indicated but are deemed inappropriate because of old age or poorly controlled medical comorbidities.

CONCLUSION

Endoscopic procedures are expected to extend spine care to the very young and the very old by offering simplified, less burdensome procedures. It may also allow for treating patients at the earlier stage of the degenerative spine disease since approach-related problems such as postoperative scarring or instability are much less likely to occur. Direct visualization of spinal pain generators at high magnification within a diseased spinal motion segment is the key element that distinguishes endoscopic from traditional spinal surgery. It enables the surgeon to diagnose and treat during the same sitting. Surgeon's skill level will determine the extent of endoscopic treatments to be attempted. On average, it will take an inexperienced novice spine surgeon five years to become proficient enough to transition the majority of their practice into endoscopic spine care [10].

CONSENT FOR PUBLICATION

Not applicable.

CONFLICT OF INTEREST

The authors declare no conflict of interest, financial or otherwise.

ACKNOWLEDGEMENT

Declared none.

REFERENCES

[1]   Borenstein DG, O'Mara JW Jr, Boden SD, *et al.* The value of magnetic resonance imaging of the lumbar spine to predict low-back pain in asymptomatic subjects : a seven-year follow-up study. J Bone Joint Surg Am 2001; 83(9): 1306-11.
[http://dx.doi.org/10.2106/00004623-200109000-00002] [PMID: 11568190]

[2]   Higgins JP, Altman DG, Gøtzsche PC, *et al.* Cochrane Statistical Methods Group. The Cochrane Collaboration's tool for assessing risk of bias in randomised trials. BMJ 2011; 343: d5928.

[3]   Chou R, Deyo R, Friedly J, *et al.* Systematic pharmacologic therapies for low back pain: A systematic review of an American College of Physicians clinical practice guideline. Ann Intern Med 2017; 166(7): 480-92.
[http://dx.doi.org/10.7326/M16-2458] [PMID: 28192790]

[4]   Al-Tamimi P. The functional and economic outcome of lumbar discectomy: A comparative study of fenestration discectomy *versus* hemilaminectomy and discectomy. J Spine 2017; 6(4): 1-8.
[http://dx.doi.org/10.4172/2165-7939.1000379]

[5]   Yeung AT. The yeung percutaneous endoscopic lumbar decompressive technique (YESSTM). J Spine 2018; 7(1): 408.
[http://dx.doi.org/10.4172/2165-7939.1000408]

[6]   Yeung AT. Transforaminal endoscopic decompression for painful degenerative conditions of the lumbar spine: A review of one surgeon's experience with over 10,000 cases since 1991. J Spine Neurosurg 2017; 6: 266.

[7]   Yeung AT, Kotheeranurak V. Transforaminal endoscopic decompression of the lumbar spine for stable degenerative spondylolisthesis as the least invasive surgical treatment using the YESS surgery technique. Int J Spine Surg 2018; 12(3): 408-14.
[http://dx.doi.org/10.4172/2165-7939.1000407]

[8]   Lewandrowski KU. Successful outcome after outpatient transforaminal decompression for lumbar foraminal and lateral recess stenosis: The positive predictive value of diagnostic epidural steroid injection. Clin Neurol Neurosurg 2018; 173: 38-45.
[http://dx.doi.org/10.1016/j.clineuro.2018.07.015] [PMID: 30075346]

[9]   Lewandrowski KU. Readmissions After Outpatient Transforaminal Decompression for Lumbar Foraminal and Lateral Recess Stenosis. Int J Spine Surg 2018; 12(3): 342-51.
[http://dx.doi.org/10.14444/5040] [PMID: 30276091]

[10]   Yeung AT. *In-vivo* endoscopic visualization of pain generators in the lumbar spine. J Spine 2017; 6(4): 385.
       [http://dx.doi.org/10.4172/2165-7939.1000385]

[11]   Yeung A, Yeung CA. Endoscopic identification and treating the pain generators in the lumbar spine that escape detection by traditional imaging studies. J Spine 2017; 6: 369.

[12]   Yeung AT, Yeung CA, Salari N, Field J, Navratil J, Maio H. Lessons learned using local anesthesia for minimally invasive endoscopic spine surgery. J Spine 2017; 6(4): 377.
       [http://dx.doi.org/10.4172/2165-7939.1000377]

[13]   Mitus AJ. The birth of InterQual: evidence-based decision support criteria that helped change healthcare. Prof Case Manag 2008; 13(4): 228-33.
       [http://dx.doi.org/10.1097/01.PCAMA.0000327413.01849.04] [PMID: 18636008]

[14]   Zolot J. A Worsening Opioid Epidemic Prompts Action. Am J Nurs 2017; 117(10): 15.
       [http://dx.doi.org/10.1097/01.NAJ.0000525858.52569.e6] [PMID: 28957912]

[15]   Cheatle MD. Facing the challenge of pain management and opioid misuse, abuse and opioid-related fatalities. Expert Rev Clin Pharmacol 2016; 9(6): 751-4.
       [http://dx.doi.org/10.1586/17512433.2016.1160776] [PMID: 26933873]

[16]   Hupp JR. The surgeon's roles in stemming the prescription opioid abuse epidemic. J Oral Maxillofac Surg 2016; 74(7): 1291-3.
       [http://dx.doi.org/10.1016/j.joms.2016.05.001] [PMID: 27156949]

[17]   Kee JR, Smith RG, Barnes CL. Recognizing and reducing the risk of opioid misuse in orthopaedic practice. J Surg Orthop Adv 2016; 25(4): 238-43.
       [PMID: 28244866]

[18]   Lurie JD, Tosteson TD, Tosteson A, *et al.* Long-term outcomes of lumbar spinal stenosis: eight-year results of the Spine Patient Outcomes Research Trial (SPORT). Spine 2015; 40(2): 63-76.
       [http://dx.doi.org/10.1097/BRS.0000000000000731] [PMID: 25569524]

[19]   Devin CJ, Chotai S, Parker SL, Tetreault L, Fehlings MG, McGirt MJ. A cost-utility analysis of lumbar decompression with and without fusion for degenerative spine disease in the elderly. Neurosurgery 2015; 77 (Suppl. 4): S116-24.
       [http://dx.doi.org/10.1227/NEU.0000000000000949] [PMID: 26378349]

[20]   Adogwa O, Parker SL, Shau DN, *et al.* Cost per quality-adjusted life year gained of revision neural decompression and instrumented fusion for same-level recurrent lumbar stenosis: defining the value of surgical intervention. J Neurosurg Spine 2012; 16(2): 135-40.
       [http://dx.doi.org/10.3171/2011.9.SPINE11308] [PMID: 22054639]

[21]   Piper K, DeAndrea-Lazarus I, Algattas H, *et al.* Risk factors associated with readmission and reoperation in patients undergoing spine surgery. World Neurosurg 2017; 110: e627-35.

[22]   Su AW, Habermann EB, Thomsen KM, Milbrandt TA, Nassr A, Larson AN. Risk Factors for 30-Day Unplanned Readmission and Major Perioperative Complications After Spine Fusion Surgery in Adults: A Review of the National Surgical Quality Improvement Program Database. Spine 2016; 41(19): 1523-34.
       [http://dx.doi.org/10.1097/BRS.0000000000001558] [PMID: 26967124]

[23]   Kim BD, Smith TR, Lim S, Cybulski GR, Kim JY. Predictors of unplanned readmission in patients undergoing lumbar decompression: multi-institutional analysis of 7016 patients. J Neurosurg Spine 2014; 20(6): 606-16.
       [http://dx.doi.org/10.3171/2014.3.SPINE13699] [PMID: 24725183]

[24]   Modhia U, Takemoto S, Braid-Forbes MJ, Weber M, Berven SH. Readmission rates after decompression surgery in patients with lumbar spinal stenosis among Medicare beneficiaries. Spine 2013; 38(7): 591-6.
       [http://dx.doi.org/10.1097/BRS.0b013e31828628f5] [PMID: 23324923]

[25]   Kocher KE, Nallamothu BK, Birkmeyer JD, Dimick JB. Emergency department visits after surgery are common for Medicare patients, suggesting opportunities to improve care. Health Aff (Millwood) 2013; 32(9): 1600-7.
[http://dx.doi.org/10.1377/hlthaff.2013.0067] [PMID: 24019365]

[26]   Yeung AT. Endoscopic decompression for degenerative and isthmic spondylolisthesis. J Neurol Disord 2017; 5(6): 371.
[http://dx.doi.org/10.4172/2329-6895.1000371]

[27]   Yeung AT. The role of endoscopic surgery in the treatment of painful conditions of an aging spine: State of the Art. J Neurol Disord 2017; 5(6): 372.
[http://dx.doi.org/10.4172/2329-6895.1000372]

[28]   Yeung AT. Selective endoscopic discectomy™ twelve years' experience. In: Kambin P, Ed. Atlas of Arthroscopic and Endoscopic Spinal Surgery, Text and Atlas. 2nd ed., Totowa, NJ, USA: Humana Press, Inc. 2006.

[29]   Yeung AT, Yeung CA, Zheng Y. Endoscopic decompression, ablation and irrigation: A minimally invasive surgical technique for painful degenerative conditions of the lumbar spine. 2010.

[30]   Gore S, Yeung A. The "inside out" transforaminal technique to treat lumbar spinal pain in an awake and aware patient under local anesthesia: results and a review of the literature. Int J Spine Surg 2014; 8: 28.
[http://dx.doi.org/10.14444/1028] [PMID: 25694940]

CHAPTER 3

How to Generate the Superiority Evidence for Endoscopic Surgery for Common Lumbar Degenerative Conditions

Kai-Uwe Lewandrowski[1,2,3,*], **Jorge Felipe Ramírez León**[4] and **Anthony Yeung**[5]

[1] *Center for Advanced Spine Care of Southern Arizona and Surgical Institute of Tucson, Tucson AZ, USA*

[2] *Associate Professor of Orthopaedic Surgery, Universidad Colsanitas, Bogota, Colombia, USA*

[3] *Visiting Professor, Department Orthopaedic Surgery, UNIRIO, Rio de Janeiro, Brazil*

[4] *Centro de Columna – Cirugía Mínima Invasiva. Bogotá, D.C., Colombia, Clínica Reina Sofía – Clínica Colsanitas. Bogotá, D.C., Colombia, Fundación Universitaria Sanitas , Bogotá, D.C., Colombia, USA*

[5] *Clinical Professor, University of New Mexico School of Medicine, Albuquerque, New Mexico Desert Institute for Spine Care, Phoenix, AZ, USA*

Abstract: Endoscopic spinal surgery affords the patient simplified and less burdensome spine care. Its superiority over open decompression surgeries has been long debated, and the current evidence is incomplete. The innovators and proponents of this procedure carry the burden of proof. The targeted endoscopic treatment of common spinal pain generators produces higher perioperative patient satisfaction than traditional spine surgery. This chapter discusses conventional spine surgery research's pros and cons of employing patient-reported outcome measures (PROM). They offer an alternative approach to establishing a better value proposition with the endoscopic *versus* open spinal surgery - the concept of durability analysis.

Keywords: Clinical evidence, Outcome analysis, Spinal endoscopy, Statistics.

THE BURDEN OF PROOF

Endoscopic spine surgery is undoubtedly on the rise in many developed countries [1 - 3]. This trend is fueled by technological advances and favorable clinical

* **Corresponding author Kai-Uwe Lewandrowski:** Center for Advanced Spine Care of Southern Arizona and Surgical Institute of Tucson, Tucson, AZ, USA, Department of Orthopaedic Surgery, UNIRIO, Rio de Janeiro, Brazil and Department of Orthoapedic Surgery, Fundación Universitaria Sanitas, Bogotá, D.C., Colombia, USA; Tel: +1 520 204-1495; Fax: +1 623 218-1215; E-mail: business@tucsonspine.com

Kai-Uwe Lewandrowski, Jorge Felipe Ramírez León, Anthony Yeung, Gun Choi, Stefan Hellinger and Álvaro Dowling (Eds.)

studies supporting its routine clinical use [4]. However, its critics still torment the lack of sufficient high-grade evidence to acknowledge its role in a modern degenerative spine practice, and some of them may never embrace it regardless [5, 6]. Since the burden of proof is on the proponents of endoscopic spinal surgery, the question raises how to demonstrate its efficacy and perhaps even areas of superiority over traditional open and other forms of minimally invasive spinal surgery techniques. Typically, there is a call for prospective randomized trials to deliver on the request for high-grade clinical evidence [5]. However, as we will outline below, this is not all that practical at times, and even the well-funded multicenter studies around the Spine Outcome Research Trial (SPORT) [7 - 10] or the Surgical Timing In Acute Spinal Cord Injury Study (STASCIS) [11] failed to provide the high-grade evidence they were designed to provide. Nevertheless, this type of evidence is frequently requested by payors and review boards to establish the medical necessity for endoscopic surgery. Repeated calls for this high-grade clinical evidence reappear when the cost of capital equipment purchases, disposables, and additional training is considered, which seemingly contributes to the escalating cost of spine care. This gap between the available clinical evidence - most of which is level III evidence comprised of retrospective endoscopic case series and a few Level I and II prospective randomized trials published comparing endoscopic- *versus* microsurgical decompression - and the need to demonstrate the clinical value preposition in endoscopic surgery poses the question how to accomplish that best.

Several authors have attempted to bridge this evidence gap by orchestrating high-grade evidence studies. For example, Ruetten [12 - 14], Komp [15, 16], and their respective team have published their results with the full endoscopic lumbar decompression for lateral recess stenosis *versus* conventional microsurgical technique 2009 [12]. In their randomized prospective controlled trial, which included some 161 patients, they were able to show similar clinical outcomes employing the German version of the North American Spine Society instrument and the Oswestry low back pain disability questionnaire. In different studies on 178 patients, the same authors reported complete leg pain relief in 82% of the patients' two-year follow-up. Only 14% of their patients complained of some occasional pain, with the overall clinical outcomes being similar between traditional microdiscectomy and full endoscopic discectomy, including recurrence rates of 6.2%. Hence, they believed that full-endoscopic techniques are of higher value than conventional decompression techniques since it provides significant advantages, including less back pain, improved rehabilitation, fewer complications, and less traumatization. However, they also recognized the need for objective data to support this notion. In 2011, Ruetten and his team attempted to close that gap by reporting on 87 patients with recurrent herniation after conventional discectomy. These patients underwent full-endoscopic or microsurgical intervention, and again similar clinical outcomes with a 79% success rate and re-recurrence rate of 5.7% were reported [16].

Several authors employed the meta-analysis tool in an attempt to provide high-grade evidence on spinal endoscopy. For example, Birkenmeier et al. compared controlled clinical trials on endoscopic and microsurgical standard procedures [17]. In 2013, his review of full-endoscopic interlaminar and transforaminal approaches for all spinal regions initially included 504 PubMed and Embase listed articles. Ultimately, four randomized controlled trials (RCTs) and one controlled study (CS) were identified that met the inclusion eligibility criteria. Stratifying these studies for randomization, inclusion and exclusion criteria, clinical outcomes, and complications, Birkenmeier was able to show that shorter surgeries, decreased blood loss, less surgical wound pain, and faster postoperative rehabilitation, shorter hospital stay, earlier return to work when patients had surgery with the endoscopic techniques *versus* the microsurgical techniques were reported [17]. Clinical outcomes were similar between the endoscopic and the microsurgical methods in any of the trials. The complication rate was lower in all five studies when patients underwent endoscopic *versus* microsurgical discectomy. Revision conversion to fusion was reported by one study to be lower with the endoscopic procedure.

Another comparative study on endoscopic lumbar discectomy *versus* microsurgical laminotomy was published by Kong et al. in 2018 [18]. Although this study included only 40 patients with available two-year follow-up data, it was able to show equivalent numbers for ODI and VAS for back pain and leg reductions with either. This finding was corroborated by a treatment open-label randomized single-center trial conducted by Limin Rong et al. These authors compared the transforaminal endoscopic discectomy to translaminar microdiscectomy [19]. This study included 153 patients who were randomized to either of these two treatments. Clinical outcomes were analyzed to reduce the ODI, VAS back and VAS leg, SF-36, and the EuroQol Group's EQ-5D. Besides the length of surgery, hospital stay, mobilization time, surgery- and total hospital cost, the authors evaluated complications-, and reoperations rates. The clinical result differences between the two treatments showed equal ODI outcomes, but in medial disc herniations, endoscopy rendered less favorable results (p = 0.027). On the contrary, far lateral disc herniation treated with translaminar microsurgical decompression was associated with less favorable ODI outcomes at three months (p = 0.008), six months (p = 0.028), and one year (p = 0.028). An increasing distance of the pathology from the surgical access point was a predictor of deteriorating outcomes. There was no difference in the complication rates - 13.75% in the endoscopic surgery group and 16.44% in the microsurgical tubular retractor group (p = 0.642). At 1-year follow-up, the endoscopic surgery approach's superiority regarding clinical outcomes could not be demonstrated, and that it was not necessarily safer either [19].

THE PROBLEM WITH TRADITIONAL OUTCOME TOOLS

At present, clinical evidence suggests that endoscopic surgery outcomes are no worse than microdiscectomy. However, the replacement of traditional spinal surgery protocols with their endoscopic counterparts can only occur when superiority can be demonstrated in patient satisfaction, cost, and long-term durability of the procedure. Do the functional outcome scores commonly used nowadays truly reflect what matters most to patients? One could argue that the ODI, VAS, Roland Morris, or SF36 outcome tools do not adequately reflect the factors impacting patient satisfaction. For example, none of these scores capture the procedure's burden or the ease of going through the entire treatment cycle. While many patients may adjust expectations for an endoscopic surgery program targeting the predominant pain generator instead of treating all possible sources of pain suggested by MRI or CT by fusion, this potential reporting bias by patients in describing their clinical outcomes which play out in a different clinical context in an ambulatory *versus* hospital setting may escape these traditional outcomes tools. A direct comparison by using the same conventional outcome tools may be misleading or fail to demonstrate the benefit to patients and society as a whole [20]. The shorter return to work time, lower utilization of health services, decreased narcotic use, and enhanced social reintegration may show such benefits [20].

THE TROUBLES OF ORCHESTRATING HIGH-LEVEL EVIDENCE SPINE OUTCOME STUDIES

In general, randomization in spine care is a difficult pursuit. Although orchestrating prospective randomized controlled trials (RCTs) on paper seems simple and conceptionally not different from multi-arm drug trials. However, the outcome for patients in pain is always known. When randomized to an ineffective treatment arm, patients recognize the lack of benefit at any point in the study if the pain persists. Getting patients to remain in a study group or not cross over from one group to another may prove very difficult. Considering the high cost of such randomized trials are few and far between, with some exceptions. An example of this dilemma is the Spine Patient Outcome Research Trial (SPORT). Funded with 13.5 Million dollars and conducted at 13 centers in 11 states simultaneously, the study ran from 2000 to 2004 and enrolled some 2500 patients. The first study reported on clinical outcomes with surgical *versus* non-surgical treatment for a herniated disc [21]. Other indications were studied later included spinal stenosis [22] and spondylolisthesis [10]. It was supported by the United

States National Institute of Health (NIH). The SPORT trial could not provide conclusive clinical evidence on surgical treatment's superiority over non-operative therapy for these indications based on the intent-to-treat analysis results due to cross-over problems. Fifty percent of randomized patients did not want surgery, and thirty percent did not wish for non-surgical treatment [21].

The use of placebo and control groups is another common problem that plaques investigational spine research trials. Most Institutional Review Boards (IRB) may not approve study designs, including a placebo control group without any treatment since this in effect amounts to letting the natural history of the underlying degenerative disorder play out. At the same time, one could not assume that this would not harm the patient. The latter problem has been addressed by the Council of International Organizations of Medical Sciences' (CIOMS), which published ethical guidelines for clinical study design [23]. CIOMS only allows placebo controls in randomized trials when: a) there is no effective treatment, or b) if denying effective care poses no harm to participants or a cure does not exist. Both of these latter scenarios do generally not apply to spine outcome research. In short, placebo control groups are largely impractical in spine care investigational trials. It may be presumptuous to pretend that prospective randomized clinical trials comparing endoscopic surgery to conventional spinal surgery techniques may suffer from the same fate as the SPORT trials. Nevertheless, straightforward level III case-control studies will likely be the backbone of clinical outcome research most surgeons can do to prove the benefit of endoscopic spinal surgery without much infrastructure and support at their disposal. Most of these studies will presumably be carried out in busy, highly specialized niche private practices where many patients can be quickly enrolled between different sites in the various study arms. These practices are likely to be the seed of future innovation as every innovation starts with level 5 evidence - an observation and personal communication.

THE ROLE OF EVIDENCE IN CLINICAL DECISION MAKING

When it comes right down to it, the real-life clinical scenarios are such that there may never be sufficient high-grade evidence to make superiority statements of one intervention over another, emphasizing the need to foremost rely on sound clinical judgment when deciding on intervention and not to abolish basic principles of critical decision-making. Only because a problem has not been investigated in every aspect of modern spine care or the clinical data lacked statistical power does not mean that the perceived benefit is not real. This point has been made by Mattei et al. in a recent article published in the NASS Journal [24]. Among several other examples, he illustrated how this played out in the Surgical Timing In Acute Spinal Cord Injury Study (STASCIS) trial [11]. This trials methodology has been criticized for lack of power analysis, randomization, of a fixed protocol of methylprednisolone and hypertensive therapy and lack of proper matching of demographic and neurological function between early and late surgery groups and heterogeneity surgical approach and the type of spinal cord/spinal column injury [25]. Despite these limitations, this study to date provides the best level 2 evidence in support of early intervention for spinal cord injury. The author points out not to rigidly rely on evidence-based medicine (EBM) standards entirely and calls out spine surgeons' responsibility to pursue high-quality scientific evidence for daily decision-making [26]. Furthermore, he states that the lack of high-grade clinical evidence does not exempt spine surgeons from the inherent responsibility of employing our best clinical judgment based on a critical and individualized risk-benefit analysis of available treatment options for each patient. There is no doubt that this drives the supporters of endoscopic spinal surgery who observe their patients improved functioning and higher satisfaction when employing a staged targeted management style of common pain generators in the spine with this minimally invasive procedure compared to conventional spine surgery relying more on image-based medical necessity criteria for surgery. What is described in the following may be a more practical way to go about the EBM analysis.

OUTCOME STUDY BY DURABILITY & UTILIZATION ANALYSIS

Cross-sectional retrospective or longitudinal prospective case series are ranked level III (cohort and case-control studies, or systematic review of these studies). Level IV studies are case series, and level V reports are expert opinion, case reports, or clinical examples. First-principles bench research is another example of level V evidence [26]. The level III clinical outcome study design commonly employed in investigational spine care may suffer from additional limitations. Patient selection criteria and the use of preoperative prognosticators of a successful outcome with the endoscopic intervention may be biased and vary widely. Short-term follow-up is another logistical consideration since not all patients enter and exit the study simultaneously. One must also consider that enrolling a patient into a study may not coincide with the beginning of treatment. Recall and hindsight biases on the surgeon's or the patient's part may influence the interpretation of a clinical outcome with intervention. It may be even more challenging to adjust for these factors with endoscopic spine surgery because of its outpatient nature. The surgery is typically short and uneventful, and the surgeon-patient interaction may be brief, limiting the amount of postoperative coaching of the patient by the surgeon. It may not be evident to the patient to link any postoperative problems during rehabilitation in the short-term or any long-term problems to the endoscopic surgery, mainly if the surgeon's follow-up is sparse. The most valuable follow-up information that may help understand the long-term outcomes and any confounding factors is a clinical and radiographic reevaluation of the patient when they are asymptomatic. Abnormal imaging findings in an asymptomatic patient may prevent overreaction in recommending aggressive intervention with more surgery at a later point in follow-up if the same patient presents with unchanged imaging findings but with more pain. In other words, one must be aware of the underlying disease progression with or without symptoms and tailor the individual patient care in a staged manner focusing on treating validated pain generators rather than imaging findings. From this vantage point, one could apply an endpoint analysis as a measure of clinical success with one procedure over another meaning: if the endoscopic treatment stopped benefitting the patient (endpoint) – the censoring event - and the patient starts utilizing additional services for the same problem a measure of the durability of the treatment effect can be derived. In statistical analysis terms – it is the cornerstone of survival analysis.

In 1958, Edward L. Kaplan and Paul Meier revealed their statistical analysis method of estimates of survival data. They studied different survival times, i.e., the duration of treatment benefit. Their analysis was motivated by the fact that patients enter and exit a clinical study at other times and may have a variable duration of clinical benefit (time-to-event) [27]. Patients in whom the clinical outcome is not known are also eliminated from the study. They are censored because their exact survival time could not be determined. Patients may also be censored and eliminated from the survival calculation when they are still doing well because it is unknown how long into the future, their treatment benefit would have lasted. The time from entering the study to censoring is called the serial time in contrast to the calendar or secular time. Calendar time describes the traditional design of clinical trials. The construction of Kaplan-Meier (KM) survival curves may better suit the clinical outcome analysis of the staged management approach heavily employed in endoscopic spine surgery. Prognosticators of favorable clinical outcomes could be derived that may otherwise not be as obvious with descriptive crosstabulation- or analysis of variance statistics typical of case-control studies. If each patient was defined by their status at the end of their serial time - event occurrence or censored - and their study group assignment, the graphic depiction of the KM survival curves illustrates the postoperative duability dynamic. The construction of survival time probabilities results from arranging the serial times for each patient from the shortest to the longest, without regard to when they entered the study. Hence, all patients within a treatment group start the analysis at the same point. They are surviving until a) the endoscopic surgery treatment benefit has disappeared - the event of interest, or b) they have been censored. In other words, only the duration of known survival is measured.

The durability intervals are charted in horizontal lines along the x-axis. Their length symbolizes the duration of the treatment benefit of the endoscopic surgery. The vertical lines are drawn to connect the horizontal lines to create a curve. The distance between the vertical lines denotes the change in the cumulative probability of durability. The follow-up is plotted on the y-axis. Hence, the Kaplan-Meier curves are non-continuous. They are nothing more than a depiction of step-wise estimates of endoscopic treatment benefit durability. These estimates comparative study groups are most accurate if all patients meet the minimum follow-up criteria - typically two years - because each patient's status is known. When the first patient is censored, it becomes an estimate. Its accuracy deteriorates further on the curve's right side as fewer patients remain in the study group. The curve's reliability deteriorates the more patients are censored. Therefore, the curves are not a prediction, and extrapolation to predict future functioning with endoscopic procedures should be avoided.

THE COMPARATIVE DURABILITY ANALYSIS

As discussed earlier, the superiority analysis may be difficult to execute by traditional clinical outcome measures. Durability analysis takes a different approach. The time after an endoscopic spinal surgery during which a patient does not utilize medical services may be considered the serial time. Serial times can also be determined for alternative minimally invasive or conventional open spinal surgeries. Kaplan-Meier curves can now be constructed as a graphic depiction of the "survival" or the procedure's durability. Statistical difference testing can now be performed by log-rank testing. It calculates the chi-square (χ^2) for each event time for each group and sums the results. These are added to obtain the ultimate χ^2 to compare the full curves of each group. This approach's significant upside is that problems with self-reported patient outcome measures (PROMs) are no longer relevant. The longer an endoscopic surgery provided pain relief making utilization of other medical services unnecessary, the better its value to society. Despite increasingly inaccurate estimates of the treatment benefit duration, KM curves provide an easy-to-understand visualization of the endoscopic surgery's durability compared to other spinal surgery protocols.

The authors have applied durability testing in several of their recently published clinical studies. They illustrated the durability difference between non-visualized percutaneous laser decompression *versus* directly visualized transforaminal endoscopic decompression in herniated disc treatment. Traditional comparative study examination would have to account for many confounding factors such as the extent of degenerative changes signified by reduced posterior disc or neuroforaminal height. To avoid such criticism that these degenerative changes could impact the clinical outcome of the 248 patients enrolled in this investigation, the authors employed the Kaplan-Meier technique to analyze the durability of clinical benefit between the two techniques. Surprisingly, the exact opposite effect was found (Fig. 1).

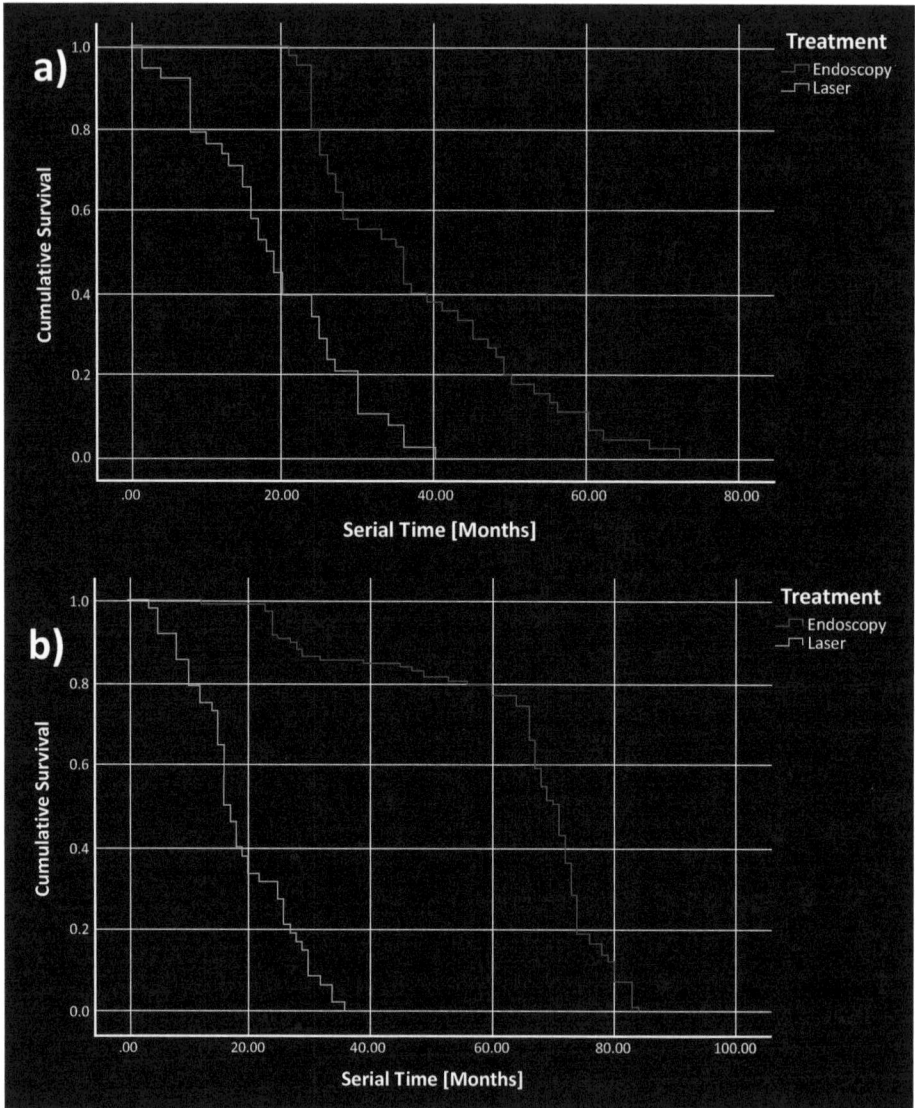

Fig. (1). Kaplan-Meier (K-M) Survival time in patients treated for contained herniated disc (n = 248) with either visualized endoscopic surgical- *versus* percutaneous laser decompression stratified by lateral recess height > 3 mm (a) and < 3 mm (b). The log-rank test calculated an ultimate chi-squares (χ2) for all comparisons of 174.778 at a statistically significant level (p < 0.0001).

In patients with relatively well-preserved posterior disc height (> 3 mm), the median durability (50 percentile) was 36 months for endoscopy patients (95% confidence interval lower boundary of 29.5 and upper boundary of 42.49 months; Figure 1a) *versus* 18 months for laser patients (95% confidence interval lower boundary of 14.38 and upper boundary of 21.63 months). The median (50 percentile) durability of the endoscopic decompression in patients with a posterior disc height of less than 3 mm (advanced degenerative changes) was 71 months (95% confidence interval lower boundary of 68.79 and upper boundary of 73.2 months; Figure 1b). The corresponding median durability in the laser-treated patients was 16 months (95% confidence interval lower boundary of 14.03 and upper boundary of 17.69 months). While these seemingly contradictory findings may not be obvious but understandable considering that a less degenerated disc with preserved disc height may still have significant potential for further degeneration *versus* a lumbar motion segment at the end-stage of the degenerative cascade where the process has basically arrested, the Kaplan-Meier analysis did clearly demonstrate that the clinical treatment benefit from the endoscopic decompression is much more durable than the laser treatment. The explanation seems obvious. Because the advanced bony and soft tissue decompression achieved by the transforaminal endoscopic surgery under direct visualization can accomplish a better decompression than the non-visualized percutaneous laser procedure, the durability of the treatment effect is longer. Endoscopic spinal decompression is a better value proposition than laser in the long-run.

CONCLUSION

Endoscopic spine surgeons are invested in the procedure because they believe in its inherent advantages and their patients' benefit. It implies superiority over traditional spinal surgeries, many of which entail spinal fusion. While patients' expectations and demands may be the driving force behind this ongoing paradigm shift, proving the value proposition of endoscopic spine surgery with higher patient satisfaction and fewer complications and reoperations is not a trivial task. To generate high-grade clinical evidence with randomization protocols is typically hampered by the crossing over of patients from one study group to another. The durability analysis is a straightforward way of demonstrating which procedure wins the competition of lower long-term societal cost. The ultimate measures of such benefit should be longer treatment benefit duration, lower utilization of medical services, fewer iatrogenic problems requiring follow-up revision surgeries, and better return to work rates.

CONSENT FOR PUBLICATION

Not applicable.

CONFLICT OF INTEREST

The authors declare no conflict of interest, financial or otherwise.

ACKNOWLEDGEMENT

Declared none.

REFERENCES

[1]   Ruetten S, Komp M. [The trend towards full-endoscopic decompression : Current possibilities and limitations in disc herniation and spinal stenosis]. Orthopade 2019; 48(1): 69-76.
[http://dx.doi.org/10.1007/s00132-018-03669-3] [PMID: 30535764]

[2]   Chen KT, Jabri H, Lokanath YK, Song MS, Kim JS. The evolution of interlaminar endoscopic spine surgery. J Spine Surg 2020; 6(2): 502-12.
[http://dx.doi.org/10.21037/jss.2019.10.06] [PMID: 32656388]

[3]   Lin GX, Kotheeranurak V, Mahatthanatrakul A, *et al.* Worldwide research productivity in the field of full-endoscopic spine surgery: a bibliometric study. Eur Spine J 2020; 29(1): 153-60.
[http://dx.doi.org/10.1007/s00586-019-06171-2] [PMID: 31642995]

[4]   Tieber F, Lewandrowski KU. Technology advancements in spinal endoscopy for staged management of painful spine conditions. J Spine Surg 2020; 6(S1) (Suppl. 1): S19-28.
[http://dx.doi.org/10.21037/jss.2019.10.02] [PMID: 32195410]

[5]   Lewandrowski KU, Yeung A. Meaningful outcome research to validate endoscopic treatment of common lumbar pain generators with durability analysis. J Spine Surg 2020; 6(S1) (Suppl. 1): S6-S13.
[http://dx.doi.org/10.21037/jss.2019.09.07] [PMID: 32195408]

[6]   Held U, Burgstaller JM, Wertli MM, *et al.* Prognostic function to estimate the probability of meaningful clinical improvement after surgery - Results of a prospective multicenter observational cohort study on patients with lumbar spinal stenosis. PLoS One 2018; 13(11): e0207126.
[http://dx.doi.org/10.1371/journal.pone.0207126] [PMID: 30408081]

[7]   Abdu WA, Sacks OA, Tosteson ANA, *et al.* Long-term results of surgery compared with nonoperative treatment for lumbar degenerative spondylolisthesis in the spine patient outcomes research trial (SPORT). Spine 2018; 43(23): 1619-30.
[http://dx.doi.org/10.1097/BRS.0000000000002682] [PMID: 29652786]

[8]   Rihn JA, Hilibrand AS, Zhao W, *et al.* Effectiveness of surgery for lumbar stenosis and degenerative spondylolisthesis in the octogenarian population: analysis of the Spine Patient Outcomes Research Trial (SPORT) data. J Bone Joint Surg Am 2015; 97(3): 177-85.
[http://dx.doi.org/10.2106/JBJS.N.00313] [PMID: 25653317]

[9]   Pearson AM, Lurie JD, Tosteson TD, Zhao W, Abdu WA, Weinstein JN. Who should undergo surgery for degenerative spondylolisthesis? Treatment effect predictors in SPORT. Spine 2013; 38(21): 1799-811.
[http://dx.doi.org/10.1097/BRS.0b013e3182a314d0] [PMID: 23846502]

[10]   Weinstein JN, Lurie JD, Tosteson TD, *et al.* Surgical compared with nonoperative treatment for lumbar degenerative spondylolisthesis. four-year results in the Spine Patient Outcomes Research Trial (SPORT) randomized and observational cohorts. J Bone Joint Surg Am 2009; 91(6): 1295-304.
[http://dx.doi.org/10.2106/JBJS.H.00913] [PMID: 19487505]

[11]   Fehlings MG, Vaccaro A, Wilson JR, *et al.* Early *versus* delayed decompression for traumatic cervical spinal cord injury: results of the Surgical Timing in Acute Spinal Cord Injury Study (STASCIS). PLoS One 2012; 7(2): e32037.
[http://dx.doi.org/10.1371/journal.pone.0032037] [PMID: 22384132]

[12]   Ruetten S, Komp M, Merk H, Godolias G. Surgical treatment for lumbar lateral recess stenosis with the full-endoscopic interlaminar approach *versus* conventional microsurgical technique: a prospective, randomized, controlled study. J Neurosurg Spine 2009; 10(5): 476-85.
[http://dx.doi.org/10.3171/2008.7.17634] [PMID: 19442011]

[13]   Ruetten S, Komp M, Merk H, Godolias G. Full-endoscopic interlaminar and transforaminal lumbar discectomy *versus* conventional microsurgical technique: a prospective, randomized, controlled study. Spine 2008; 33(9): 931-9.
[http://dx.doi.org/10.1097/BRS.0b013e31816c8af7] [PMID: 18427312]

[14]   Ruetten S, Komp M, Merk H, Godolias G. A new full-endoscopic technique for cervical posterior foraminotomy in the treatment of lateral disc herniations using 6.9-mm endoscopes: prospective 2-year results of 87 patients. Minim Invasive Neurosurg 2007; 50(4): 219-26.
[http://dx.doi.org/10.1055/s-2007-985860] [PMID: 17948181]

[15]   Komp M, Hahn P, Oezdemir S, *et al.* Bilateral spinal decompression of lumbar central stenosis with the full-endoscopic interlaminar *versus* microsurgical laminotomy technique: a prospective, randomized, controlled study. Pain Physician 2015; 18(1): 61-70.
[http://dx.doi.org/10.36076/ppj/2015.18.61] [PMID: 25675060]

[16]   Komp M, Hahn P, Merk H, Godolias G, Ruetten S. Bilateral operation of lumbar degenerative central spinal stenosis in full-endoscopic interlaminar technique with unilateral approach: prospective 2-year results of 74 patients. J Spinal Disord Tech 2011; 24(5): 281-7.
[http://dx.doi.org/10.1097/BSD.0b013e3181f9f55e] [PMID: 20975592]

[17]   Birkenmaier C, Komp M, Leu HF, Wegener B, Ruetten S. The current state of endoscopic disc surgery: review of controlled studies comparing full-endoscopic procedures for disc herniations to standard procedures. Pain Physician 2013; 16(4): 335-44.
[http://dx.doi.org/10.36076/ppj.2013/16/335] [PMID: 23877449]

[18]   Kong L, Shang XF, Zhang WZ, *et al.* Percutaneous endoscopic lumbar discectomy and microsurgical laminotomy : A prospective, randomized controlled trial of patients with lumbar disc herniation and lateral recess stenosis. Orthopade 2019; 48(2): 157-64.
[http://dx.doi.org/10.1007/s00132-018-3610-z] [PMID: 30076437]

[19]   Chen Z, Zhang L, Dong J, *et al.* Percutaneous transforaminal endoscopic discectomy compared with microendoscopic discectomy for lumbar disc herniation: 1-year results of an ongoing randomized controlled trial. J Neurosurg Spine 2018; 28(3): 300-10.
[http://dx.doi.org/10.3171/2017.7.SPINE161434] [PMID: 29303469]

[20]   Roos EM, Boyle E, Frobell RB, Lohmander LS, Ingelsrud LH. It is good to feel better, but better to feel good: whether a patient finds treatment 'successful' or not depends on the questions researchers ask. Br J Sports Med 2019; 53(23): 1474-8.
[http://dx.doi.org/10.1136/bjsports-2018-100260] [PMID: 31072841]

[21]   Weinstein JN, Lurie JD, Tosteson TD, *et al.* Surgical vs nonoperative treatment for lumbar disk herniation: the Spine Patient Outcomes Research Trial (SPORT) observational cohort. JAMA 2006; 296(20): 2451-9.
[http://dx.doi.org/10.1001/jama.296.20.2451] [PMID: 17119141]

[22]   Lurie JD, Tosteson TD, Tosteson A, *et al.* Long-term outcomes of lumbar spinal stenosis: eight-year results of the Spine Patient Outcomes Research Trial (SPORT). Spine 2015; 40(2): 63-76.
[http://dx.doi.org/10.1097/BRS.0000000000000731] [PMID: 25569524]

[23]   Millum J, Grady C. The ethics of placebo-controlled trials: methodological justifications. Contemp Clin Trials 2013; 36(2): 510-4.
[http://dx.doi.org/10.1016/j.cct.2013.09.003] [PMID: 24035802]

[24]   Mattei TA. Evidence-based medicine and clinical decision-making in spine surgery. North American Spine Society Journal 2020; p. 3.

[25]   O'Toole JE. Timing of surgery after cervical spinal cord injury. World Neurosurg 2014; 82(1-2): e389-90.
[http://dx.doi.org/10.1016/j.wneu.2013.02.024] [PMID: 23403350]

[26]   Wilson JR, Singh A, Craven C, *et al.* Early *versus* late surgery for traumatic spinal cord injury: the results of a prospective Canadian cohort study. Spinal Cord 2012; 50(11): 840-3.
[http://dx.doi.org/10.1038/sc.2012.59] [PMID: 22565550]

[27]   Kaplan E, Meier P. Nonparametric estimation from incomplete observations. J Am Stat Assoc 1958; 53(282): 457-81.
[http://dx.doi.org/10.1080/01621459.1958.10501452]

CHAPTER 4

Artificial Intelligence Algorithms in the Identification and Demonstrating of Pain Generators Treated with Endoscopic Spine Surgery

Sandeep Shah[1], Narendran Muraleedharan Basme[2], Vikram Sobti[3], Jorge Felipe Ramírez León[4] and Kai-Uwe Lewandrowski[5,6,7,*]

[1] *Multus Medical, LLC, Phoenix, Arizona, USA*

[2] *Aptus Engineering, Inc, Scottsdale, Arizona, and Multus Medical, LLC, Phoenix, Arizona, USA*

[3] *Innovative Radiology, PC, River Forest, Illinois, USA*

[4] *Centro de Columna – Cirugía Mínima Invasiva. Bogotá, D.C., Colombia, Clínica Reina Sofía – Clínica Colsanitas. Bogotá, D.C., Colombia, Fundación Universitaria Sanitas , Bogotá, D.C., Colombia, USA*

[5] *Center for Advanced Spine Care of Southern Arizona and Surgical Institute of Tucson, Tucson AZ, USA*

[6] *Departmemt of Orthopaedics, Fundación Universitaria Sanitas, Bogotá, D.C., Colombia, USA*

[7] *Visiting Professor, Department of Orthopaedics, Fundación Universitaria Sanitas, Bogotá, D.C., Colombia, USA*

Abstract: Identifying pain generators in multilevel lumbar degenerative disc disease focuses on artificial intelligence (AI) applications in endoscopic spine care to assure adequate symptom relief with the targeted endoscopic spinal decompression surgery. Artificial intelligence (AI) applications of deep learning neural networks to analyze routine lumbar MRI scans could improve clinical outcomes. One way to accomplish this is to apply AI management of patient records using a highly automated workflow, highlighting degenerative and acute abnormalities using unique three-dimensional patient anatomy models. These models help with the identification of the most suitable endoscopic treatment protocol. Radiology AI bots could help primary care doctors, specialists including surgeons and radiologists to read the patient's MRI scans and more accurately and transcribe radiology reports.

* **Corresponding author Kai-Uwe Lewandrowski:** Center for Advanced Spine Care of Southern Arizona and Surgical Institute of Tucson, Tucson, AZ, USA, Department of Orthopaedic Surgery, UNIRIO, Rio de Janeiro, Brazil and Department of Orthoapedic Surgery, Fundación Universitaria Sanitas, Bogotá, D.C., Colombia, USA; Tel: +1 520 204-1495; Fax: +1 623 218-1215; E-mail: business@tucsonspine.com

In this chapter, the authors introduce the concept of AI applications in endoscopic spine care and present some initial feasibility data validating its use based on intraoperatively visualized pathology. This research's ultimate objective is to assist in the development of AI algorithms predictive of the most successful and cost-effective outcomes with lumbar spinal endoscopy by using the radiologist's MRI grading and the grading of an AI deep learning neural network (Multus Radbot™) as independent prognosticators.

Keywords: Artificial intelligence, Endoscopic spinal surgery, Magnetic resonance imaging, Pain generator prognostication.

INTRODUCTION

The role of digital health applications is improving health and patient care. In endoscopic spine care, this translates into a better understanding of the relevant pain generator. The typical multilevel degenerative spine disease with nerve root entrapment due to spinal stenosis is of particular relevance. Deep learning neural networks – artificial intelligence (AI) – have been applied in routine lumbar MRI scan assessment to improve diagnostic accuracy and reliability [1 - 3]. Additional benefit may be in improving information- and workflow in managing symptomatic patients suffering from sciatica-type low back and leg pain [4 - 6]. The diagnostic gap in routine lumbar MRI reporting has been estimated to be as high as 35% when basing clinical decision making in lumbar spine care solely on images [7]. While one approach is to take additional diagnostic tests and protocols into account [8], another one is to think of ways to improve the prognostic value of the information extracted from the MRI scan. This involves extending the routine lumbar MRI scan beyond merely assessing mechanical compression and correlating directly visualized pathology with information buried within the DICOM data set of the MRI scan [9].

Traditionally, the radiologist provides a severity grading by subjective visual analysis of advanced cross-sectional MRI imaging of the spine [10 - 12]. Rarely, actual objective measurements of the diseased spinal motion segments' dimensions are provided in routine reporting. These omissions leave room for errors, which may stall the referral to specialists for appropriate care and overutilization in other areas [13], rarely addressing the patients' disability definitively stemming from the underlying structural abnormality [14 - 19]. The personal [14, 16 - 21] and professional burden of poorly controlled pain, lack of strength, coordination, or insufficient endurance is immense [20, 22]. Rather than continuing on the path of escalating costs, which will likely prompt rationing of medical services [23 - 26], AI aims to [27 - 34] provide targeted care to those patients who will likely benefit from it. To provide such targeted care more consistently, a higher-level of accuracy is required in the utilization of the routine MRI scan.

The endoscopic spine surgeon authors of this chapter became interested in collaborating with the other authors on AI applications for several reasons. There is a need for better prognosticators in the preoperative diagnostic process to steer this minimally invasive targeted decompression procedure at the pain generators causing the patient's symptoms [1]. Since this involves ignoring other potential abnormal findings on preoperative imaging studies, the diagnostic value of the AI prognosticators used needs to be higher than routine reporting, which often may underrepresent clinical pathology and therefore not trigger appropriate referrals to specialists and, thus, delay initiation of definitive spine care beyond the scope of generic referrals to physical therapy, and pain management regardless of whether or not successful or even needed. Frustrated with the frequent delay in appropriate spine care delivery, the authors of this chapter also aimed to investigate the merits of AI applications in endoscopic spine care based on workflow improvements. Automatically generated MRI reports could initiate the most appropriate referral to non-surgical and surgical specialists.

This chapter presents some initial feasibility and reliability data of clinical application of these AI concepts in endoscopic spine care of patients suffering from sciatica due to herniated disc. Ultimately, the author's goal was to develop more useful diagnostic tools to isolate pain generators in the lumbar spine and illustrate them to patients with 3D illustrations and animations to solidify the rationale for simplified yet effective targeted endoscopic treatments - a stark contrast to image-based medical necessity criteria which often lead to extensive open surgeries in the thoracolumbar spine.

WORKFLOW AUTOMATION

The AI optimization of workflow dynamics of patient care related information focuses on better management of effort, time, and accuracy. With the advent of AI and cloud technologies, it is becoming technically feasible to store and access patient data in secure cloud storage. Patient data can be easily accessed by multiple providers also located in remote locations. Patient data consists of administrative data and medical data. The administrative data includes data fields like name, date of birth, gender, address, insurance, facility name, and referring physician information. The medical data can include images, scans, and medical reports. For each patient for every medical procedure, numerous documents need to be created, stored, accessed, read, verified, edited, and approved as it works through the medical system. The manual system of managing these documents is inefficient and prone to human error and inaccuracies.

Concerning MRI DICOM data management, the authors' commercialization of AI imaging processing technology (Multus Medical, Inc., Phoenix AZ, USA) automated the workflow by taking DICOM datasets from participating MRI centers at the origin and automatically reading them into its portal through the PACS system. Thru AI tools, it scans and analyzes the DICOM data documents, converts them into digital format, and uploads the information to the cloud storage for all the patient data. Once the information is securely stored in the cloud, multiple healthcare providers can access the information through cloud technologies. For example, data acquired at the scanning center can easily be accessed by the primary care physician, radiologists, surgeon, and staff responsible for managing patient care. The hardware and software have been set up to compute and storage infrastructure to help manage the patient information as it goes thru multiple stages of the AI analysis and automated reporting in real-time to improve availability and utilization of the time-sensitive medical information by involved providers and to improve the patients' experience throughout the entire process.

THREE-DIMENSIONAL DEMONSTRATION

Two-dimensional MRI or CT scans typically presented in the axial, coronal, and sagittal planes may be challenging to understand to health care providers and the layperson patient. Thus, understanding the plan of care may be hindered. With patent satisfaction gaining more importance and patient education, a growing need to have a patient-specific 3D model that shows patient anatomy and its degeneration and injuries exists. The authors have developed an MRI model matching utility designed to work with a generic 3D model manipulation and matching philosophy. This generic capability makes it easy to scale with different anatomy and pathologies for the patient. This capability is enhanced using AI algorithms. The operating time to manipulate the model and custom fit for a patient and its injuries is significantly reduced, and the accuracy is higher. Given the high-performance graphics engine required, the development was done using high-performance OpenGL and OpenSceneGraph-based graphical visualization and manipulation toolsets written in C++ - a high performance, low-level language. The design communicates seamlessly with the automated workflow infrastructure referenced previously. It integrates the patient portal, DICOM images from the PACS system, interaction with primary care, radiologists, specialists, and surgeons. The 3D interactive model also has a custom renderer built-in, which provides more freedom and control of the output rendering. The model can be an interactive model when discussing with the patient (Fig. **1**).

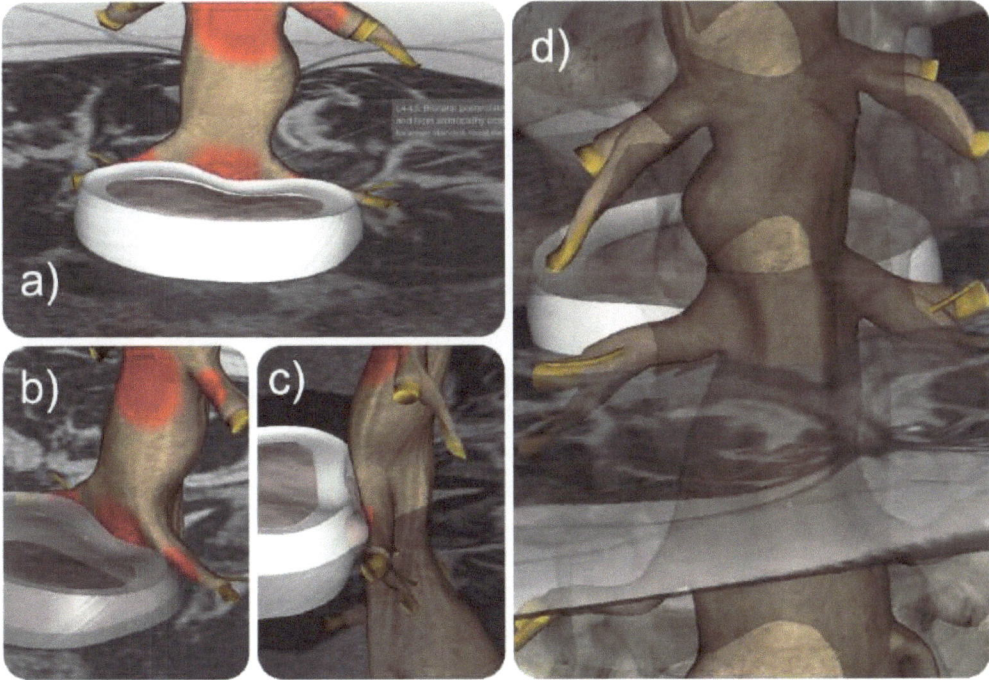

Fig. (1). OpenSceneGraph-based graphical visualization of identified pain generators due to compression and inflammation of the neural elements from a painful L4/5 herniated disc. The axial MRI scans (a-d) are projected into the rendering of the patient's spinal anatomy. The resulting graphic depiction may aid in surgical planning and communication of the plan of care to patients.

THE RADIOLOGY BOT

The authors have developed a deep learning algorithm for routine reporting in spine magnetic resonance imaging to improve the accuracy and predictive value of the magnetic resonance imaging (MRI) scan when applied to the preoperative planning of targeted minimally invasive spinal surgeries on lumbar foraminal and lateral recess stenosis. These targeted procedures often ignore most pathologies reported on routine lumbar MRI scans of patients with injuries or degenerative spine conditions and only focus treatment on the validated painful pathologies. The preoperative MRI scan is an integral part of the diagnostic work-up besides history, physical examination, electrodiagnostic studies, and confirmative diagnostic spinal injections. Also, Multus Medical has developed a deep learning algorithm that automatically identifies suspected findings suggestive of neural compression and vertebral compression fractures on spine MRI scans and provides a passive notification to the workstation of this finding's presence in the scan. This notification is received by the application, flagging the identified scan and helps clinicians engaged in bone-health management to view the scan ahead of others. The device prioritizes and triage radiological medical images only and does not provide diagnostic information beyond triage. The software uses an artificial intelligence algorithm to analyze spine MRI scans automatically. Suppose a suspected foraminal stenosis injury is found in a scan. In that case, the alert is automatically sent to the application on the bone-health clinician's workstation in parallel with the ongoing standard of care within the bone health setting. The standard of care radiology workflow (*i.e.,* reviewing and reporting the findings that initiated the request for MRI) continues unaffected by the bone health program's parallel workflow. For clarity, the RadBot device does not flag/prioritize cases within this radiology workflow. The standalone desktop application, Radbot Worklist, includes three sagittal preview images meant for informational purposes only and is not intended for diagnostic use. The Radbot Worklist presents all cases processed by the algorithm and flags those with a suspected finding.

The Radbot device works in parallel to conjunction with the standard care workflow within spine health programs and utterly independent of the standard of care workflow within the radiology department. After a spine MRI scan has been performed, a copy of the study is automatically retrieved and processed by the RadBot device. The device performs the study analysis and returns a notification about a suspected foraminal stenosis injury to the Radbot Worklist to notify the Spine- and Bone Health and Fracture Prevention Programs clinicians reviewing the Spine MRI scans. Any provider may review the study instantly or later for further analysis. Significant time savings are realized until the critical MRI image information is presented to the physician taking care of the patient whose MRI scan was flagged for critical findings warranting expedited review *versus* routine degenerative scan who slip further down the priority list and are read out routinely. The software does not recommend treatment or provide a diagnosis. However, it does prioritize scans by their importance and is therefore meant to assist in improved workload prioritization of cases busy spine care and bone health programs. A clinician provides the final diagnosis after reviewing the scan itself.

SURGICAL ANIMATION

Leveraging the software design developed for 3D representation and the automated workflow, a surgical animation framework was developed using the patient-specific models which specific anatomical objects as 3D geometrical model objects (comprised of vertices, triangles/faces, textures), injury objects as 3D geometrical models along with modified textures to represent discoloration, and labels corresponding to injuries based on medical reports and diagnosis. The model also includes specific medical devices and surgical instruments used in the patient-specific medical procedure as 3D geometrical model objects (comprised of vertices, triangles/faces, textures), along with modified textures. A medical procedure animation rendering project is created from an anatomical segmented 3D model and the 3D model of the medical devices for patient-specific and medical process specific. The medical device models interact with the anatomical models to highlight patient-specific medical procedures *via* a custom "storyboarding" process. The project contains patient and medical process-specific anatomical objects, injury objects, labels, medical devices, and a storyboard. The storyboard consists of multiple animation key-frames. Each key-frame has information representing states of the patient and medical procedure-specific 3D models (anatomical/injury objects, labels, medical devices and their interactions with each other.

The key-frame state also consists of custom position and orientation of one or multiple (port/auxiliary) cameras and the following parameters for each object (anatomical, injury, medical devices, and any other imported 3D objects): The storyboard consists of information representing relative state changes between animation key-frames for the custom patient and medical procedure. An animation is made of multiple key-frames at varying time steps for the desired length of custom rendering. The final video is generated by rendering each time step (at 16.7ms intervals for a 60fps video) and interpolating all parameters between the previous and next key-frame for the specific medical procedure. Different interpolation functions may be used to achieve the desired effect during state changes and transitions. Custom hardware infrastructure is implemented to create, store, access, and render the various 3-D models, key-frames, and interpolation schemes optimized for easy-to-understand patient education. Excerpts from such an animation prepared for a patient undergoing a transforaminal endoscopic discectomy is shown in Fig. (**2**).

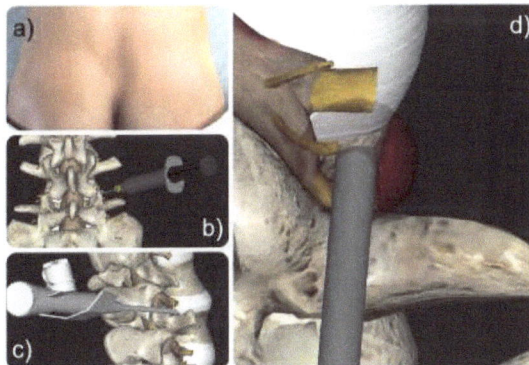

Fig. (2). Shown are multiple animation key-frames from the storyboard, with each key-frame representing states of the patient and transforaminal endoscopic procedure. These specific 3D models show anatomical structures and pain generators and the endoscopic instruments typically employed during the transforaminal decompression for herniated disc and foraminal stenosis.

AI DISC HERNIATION AND STENOSIS DETECTORS

The AI neural network graded pathologies, including circumferential and paracentral disc herniation, further subclassified as extrusion, protrusion, sequestration, fragmentation, and central canal foraminal stenosis. The operating surgeon's corresponding clinical grading was done based on the size and location of the compressive pathology by employing validated radiographic classification systems [10 - 12, 35]. MRI criteria of foraminal stenosis were 15 mm or less for neuroforaminal height, 3 mm or less for posterior disc height and 3 mm or less for neuroforaminal width [36]. Disc herniations were graded as central, paracentral, or combined central- and paracentral and as contained or extruded [11]. Diagnostic spinal injections were used to confirm the pain level [8, 37 - 41]. An independent radiologist graded the foraminal and lateral recess stenosis severity from 1 to 10, with 10 representing severe stenosis. Also, the foraminal stenotic process's location was recorded from medial to lateral into the entry-, mid-, and exit zone employing validated radiographic classification systems [10].

Previously published, the deep learning algorithms used segmentation models. The pathology detectors were able to assign a severity score, for example, by assessing the posterior annulus' deformity. Deformity value of greater than 50% triggered the respective diagnosis of disc herniation or stenosis. The herniation detector was trained to identify posterior-, central-, and paracentral disc herniations and classify them as protrusions, extrusions, or contained circumferential bulges. In comparison, the central canal and foraminal detectors were trained to identify stenosis. Each of the three detectors has a remapped contiguous confidence level ranging between 0 and 10 to determine whether or not a particular pathology is, in fact, present in the patient's MRI scan. These performance characteristics were validated by analyzing training data sets. The AI detectors auto-tune the confidence level threshold to 50% by referring to the training data set. The detectors were auto-tuning with a combination of functions, including sigmoids, softmax for final layer activations, and rectified linear unit (ReLU) for the image kernel layers. These were non-linear detector functions [42]. These non-linear activation functions learn and predict various outcomes. This results in the confidence level output from the algorithm for each class having a very non-linear relationship to the pathology's severity.

CLINICAL SERIES

Sixty-five patients with an average age of 62.54 years underwent endoscopic transforaminal decompression for herniated disc. The average follow-up was 57.4 months. The inclusion criteria were: 1) lumbar radiculopathy, 2) MRI evidence of foraminal- or lateral recess stenosis, 3) failed non-operative care. The exclusion criteria were: 1) spondylolisthesis greater than Grade 1, 2) severe central stenosis, 3) end-stage facet arthropathy, 4) infection; and 5) metastatic disease. The MRI scans of these 65 patients including 383 levels were analyzed by the deep learning neural network models and compared to the reports provided by board-certified radiologists. To establish the indication for endoscopic surgery, disc herniations and stenosis in the spinal canal, lateral recess, and the neuroforamen were classified employing the same radiographic classification systems used during the AI training [10 - 12, 35]. Patients underwent transforaminal endoscopic surgery techniques previously published employing the "outside-in" technique [43]. The working cannula was placed in the neuroforamen following serial dilation and initial foraminoplasty [44 - 48]. The endoscopic decompression procedure was directly visualized throughout the surgery. An exemplary case of a 48-year old male who was treated with transforaminal outside-in endoscopic decompression with foraminoplasty and discectomy for failed conservative care of an L4/5 herniated disc is shown in Fig. (3).

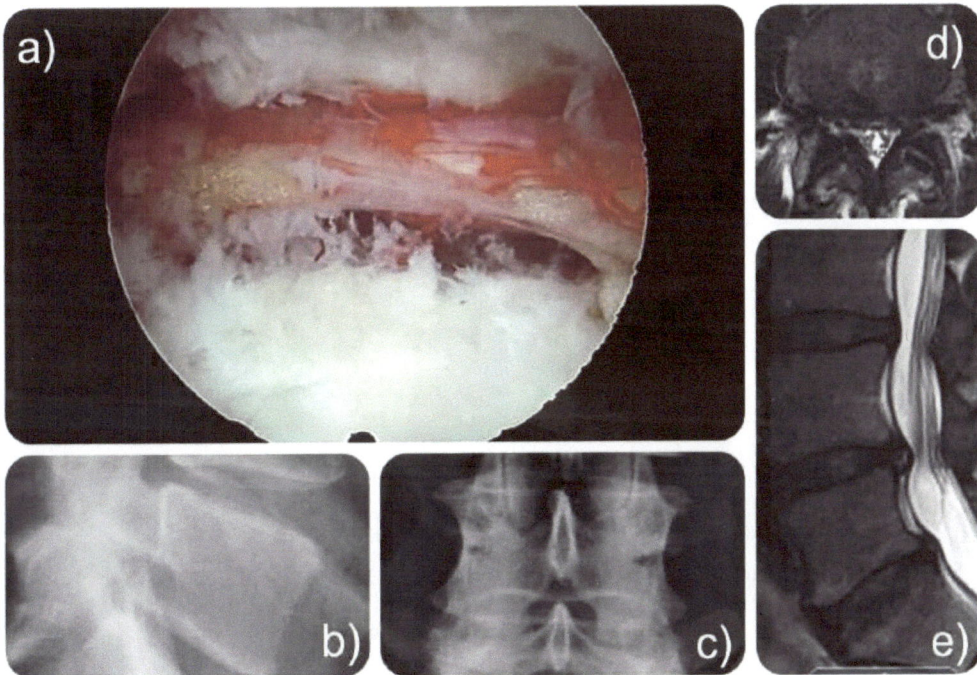

Fig. (3). An exemplary case of a 48-year-old male who underwent L4/5 transforaminal endoscopic decompression for herniated disc (**a**). The preoperative x-rays (**b, c**), and axial (**d**) MRI and sagittal (**e**) scan.

The statistical analysis of correlation between clinical outcomes and decompression of compressive pathology as predicted by the AI algorithm *versus* the radiologist report is based on the hypothesis that AI grades it more accuretly resulting in more reliable symptom relief. This was done with logistic regression analysis and the log-odds are converted to a probability by the logistic model allowing the authors to compare the predictive value of the stenosis grading provided by either the AI or the radiologist. The confidence intervals for the likelihood ratios were calculated using the "log method" according to Altman *et al.* [49] Macnab outcome analysis showed that 86.4% of the 88 foraminal decompressions resulted in Excellent and Good (Improved) clinical outcomes. The radiologist's stenosis grading showed an average severity score of 4.71 ± 2.626, and the average AI severity grading was 5.65 ± 3.73. Logit regression probability analysis of the two independent prognosticators showed that both the radiologist's grading (86.2%; odds ratio 1.264) and the AI grading (86.4%; odds ratio 1.267) were nearly equally predictive of a successful outcome with the endoscopic decompression (Fig. **4**).

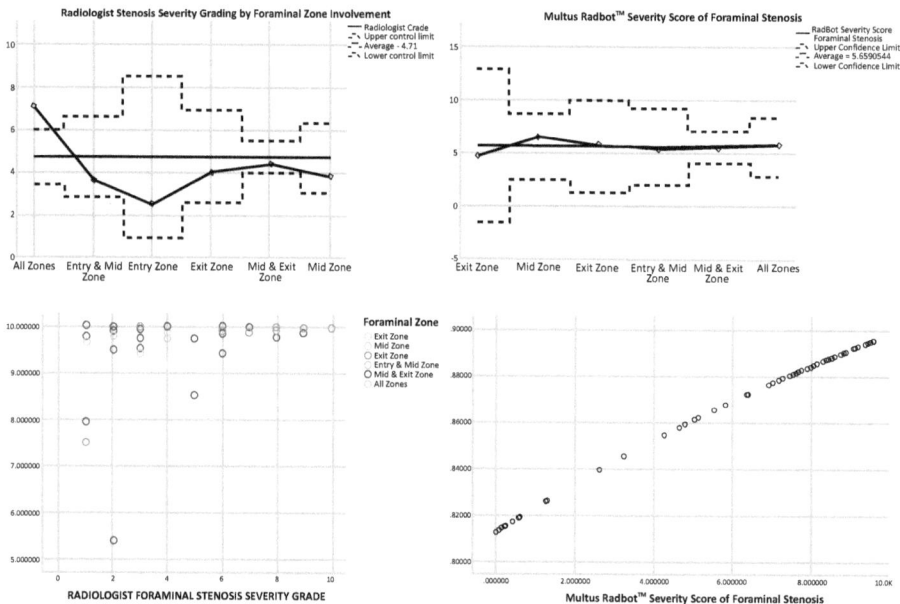

Fig. (4). Results of the logit regression analysis of AI *versus* radiologist grading are shown. The top left panel illustrates the radiologist's foraminal severity grading plotted for the different foraminal zones with an average score of 4.71 ± of 2.62 and variable grading across all zones. In comparison (top right panel), the AI severity grading plotted was less variable, with an average of 5.65 ± 3.73. This comparison suggests less accurate reporting and underreporting of the disease severity by routine MRI reporting illustrating its diagnostic gap to identify painful pathology directly visualized by endoscopy correctly. In the bottom left panel, the scatter plot of the severity grading (continuous scale) provided by the AI algorithm *versus* the radiologist grading (ordinal scale) shows a non-linear relationship between these two independent predictor variables, with the AI consistently grading higher in nearly all foraminal zones. In the bottom right panel, the non-linear logit model's scatterplot describes the probability of improved clinical outcomes as defined by the dichotomized Macnab criteria predicted by the contiguous AI grading.

DISCUSSION

The authors' deep learning network is capable of identifying compressive pathology at a similar probability level as the radiologists and treating the pathology suggested by the AI surgically with the endoscopic discectomy procedure providing clinical evidence that the algorithm successfully identified relevant pain generators that caused the patients symptoms in the context and at the time when the patient presented in consultation for surgical evaluation. While the clinical outcomes with the endoscopic spine surgery found in this small feasibility study of correlating AI predictions and clinical improvements, there are many additional advantages to AI application in spine care other than more accurately predicting clinical improvement with surgery.

The OpenSceneGraph-based graphical visualization of identified pain generators due to compression and inflammation of the neural elements from painful disc herniations provides an easy-to-understand individualized educational means for patients who now may better understand the source of their spinal pain and the plan of care required to correct the problem to achieve pain relief. This demonstration may be further aided with surgical animation illustrating the steps involved and, more importantly, making visually apparent to the patient the scope of surgery, the risk, and the burden involved to go through them with treatment. Many patients hesitate to proceed with the suggested spine surgery because they are afraid and often rely more on second-hand information from peers in their family and friend circles rather than objective information. Other advantages related to the improvement of the workflow. With the RadBot™ AI software and hardware solutions developed by the authors, the patients' MRI study is automatically retrieved and processed. It notifies the physicians involved in an individual patient's care about a suspected painful degenerative pathology or injury. While the software does not diagnose or recommends, it does reprioritize scans by their importance as they come in and, therefore, helps improve workload prioritization of cases in busy spine care and bone health programs.

CONCLUSION

AI deep learning network application may be effectively used to assist in utilizing the lumbar MRI scan as a prognosticator of favorable clinical outcomes with the endoscopic spine surgery for foraminal stenosis due to a herniated disc. AI may also aid in a visual demonstration of the painful pathology by superimposing the patient's actual MRI scans into a spine model and animating the proposed endoscopic decompression. Further translational clinical studies should teach the AI algorithms how to correctly identify the litany of validated pain generators directly visualized during spinal endoscopy. Many common pain generators, including toxic annular tears, entrapped annular disc herniations, foraminal ligament scaring, nerve root tethering, adhesions, and intradiscal abnormalities ranging from fissures to cavitation and delamination of endstage degenerated disc routinely escape detection with currently employed MRI interpretation protocols. Future AI algorithms may be capable of extracting the respective correlates from the DICOM data sets.

CONSENT FOR PUBLICATION

Not applicable.

CONFLICT OF INTEREST

The authors declare no conflict of interest, financial or otherwise.

ACKNOWLEDGEMENT

Declared none.

REFERENCES

[1]   Joshi RS, Haddad AF, Lau D, Ames CP. Artificial intelligence for adult spinal deformity. Neurospine 2019; 16(4): 686-94.
[http://dx.doi.org/10.14245/ns.1938414.207] [PMID: 31905457]

[2]   Han XG, Tian W. Artificial intelligence in orthopedic surgery: current state and future perspective. Chin Med J (Engl) 2019; 132(21): 2521-3.
[http://dx.doi.org/10.1097/CM9.0000000000000479] [PMID: 31658155]

[3]   Galbusera F, Casaroli G, Bassani T. Artificial intelligence and machine learning in spine research. JOR Spine 2019; 2(1): e1044.
[http://dx.doi.org/10.1002/jsp2.1044] [PMID: 31463458]

[4]   LewandrowskI KU, Muraleedharan N, Eddy SA, *et al.* Feasibility of deep learning algorithms for reporting in routine spine magnetic resonance imaging. Int J Spine Surg 2020; 14(s3): S86-97.
[http://dx.doi.org/10.14444/7131] [PMID: 33298549]

[5]   Lewandrowski KU, Muraleedharan N, Eddy SA, *et al.* Artificial intelligence comparison of the radiologist report with endoscopic predictors of successful transforaminal decompression for painful conditions of the lumber spine: application of deep learning algorithm interpretation of routine lumbar magnetic resonance imaging scan. Int J Spine Surg 2020; 14(s3): S75-85.
[http://dx.doi.org/10.14444/7130] [PMID: 33208388]

[6]   Lewandrowski KU, Muraleedharan N, Eddy SA, *et al.* Reliability analysis of deep learning algorithms for reporting of routine lumbar MRI scans. Int J Spine Surg 2020; 14(s3): S98-S107.
[http://dx.doi.org/10.14444/7131] [PMID: 33122182]

[7]   Yeung AT, Lewandrowski KU. Retrospective analysis of accuracy and positive predictive value of preoperative lumbar MRI grading after successful outcome following outpatient endoscopic decompression for lumbar foraminal and lateral recess stenosis. Clin Neurol Neurosurg 2019; 181: 52.
[http://dx.doi.org/10.1016/j.clineuro.2019.03.011] [PMID: 30986727]

[8]   Lewandrowski KU. Successful outcome after outpatient transforaminal decompression for lumbar foraminal and lateral recess stenosis: The positive predictive value of diagnostic epidural steroid injection. Clin Neurol Neurosurg 2018; 173: 38-45.

[http://dx.doi.org/10.1016/j.clineuro.2018.07.015] [PMID: 30075346]

[9]   Kusunose K, Haga A, Inoue M, Fukuda D, Yamada H, Sata M. Clinically Feasible and Accurate View Classification of Echocardiographic Images Using Deep Learning. Biomolecules 2020; 10(5): E665.
[http://dx.doi.org/10.3390/biom10050665] [PMID: 32344829]

[10]   Lee CK, Rauschning W, Glenn W. Lateral lumbar spinal canal stenosis: classification, pathologic anatomy and surgical decompression. Spine 1988; 13(3): 313-20.
[http://dx.doi.org/10.1097/00007632-198803000-00015] [PMID: 3388117]

[11]   Lee S, Kim SK, Lee SH, *et al.* Percutaneous endoscopic lumbar discectomy for migrated disc herniation: classification of disc migration and surgical approaches. Eur Spine J 2007; 16(3): 431-7.
[http://dx.doi.org/10.1007/s00586-006-0219-4] [PMID: 16972067]

[12]   Pfirrmann CW, Metzdorf A, Zanetti M, Hodler J, Boos N. Magnetic resonance classification of lumbar intervertebral disc degeneration. Spine 2001; 26(17): 1873-8.
[http://dx.doi.org/10.1097/00007632-200109010-00011] [PMID: 11568697]

[13]   Lewandrowski KU. Retrospective analysis of accuracy and positive predictive value of preoperative lumbar MRI grading after successful outcome following outpatient endoscopic decompression for lumbar foraminal and lateral recess stenosis. Clin Neurol Neurosurg 2019; 179: 74-80.
[http://dx.doi.org/10.1016/j.clineuro.2019.02.019] [PMID: 30870712]

[14]   Yeung AT, Gore S. *In-vivo* endoscopic visualization of patho-anatomy in symptomatic degenerative conditions of the lumbar spine II: Intradiscal, foraminal, and central canal decompression. Surg Technol Int 2011; 21: 299-319.
[PMID: 22505004]

[15]   Fischgrund JS, Rhyne A, Franke J, *et al.* Intraosseous basivertebral nerve ablation for the treatment of chronic low back pain: 2-year results from a prospective randomized double-blind sham-controlled multicenter study. Int J Spine Surg 2019; 13(2): 110-9.
[http://dx.doi.org/10.14444/6015] [PMID: 31131209]

[16]   Yeung A, Roberts A, Zhu L, Qi L, Zhang J, Lewandrowski KU. Treatment of soft tissue and bony spinal stenosis by a visualized endoscopic transforaminal technique under local anesthesia. Neurospine 2019; 16(1): 52-62.
[http://dx.doi.org/10.14245/ns.1938038.019] [PMID: 30943707]

[17]   Lewandrowski KU, de Carvalho PST, Calderaro AL, *et al.* Outcomes with transforaminal endoscopic *versus* percutaneous laser decompression for contained lumbar herniated disc: a survival analysis of treatment benefit. J Spine Surg 2020; 6 (Suppl. 1): S84-99.
[http://dx.doi.org/10.21037/jss.2019.09.13] [PMID: 32195418]

[18]   Yeung A, Lewandrowski KU. Five-year clinical outcomes with endoscopic transforaminal foraminoplasty for symptomatic degenerative conditions of the lumbar spine: a comparative study of inside-out *versus* outside-in techniques. J Spine Surg 2020; 6 (Suppl. 1): S66-83.
[http://dx.doi.org/10.21037/jss.2019.06.08] [PMID: 32195417]

[19]   Yeung A, Lewandrowski KU. Early and staged endoscopic management of common pain generators in the spine. J Spine Surg 2020; 6 (Suppl. 1): S1-5.
[http://dx.doi.org/10.21037/jss.2019.09.03] [PMID: 32195407]

[20]   Lewandrowski KU, Ransom NA, Yeung A. Return to work and recovery time analysis after outpatient endoscopic lumbar transforaminal decompression surgery. J Spine Surg 2020; 6 (Suppl. 1): S100-15.
[http://dx.doi.org/10.21037/jss.2019.10.01] [PMID: 32195419]

[21]   Lewandrowski KU. The strategies behind "inside-out" and "outside-in" endoscopy of the lumbar spine: treating the pain generator. J Spine Surg 2020; 6 (Suppl. 1): S35-9.
[http://dx.doi.org/10.21037/jss.2019.06.06] [PMID: 32195412]

[22]   Yeung A, Wei SH. Surgical outcome of workman's comp patients undergoing endoscopic foraminal decompression for lumbar herniated disc. J Spine Surg 2020; 6 (Suppl. 1): S116-9.

[http://dx.doi.org/10.21037/jss.2019.11.03] [PMID: 32195420]

[23] Faciszewski T. Spine policy. What's in a name? Spine J 2001; 1(4): 300.
[http://dx.doi.org/10.1016/S1529-9430(01)00124-3] [PMID: 14588335]

[24] Thorsteinsdottir B, Beck A, Tilburt JC. Grow a spine, have a heart: responding to patient requests for marginally beneficial care. AMA J Ethics 2015; 17(11): 1028-34.
[http://dx.doi.org/10.1001/journalofethics.2015.17.11.ecas2-1511] [PMID: 26595243]

[25] Inglis T, Schouten R, Dalzell K, Evison J, Inglis G. Access to orthopaedic spinal specialists in the Canterbury public health system: quantifying the unmet need. N Z Med J 2016; 129(1442): 19-24.
[PMID: 27657155]

[26] Mok JK, Sheha ED, Samuel AM, *et al.* Evaluation of current trends in treatment of single-level cervical radiculopathy. Clin Spine Surg 2019; 32(5): E241-5.
[http://dx.doi.org/10.1097/BSD.0000000000000796] [PMID: 30762836]

[27] Weir S, Samnaliev M, Kuo TC, *et al.* Persistent postoperative pain and healthcare costs associated with instrumented and non-instrumented spinal surgery: a case-control study. J Orthop Surg Res 2020; 15(1): 127.
[http://dx.doi.org/10.1186/s13018-020-01633-6] [PMID: 32238173]

[28] Marrache M, Harris AB, Raad M, *et al.* Preoperative and postoperative spending among working-age adults undergoing posterior spinal fusion surgery for degenerative disease. World Neurosurg 2020; 138: e930-9.
[http://dx.doi.org/10.1016/j.wneu.2020.03.143] [PMID: 32251816]

[29] Jain A, Yeramaneni S, Kebaish KM, *et al.* Cost-utility analysis of rhbmp-2 use in adult spinal deformity surgery. Spine 2020; 45(14): 1009-15.
[http://dx.doi.org/10.1097/BRS.0000000000003442] [PMID: 32097274]

[30] Safaee MM, Dalle Ore CL, Zygourakis CC, Deviren V, Ames CP. Estimating a price point for cost-benefit of bone morphogenetic protein in pseudarthrosis prevention for adult spinal deformity surgery. J Neurosurg Spine 2019; 30(6): 1-8.
[http://dx.doi.org/10.3171/2018.12.SPINE18613] [PMID: 30849745]

[31] Jonsson E, Hansson-Hedblom A, Kirketeig T, Fritzell P, Hagg O, Borgstrom F. Cost and health outcomes patterns in patients treated with spinal cord stimulation following spine surgery-a register-based study. Neuromodulation 2020; 23(5): 626-33.
[PMID: 31667934]

[32] Hansson-Hedblom A, Jonsson E, Fritzell P, Hägg O, Borgström F. The association between patient reported outcomes of spinal surgery and societal costs: a register based study. Spine 2019; 44(18): 1309-17.
[http://dx.doi.org/10.1097/BRS.0000000000003050] [PMID: 30985570]

[33] Carr DA, Saigal R, Zhang F, Bransford RJ, Bellabarba C, Dagal A. Enhanced perioperative care and decreased cost and length of stay after elective major spinal surgery. Neurosurg Focus 2019; 46(4): E5.
[http://dx.doi.org/10.3171/2019.1.FOCUS18630] [PMID: 30933922]

[34] Ball JR, Sekhon LH. Timing of decompression and fixation after spinal cord injury--when is surgery optimal? Crit Care Resusc 2006; 8(1): 56-63.
[PMID: 16536723]

[35] Milette PC. Classification, diagnostic imaging, and imaging characterization of a lumbar herniated disk. Radiol Clin North Am 2000; 38(6): 1267-92.
[http://dx.doi.org/10.1016/S0033-8389(08)70006-X] [PMID: 11131632]

[36] Hasegawa T, An HS, Haughton VM, Nowicki BH. Lumbar foraminal stenosis: critical heights of the intervertebral discs and foramina. A cryomicrotome study in cadavera. J Bone Joint Surg Am 1995; 77(1): 32-8.

[http://dx.doi.org/10.2106/00004623-199501000-00005] [PMID: 7822353]

[37] el-Khoury GY, Ehara S, Weinstein JN, Montgomery WJ, Kathol MH. Epidural steroid injection: a procedure ideally performed with fluoroscopic control. Radiology 1988; 168(2): 554-7.
[http://dx.doi.org/10.1148/radiology.168.2.2969118] [PMID: 2969118]

[38] Geurts JW, Kallewaard JW, Richardson J, Groen GJ. Targeted methylprednisolone acetate/hyaluronidase/clonidine injection after diagnostic epiduroscopy for chronic sciatica: a prospective, 1-year follow-up study. Reg Anesth Pain Med 2002; 27(4): 343-52.
[PMID: 12132057]

[39] Valat JP. Epidural corticosteroid injections for sciatica: placebo effect, injection effect or anti-inflammatory effect? Nat Clin Pract Rheumatol 2006; 2(10): 518-9.
[http://dx.doi.org/10.1038/ncprheum0286] [PMID: 17016473]

[40] MacVicar J, King W, Landers MH, Bogduk N. The effectiveness of lumbar transforaminal injection of steroids: a comprehensive review with systematic analysis of the published data. Pain Med 2013; 14(1): 14-28.
[http://dx.doi.org/10.1111/j.1526-4637.2012.01508.x] [PMID: 23110347]

[41] Chang MC, Lee DG. Outcome of Transforaminal Epidural Steroid Injection According to the Severity of Lumbar Foraminal Spinal Stenosis. Pain Physician 2018; 21(1): 67-72.
[http://dx.doi.org/10.36076/ppj.1.2018.67] [PMID: 29357335]

[42] Olgac A, Karlik Bekir. Performance analysis of various activation functions in generalized MLP architectures of neural networks. International Journal of Artificial Intelligence And Expert Systems 2011; 1: 111-22.

[43] Lewandrowski KU. "Outside-in" technique, clinical results, and indications with transforaminal lumbar endoscopic surgery: a retrospective study on 220 patients on applied radiographic classification of foraminal spinal stenosis. Int J Spine Surg 2014; 8: 8.
[http://dx.doi.org/10.14444/1026] [PMID: 25694915]

[44] Hoogland T. Percutaneous endoscopic discectomy. J Neurosurg 1993; 79(6): 967-8.
[PMID: 8246070]

[45] Hoogland T, Scheckenbach C. Percutaneous lumbar nucleotomy with low-dose chymopapain, an ambulatory procedure. Z Orthop Ihre Grenzgeb 1995; 133(2): 106-13.
[http://dx.doi.org/10.1055/s-2008-1039420] [PMID: 7754655]

[46] Schubert M, Hoogland T. Endoscopic transforaminal nucleotomy with foraminoplasty for lumbar disk herniation. Oper Orthop Traumatol 2005; 17(6): 641-61.
[http://dx.doi.org/10.1007/s00064-005-1156-9] [PMID: 16369758]

[47] Hoogland T, Schubert M, Miklitz B, Ramirez A. Transforaminal posterolateral endoscopic discectomy with or without the combination of a low-dose chymopapain: a prospective randomized study in 280 consecutive cases. Spine 2006; 31(24): E890-7.
[http://dx.doi.org/10.1097/01.brs.0000245955.22358.3a] [PMID: 17108817]

[48] Hoogland T, van den Brekel-Dijkstra K, Schubert M, Miklitz B. Endoscopic transforaminal discectomy for recurrent lumbar disc herniation: a prospective, cohort evaluation of 262 consecutive cases. Spine 2008; 33(9): 973-8.
[http://dx.doi.org/10.1097/BRS.0b013e31816c8ade] [PMID: 18427318]

[49] Higgins JP, Thompson SG, Deeks JJ, Altman DG. Measuring inconsistency in meta-analyses. BMJ 2003; 327(7414): 557-60.
[http://dx.doi.org/10.1136/bmj.327.7414.557] [PMID: 12958120]

CHAPTER 5

Postoperative Management of Sequelae, Complications, and Readmissions Following Outpatient Transforaminal Lumbar Endoscopy

Kai-Uwe Lewandrowski[1,2,3,*], **Jorge Felipe Ramírez León**[4], **Álvaro Dowling**[5], **Stefan Hellinger**[6], **Nicholas A Ransom**[7] and **Anthony Yeung**[8]

[1] *Center for Advanced Spine Care of Southern Arizona and Surgical Institute of Tucson, Tucson AZ, USA*

[2] *Associate Professor of Orthopaedic Surgery, Universidad Colsanitas, Bogota, Colombia, USA*

[3] *Visiting Professor, Department Orthopaedic Surgery, UNIRIO, Rio de Janeiro, Brazil*

[4] *Fundación Universitaria Sanitas, Bogotá, D.C., Colombia, Research Team, Centro de Columna, Bogotá, Colombia, USA*

[5] *Centro de Cirugía de Mínima Invasión, CECIMIN - Clínica Reina Sofia, Bogotá, Colombia, USA*

[6] *Department of Orthopedic Surgery, Arabellaklinik,, Munich, Germany*

[7] *Orthopaedic Spine Surgeon, Director of Endoscopic Spine Clinic, Santiago, Chile*

[8] *Clinical Professor, University of New Mexico School of Medicine, Albuquerque, New Mexico Desert Institute for Spine Care, Phoenix, AZ, USA*

Abstract: Best management practices of complications resulting from outpatient transforaminal endoscopic decompression surgery for lumbar foraminal and lateral recess stenosis are not established. Recent advances in surgical techniques allow for endoscopically assisted bony decompression for neurogenic claudication symptoms due to spinal stenosis. These broadened indications also produced a higher incidence of postoperative complications ranging from dural tears, recurrent disc herniations, nerve root injuries, foot drop, facet and pedicle fractures, or infections. Postoperative sequelae such as dysesthetic leg pain, and infiltration of the surgical access and spinal canal with irrigation fluid causing spinal headaches and painful wound swelling, as well as failure to cure, are additional common postoperative problems that can lead to hospital readmissions and contribute to lower patient satisfaction with the procedure. In this chapter, the authors focus on analyzing the incidence of such problems and, more importantly, how to manage them. While the incidence of these problems is recogniz-

* **Corresponding author Kai-Uwe Lewandrowski:** Center for Advanced Spine Care of Southern Arizona and Surgical Institute of Tucson, Tucson, AZ, USA, Department of Orthopaedic Surgery, UNIRIO, Rio de Janeiro, Brazil and Department of Orthoapedic Surgery, Fundación Universitaria Sanitas, Bogotá, D.C., Colombia, USA; Tel: +1 520 204-1495; Fax: +1 623 218-1215; E-mail: business@tucsonspine.com

ably low, knowing the art of managing them in the postoperative recovery period can make the difference between a flourishing endoscopic outpatient spinal surgery program and one that will continue to struggle with replacing traditional open spinal surgeries.

Keywords: Lumbar endoscopy, Transforaminal decompression, Complications, Sequelae, Postoperative management.

INTRODUCTION

Endoscopy is on the verge of becoming mainstream in spinal surgery. The advantages are increasingly recognized by patients who have the internet at their fingertips and can readily find centers of excellence where innovative surgeons are pushing the envelope of technology applications in spine surgery. Besides the many immediate advantages such as less approach-related access trauma and reduced surgical pain, and diminished need for narcotic pain killers postoperatively, there are many other long-term advantages of staged context-driven endoscopic spine care where only validated predominant pain generators are being treated while ignoring many potential others. This trend away from image-based medical necessity criteria for surgical intervention deemphasizing correction of spinal malalignment, instability, and deformity not only creates the need to redefine the preoperative patient selection criteria, surgical indications, and treatments but also the postoperative management protocols.

Endoscopic spine surgery is fundamentally different from open spine surgery and many other forms of minimally invasive spine surgery. Many of the common problems that steer numerous patients away from open spine surgery, including infections, need for repeat and additional surgeries, complications from scarring, and surgical injury to the neural structures are by far less frequent with endoscopic spine surgery. In contrast, other sequelae and complications specific to endoscopic spine surgery are relevant. Not every spine surgeon is familiar with them, and perhaps even less so with how to manage them. While there is a dedicated chapter in this Bentham text series on the specific surgical complications with the endoscopic spinal surgery both in the cervical and lumbar spine, in this chapter, the authors are describing their clinical experience with their postoperative management of common problems one should be ready to encounter in their busy endoscopic spine practice. While there is no question that the long-term advantages of the endoscopic spine surgery outweigh the short-term problems, patient satisfaction may be negatively impacted if complications such as dural tears, nerve root injury, foot drop, and other sequelae including spinal headaches, dysesthesia, sensory changes, temporary motor weakness, and impaired proprioception are poorly managed during the postoperative recovery period. A recent study suggested that unavoidable side-effects from an expertly executed endoscopic spine surgery defined as sequelae are much more common than actual complications. Nearly a quarter of patients who undergo endoscopic surgery of the lumbar spine may encounter sequela-type problems during the postoperative recovery. Therefore, a text on endoscopic spinal surgery would not be complete unless these issues are openly discussed, and their management debated. This is the purpose of this chapter.

THE REFERENCE STANDARDS

The complication rates with endoscopic spinal surgery need to be discussed in comparison to established rates with the gold stand procedure – the microdiscectomy operation. Contrary to common perception, the complication rates reported in the literature for open and other forms of minimally invasive surgery are higher than one would expect. Nonetheless, they are the reference standard for comparison to endoscopic surgery (Table **1**).

Table 1. Common complications and their incidence reported with microdiscectomy [1 - 5].

Complication(s)	Rate
Dural tears	3%–4%
Cerebrospinal fistula	0.1%
Wrong level surgery	1.2%–3.3%
Wound infections	2%–3%
Spondylodiscitis	< 1%6
Significant blood loss	5%
Nerve root damage ranging from sensory dysfunction to loss of motor strength (foot drop)	0.3%
Life-threatening retroperitoneal vascular lesion	0.05%
Epidural hematoma with new neurological deficits	0.1%–0.2%
Deep venous thrombosis (DVT) even under chemical thromboprophylaxis	2.2%
Persistent leg pain after adequate decompression due to intraoperative nerve root manipulation causing Neurapraxia for days to weeks	2% [11]

What is evident from this literature review is that complications with the gold standard operation are not that uncommon and occur at an incidence between 0.1% to 5%. In the following, the authors intend to review the comparable complication rates and the incidence of unavoidable side effects of well-executed surgeries – sequelae.

SEQUELAE

Postoperative Dysesthesia

Sequelae are defined as an unavoidable consequence or side effect of an expertly executed surgery and do not include failure to cure [6]. In endoscopic spine surgery, examples include incisional pain, bone bruising of the iliac crest, infiltration of paraspinal- and the subcutaneous tissues with irrigation fluid causing distention pain, spinal headaches due to infusion of irrigation fluid into the spinal canal mainly when the surgeon works in the epidural space employing the outside-in technique, impairment of proprioception with poor effort induced weakness in the lower extremity, and dysesthesia with burning leg pain due to irritation of the dorsal root ganglion (DRG) from surgical trauma [7]. The latter problem is the most common one that causes the highest patient dissatisfaction with endoscopic surgery. Typically, the dysesthesia affects the exiting nerve root at the surgical level. Hence, the patient may complain of burning pain in a different dermatomal distribution. This type of pain is often unrelenting and constant. It is rarely affected by narcotic pain killers, patient position, or activity level, for which reason most patients find it very annoying. Several ideas were floated around to lower the incidence of postoperative DRG irritation after spinal endoscopy. De Carvalho *et al.* suggested that intraoperative neuromonitoring in patients who undergo endoscopic spinal surgery under general anesthesia may lower the rate of postoperative dysesthesia [8]. Cho *et al.* popularized the floating retraction technique concept to accomplish the same goal. In his study, Cho *et al.* had no postoperative dysesthesia in all of their 154 study patients [9]. Whether or not that is reproducible in any other spine surgeon's practice will likely depend on patient selection and skill level.

A recent study on postoperative dysesthesia following routine lumbar endoscopic decompression suggested that the incidence was related to the surgeon's skill level [10]. This study enrolled 451 patients in 7 centers from 4 countries consisting of 250 men and 201 women with an average age of 55.77 ± 15.6 years, with an average follow-up of 47.16 months. Macnab outcomes were excellent in 40.6% and good in 43.2% of patients. An uneventful postoperative recovery was observed in 78.5% of patients. The remaining 21.5% of patients reported dysesthesia leg pain with a typical onset of 5 to 10 days postoperatively. These patients were treated with transforaminal epidural steroid injections (TESI), non-steroidal anti-inflammatories, gabapentin, pregabalin, and activity modifications. The dysesthesia rates were similar between the surgical levels from L1 to S1. The dysesthesia rate was nearly identical regardless of whether the patient had a single- (21.8%) or a two-level (20.2%) operation without a statistically significant difference in endoscopic decompression (p = 0.742). Foraminal stenosis patients had a higher incidence of postoperative dysesthesia (27%) than patients with herniated discs. The highest dysesthesia rate was observed in patients with recurrent disc herniations (41.2%). The dysesthesia rates differed with statistical significance ranging from 11.6% - 33% (p = 0.002), suggesting that surgeon skill level is one of the most relevant contributing factors to the dysesthesia rates. Managing patients with dysesthesia is highly relevant to obtaining high patient satisfaction with endoscopic lumbar spine surgery. In this study, the authors demonstrated a statistically significant correlation between postoperative dysesthetic leg pain due to DRG irritation and less favorable long-term clinical outcomes (p < 0.0001). Forty-five percent of patients with fair and 61.3% of patients with poor Macnab outcomes had dysesthesia [10].

Preoperative education and reassurance postoperatively and medical and interventional management is the key to successfully managing these patients. The mere occurrence of dysesthesia in itself does not predict an unfavorable outcome. However, a complete decompression during the index endoscopy is very important. The predominant pain generator surgeons should validate preoperatively. It was evident that there are risk factors for postoperative dysesthesia, including stenosis surgery and recurrent herniated disc, suggesting progressive degenerative changes and epidural fibrosis being responsible for this finding. This observation was further corroborated by higher dysesthesia rates in those patients with more advanced degenerative changes in whom only fair and poor Macnab outcomes could be achieved. Still, there was no evidence supporting the commonly propagated perceptions that multilevel surgeries or that endoscopic surgery at L5/S1 or diabetes were putting patients at higher risk for postoperative dysesthesia [10].

Other Common Sequalae

Sequelae are defined as an unavoidable consequence or side effect of an expertly executed surgery and do not include failure to cure. In endoscopic spine surgery, examples include incisional pain, bone bruising of the iliac crest, infiltration of paraspinal- and the subcutaneous tissues with irrigation fluid causing distention pain, spinal headaches due to infusion of irrigation fluid into the spinal canal mainly when the surgeon works in the epidural space employing the outside-in technique, impairment of proprioception with poor effort induced weakness in the lower extremity, and dysesthesia with burning leg pain due to irritation of the dorsal root ganglion (DRG) from surgical trauma (Table **2**) [7]. The latter problem is the most common one that causes the highest patient dissatisfaction with endoscopic surgery [6].

Table 2. Postoperative Sequelae and deviations from normal postoperative course [6].

Deviation From Normal Postop Course	No. of 1839 Patients	Rate
Sequelae	320	Overall: 17.4%
Extravasation of irrigation fluid	69	3.75%
Spinal headaches	8	0.44%
Ecchymosis	14	0.76%
Dorsal root ganglion irritation	229	12.45%
Failure to cure	80	Overall: 4.35%
Contained disc herniation	41	2.23%
Central and lateral recess stenosis	39	2.12%
Acute-care readmissions (within 6 weeks)	16	Overall: 0.87%
Dorsal root ganglion irritation	9	0.49%
Infection	2	0.11%
Poor pain control	5	0.27%
Cumulative risk of adverse postop event	442	24.04%

Failure to Cure & Readmissions

Failure to cure following a well-intended and executed spinal surgery that met accepted medical necessity criteria for surgical indications in itself does not constitute a complication which is typically defined as any undesirable and unexpected result of an operation [11]. Failure to cure is also distinct from incomplete decompression in as much as the former relates to likely not having directed endoscopic spine care towards the patient's predominant pain generator *versus* the latter not having achieved the objectives of the operation [6]. With the success of lumbar endoscopic decompression surgery hinging heavily on correctly identifying the pain generator that causes most of the patient's disability, failure to cure may occur when the preoperative work-up was inaccurate. This scenario is common when clinical decision making for surgical intervention is solely image-based. A recent study has found that the diagnostic gap that exists with routine lumbar MRI reporting may be as high as 30% [12, 13]. Therefore, the authors recommend the additional use of diagnostic injections to confirm pain relief before endoscopic spine surgery is carried out on suspected pain generators. The combination of these two preoperative prognosticators of favorable outcomes with endoscopic decompression may raise their accuracy up to 98% [14].

Readmission after endoscopy is also an uncommon scenario. Common reasons are DRG irritation (0.49%), poor pain control (0.27%), and infection (0.11%) [15]. Exacerbation of poorly controlled medical comorbidities have led to transfers to an emergency room in 3 of 11 COPD patients that had an acute exacerbation immediately postoperatively. None of these led to readmission to a hospital for medical management of COPD. These numbers constitute an acute ER use rate of 0.16% for decompensated medical problems [6]. In addition, there were 26 (1.41%) acute unintended postoperative ER visits by patients after discharge from the ASC to their home within the first 6 postoperative weeks. Hence, the overall acute ER use rate in this study was 1.58% (29 patients). Ten of the 26 patients evaluated in the ER within 6 weeks from the index procedure were sent home after reassurance and successful management of dysesthetic leg pain (Table **3**). However, 16 (0.87%) patients were acutely readmitted to a hospital over the 9-year study period (0.87%): 9 for dysesthetic leg pain, 2 for wound infections (1 superficial and 1 discitis), and 5 for poorly controlled incisional pain. Of the 16 admitted patients, 10 patients received a postoperative MRI scan, whereas another 3 had a postoperative CT scan as part of their postoperative workup. None of these advanced imaging studies prompted any change in management [6].

Table 3. Complications & deviation from uneventful postoperative course following lumbar transforaminal endoscopy [6].

Complications	No. of 1839 Patients	Rate
Durotomy	2	0.11%
Foot drop	2	0.11%
COPD exacerbation	11	0. 6%
Superficial wound infection	1	0.05%
Discitis	1	0.05%
Reherniation after discectomy for extruded disc fragment	9	0.5%
Cumulative complications	26	1.42%

COMPLICATIONS

Complications after transforaminal endoscopic lumbar surgery are uncommon. They include dural tears, infections, herniations, incomplete decompression, and instrument failure (Table **3**). Unintended outcomes requiring reoperation per se are not "complications", but constitute a "failure to cure" even though the operation itself may have been uneventful. The authors will review the common complications and reasons for reoperation in an itemized fashion in the following.

Dural Tear

Dural tears have become more relevant, with more endoscopic surgeries of the lumbar spine being performed with the outside-in technique in the epidural space [16]. The original YESS™ technique popularized by Yeung *et al.* placed the working cannular initially inside the degenerative disc to perform the majority of the discectomy [17 - 23]. Further modification of Yeung's original method includes a foraminoplasty through an annular window with graspers, flexible shavers, and lasers [24]. Mechanized burrs and shavers have added to the increased risk of durotomy, which has been recently found to be primarily associated with such power tools. Other authors have identified additional risk factors related to durotomy during spinal endoscopy, including radiofrequency, adhesion in the spinal canal, previous surgery with cicatrix, giant disc fragments, and redundant dura [25]. While foraminoplasty has become an integral part of endoscopic lumbar decompression surgery, especially in stenosis patients, dural tears primarily occur during the transforaminal surgery's actual discectomy portion [16] and interlaminar portion during the medial facetectomy with power burrs and removal of the ligamentum flavum [25]. Therefore, surgeons and, in particular, novice surgeons who are still mastering the learning curve should be meticulously cautious during the endoscopic discectomy.

Opinions vary widely as far as managing these incidental durotomies [25]. If small, and if a small rootlet herniation obliterates the durotomy, most surgeons recommend non-surgical conservative care with 24 hours of bed rest. Intraoperative repair or conversion to open surgery did not seem to be perceived as necessary by the majority of surgeons who recently responded to an online survey orchestrated by the authors of this chapter. A few surgeons have advocated the use of a sealant or placement of a small Duragen™ patch through the endoscopic cannula. An endoscopic repair can only be executed by the most skilled surgeons [26] who have their support teams trained to deal with this complication and have the additional resources at hand when this unexpected complication occurs during routine lumbar endoscopy. In a recent surgeon survey, only a few surgeons admitted to having abandoned the operation, and most continued the discectomy decompression to accomplish the goal of the procedure in spite of durotomy [25]. In doing so, extensive retraction on the nerve roots or the dural sac should be avoided [16]. In rare cases, the disc herniation may be located in part in the dural sac due to tearing or erosion. In this case, Tamaki *et al.* performed an intentional durotomy to facilitate removal of the herniated disc followed by dural repair [27].

Many patients may not have any symptoms at all. Some patients may report spinal headaches but based on the authors' clinical observations, those are not the number one problem reported by patients [6]. However, incidental durotomy may cause postoperative radicular pain, sensory, and motor dysfunction, which may be reported by the patient immediately in the recovery room [16]. Reassurance and open discussion with the patient about what this unforeseen complication means in conjunction with a reiteration of a robust preoperative patient teaching program helps most patients cope with this problem well, particularly if no additional treatment is required. Typically, patients respond quickly to supportive non-operative care measures. Many of the authors of this chapter perform their surgeries at outpatient facilities. It comes in handy to have knee immobilizers available in the ambulatory surgery center setting just if a patient experiences motor weakness or proprioception problems. A transfer to another tertiary referral center is typically unnecessary, and patients can be sent home with specific instructions on bed rest, hydration, pain control for spinal headaches when present, and early mobilization within 48 hours. Patients who do not improve significantly within 48 hours should be reimaged with MRI and considered for admission to a hospital for an open dural repair of large tears, all at the attending surgeon's discretion [28].

Infection

In general, infections after endoscopic spinal surgery in the lumbar spine are very uncommon. The entire procedure is performed under constant irrigation, which likely is contributing to the low infection rates when comparing the endoscopic to open surgery data. A recent study in a large single-center study found the infection rate to be 0.11% [6]. This case series of 1839 patients reported two patients requiring treatment for infection after endoscopic discectomy [6]. There was superficial wound dehiscence from a stitch abscess in one patient, which resolved on its own with a short course of intravenous antibiotics with cephalexin followed by two weeks of oral antibiotics. The other patient had a history of spinal infection with L4/5 discitis some 20 years prior and developed a fever after an uneventful endoscopic stenosis decompression at the same level. While it was unclear whether this infection was new or reactivation of the dormant infection, it was treated as a new infection at the infectious disease consultant's direction, and the patient was treated with six weeks of intravenous antibiotics. Ultimately, both patients had a satisfactory outcome, and all clinical signs of infection resolved [6]. Despite these low numbers, the authors do not suggest trivializing postoperative infection risk with routine endoscopic surgery of the lumbar spine. As with any other surgery, the infection risk is dependent on patient selection criteria, the patients' underlying medical comorbidities, and indirectly on the surgeon's skill level as longer surgeries are associated with higher infection rates [29].

The overall infection risk with spine surgery ranges between 0.1% to 3.5% [30, 31]. However, infection rates may be substantially higher with the surgery's increasing complexity. It is also evident that medically complicated patients with multiple poorly controlled or managed comorbidities are at a higher risk [32]. A recent meta-analysis indicated higher risk ratios (RR) for bacterial infections in diabetics with an RR of 2.22 (95% confidence interval [95% CI] 1.38-3.60; P = 0.001), in patients having undergone surgeries longer than 3 hours with an RR of 2.16 (95% CI 1.12-4.19; P = 0.009), in patients with a body mass index of more than 35 (RR = 2.36, 95% CI 1.47-3.80; P = 0.000), and in patients whose surgery involved a posterior approach (RR = 1.22, 95% CI 1.05-1.41; P = 0.009) [33]. In lumbar endoscopic discectomy surgery, the infection rates are somewhat lower, perhaps because of the surgeries' lower complexity. Gu *et al.* only reported on one out of 209 patients who underwent percutaneous endoscopic transforaminal discectomy rendering the incidence in that series at 0.47% [34]. The one patient in Gu's series was successfully treated with intravenous antibiotics for two weeks [34]. Although uncommon, when suspected, an infection after endoscopic transforaminal decompression should be treated promptly. Laboratory workup should include erythrocyte sedimentation rate (ESR) and C-reactive protein (CRP). Advanced imaging studies, including MRI scans, may not help in the early postoperative convalescence period because of overall increased edema in the surgical area. However, it may be helpful in the delayed onset of infection by demonstrating fluid collections. The latter could be accessed via aspiration or percutaneous biopsy needles under ultrasound, fluoroscopic, or CT-guidance. Ideally, culture material can be obtained before instituting antibiotic treatment to avoid false-negative cultures and to obtain proper bacterial cultures of the species that caused the infection. The infectious disease team's consultant typically recommends culture-specific intravenous antibiotic treatment, often for a minimum of 6 weeks, followed by additional antibiotics by mouth if deemed appropriate or to achieve suppression. Endoscopic irrigation and debridement of the discectomy level should be performed in those patients with severe localized and radicular pain. In patients refractory to this care, an open debridement may become necessary. In the opinion of this team of authors, however, this is the last resort of the infection cannot be controlled since such operations bear the risk of iatrogenic instability and may prompt fusion surgeries.

Incomplete Decompression

Intraoperatively, it is often difficult to assess whether or not the decompression and the discectomy, in particular, is sufficient. The bony decompression for the foramen and the lateral recess may be straightforward to assess. Once one can directly visualize the traversing or exiting nerve root, and one has reached the lateral recess, the bony decompression is frequently complete. However, deciding when enough of a herniated disc has been removed may not be as straightforward. The herniated disc's location may further complicate this problem within the spinal motion segment and whether any extruded fragments are located in locations distant to the disc space. The size is just as important as the location of the disc herniation. Choi performed a retrospective review of some 10228 patients and found that there was incomplete decompression in 283 [35]. Risk factors included the disc herniation location that is inherently difficult for an endoscopy to reach. This outcome occurred in 95 patients. When broken down by the type and location of the herniated disc, there were 91 cases with central herniation (32.2%), 70 with migrated herniation (24.7%), 63 with axillary type herniation (22.3%), 18 with shoulder-type herniation (6.4%), and 12 with foraminal/extraforaminal herniation (4.2%). All of these 283 patients did have problems related to incomplete decompression requiring additional intervention [35]. Skill level may also play a role in central canal stenosis or a highly migrated disc herniation extending into zones distant from the intervertebral disc space beyond the reach of rigid spinal endoscopes. This problem was described by Lee *et al.*, who also recommended that disc herniations should be released entirely and delivered before attempting to remove them with graspers or rongeurs [36]. Access planning is also essential in setting up the surgery from the start to maximize the reach of the rigid endoscope.

Most importantly, though, if one is convinced that that the decompression is complete, the surgeon should take another look and carefully assess the decompression site for any incarcerated or retained disc fragments [36]. To avoid incomplete decompression, the authors of this chapter have adopted a hybridized outside-in and inside-out technique where the starting point may be different. Yeung prefers to start inside the disc (inside-out), and the other authors prefer initiating the surgery in the epidural space (outside-in). However, eventually, all endoscopic spine surgeons of this chapter arrive at the same endpoint – a complete decompression anterior to the dural sac and the posterolateral aspect of the dural sac in the epidural space [37]. In a five-year follow-up study comparing the clinical outcomes with both the outside-in and the insight-out technique, the first and senior author determined that long-term results are not only better than with this hybridized technique than with either technique alone but that the reoperation rates for incomplete decompression were a magnitude lower. This comparative study by Yeung and Lewandrowski showed excellent results according to the MacNab criteria in 52.8%, good in 35.8%, fair in 17 (9.7%), and poor in 3 (1.7%), respectively [38]. There was a higher reoperation rate in the outside-in group (35.6%) than in the inside-out group (8.1%). The secondary fusion rate was also higher with the outside-in (8.9%) than with the inside-out technique (2.3%). Ultimately, the long-term clinical outcomes with the endoscopic transforaminal decompression procedure were favorable regardless of whether the inside-out or outside-in technique was used. The authors' fusion rate was 3.2 times decreased at 5-year follow-up compared to recently reported reoperation rates for traditional decompression/fusion [38]. Long-term clinical outcomes with the inside-out technique were presumably better because of the ability to visualize and decompress underneath the dural sac, the ventral facet, and the axilla between the exiting and traversing nerve root known as the hidden zone of MacNab [38]. When the decompression is considered complete, the surgeon should carefully check for any entrapped, hidden, or residual fragments that should be removed. Sometimes massaging the disc fragments with the working cannula's bevel may deliver it into the field and facilitate its removal. Ultimately, a pulsating nerve with a free-floating epidural root is the best judgment of an appropriately decompressed painful nerve root [39, 40]

Recurrent Disc Herniation

The question as to how much disc tissue to remove during routine lumbar discectomy has always been controversial. Some surgeons employ chromodiscography with indigo carmine during endoscopic surgery to distinguish between diseased and normal tissue more accurately [41]. On the one hand, the operation's goal is to decompression the neural element and eliminate neurogenic pain. On the other hand, removing too much possibly healthy from the nucleus pulposus may accelerate the degenerative cascade and propagate recurrence of symptoms due to asymmetric vertical collapse and weight-bearing through the diseased lumbar motion segment [42]. Therefore, after discectomy, recurrent symptoms are not just a function of incomplete discectomy but are dependent on the overall functional status of the lumbar motion segment. Underlying anterolateral and vertical instability could lead to new [43], contained disc bulges or extruded disc herniations, particularly in patients with endstage degenerative vacuum disc disease [44 - 50]. Such hollow vacuum discs are likely mechanically incompetent. The same surgical intervertebral disc could develop another disc herniation even though the discectomy was deemed adequate during the index discectomy procedure. Typically, patients with such advanced vacuum disc motion segments have short-term pain relief from a straightforward laminotomy microdiscectomy procedure and may ultimately be candidates for a fusion surgery with interbody fusion to obtain more reliable intervertebral and neuroforaminal height restoration producing more durable clinical outcomes.

Several risk factors have been identified for the recurrence of disc herniations after microsurgical discectomy [40, 51 - 60]. The only available randomized trial comparing outcomes and complications including recurrence rates between the traditional microsurgical and endoscopic discectomy indicated no statistical difference in the recurrence rates of symptomatic herniated discs requiring additional treatments including surgery between the two types of surgical treatments. Therefore, it is reasonable to assume that endoscopic transforaminal discectomy in the lumbar spine has similar risk factors that have been validated with routine microsurgical discectomy. Risk factors are male gender [53], obesity (BMI $\geq$ 25) [57, 58], old age ($\geq$ 50 years) [52, 58], previous lumbar trauma, and presence of a central disc herniation [61] which is believed to represent a motion segment with more advanced degenerative changes [61]. In addition to these generic risk factors, there are likely some risk factors that are specific to the endoscopic transforaminal discectomy procedure. There is no doubt that there is a learning curve with spinal endoscopy surgery. A recent study by Ransom *et al.* suggested that even established spine surgeons with many years of surgical experience may have an initial learning curve of 15 cases before their clinical outcomes with the endoscopic lumbar discectomy may be equivalent to those they traditionally can obtain with open or minimally invasive microdiscectomy [62]. Surgeon skill level may definitively be of concern when rationalizing the variations in recurrence rates. An additional consideration is the availability of sophisticated endoscopic instruments. Before 2010, motorized decompression tools and more reliable and larger graspers and Kerrison rongeurs were not as widely available as nowadays [40, 61]. Yin *et al* found that the recurrence rate after endoscopic lumbar discectomy was significantly higher at the higher lumbar disc levels (5.4%) than that at L4-5 (2.7%) and L5-S1 (3.1%). The recurrent rates in far-lateral disc herniations was 4.7%, and in migrated herniations was 3.8%. Nearly two-thirds (61.7%) of recurrent disc herniations occurred at 6 months following the index operation. Patient education protocols should be established, and patients should be carefully instructed as to what to expect postoperatively and which instructions to follow to avoided early recurrence [63, 64]. While the data on how postoperative rehabilitation programs may positively impact patients recovery and functioning and lower the recurrence rate following the endoscopic surgery, it seems obvious that protocols should be established to manage patients postoperatively to allow for the natural healing process to play out while maximizing benefit with rehabilitation programs [65].

Foot Drop

Fortunately, this complication is not common. This chapter's authors could not find any specific published reports dedicated to investigating foot drop incidence after lumbar endoscopic spine surgery Footdrop, however, may occur when there are pre-existing pre-operative co morbidities. Instead, there are a few reports on employing endoscopy to treat foot drop that develops due to nerve root compression from a herniated disc. For example, Telfeian *et al.* reported his consecutive series of 211 patients treated with transforaminal endoscopic treatment for lumbar radiculopathy [66]. The authors performed 77 endoscopic surgeries at the L5-S1 level for far lateral extraforaminal disc herniations. Five of these 77 patients developed a postoperative foot drop. While clinical outcomes were favorable and seemingly unaffected by the preoperative foot drop, the tibialis's mean motor strength score improved from a preoperative value of 2.6 to 4.8 postoperatively at one-year follow-up [66]. In another application, the author presented a case where he employed endoscopy for foot drop that developed 12 years after a total disc arthroplasty [66]. Adsul *et al.* also presented a case of a patient with acute onset of foot drop, which was successfully treated with the transforaminal endoscopic decompression for far lateral disc herniation at L4/5, and L5/S1 [67]. A similar case was presented by Chun *et al.* [68]

One article reported on two patients who developed a foot drop postoperatively, rendering the incidence in that series 0.11%. Both of these complications occurred after L4-5 decompression surgery for lateral recess stenosis. Both of these patients were sent home from the ambulatory surgery center without problems. The patients were treated conservatively with an ankle-foot orthosis and physical therapy. One of the two patients had non–insulin-dependent diabetes mellitus. The diabetic patient improved somewhat from a 2/5 motor strength examination for extensor hallucis longus and tibialis anterior muscles shortly after surgery to 4/5 motor strength at nine months follow-up visit. The other patient's transitory weakness with extensor hallucis longus and tibialis anterior weakness (4/5) normalized within six weeks [6].

Reoperation

Causes of reoperation vary from residual fragments, LDH recurrence, discogenic back pain to discitis, and postoperative hematoma. In their retrospective study comparing percutaneous transforaminal endoscopic discectomy (n = 301) and microscopic discectomy (n = 614), Kim *et al.* found that 28 cases (9.5%) in the endoscopy group and 38 cases (6.3%) in the microdiscectomy group experienced reoperation, and the difference was of no statistical significance [69]. A study reported by Cheng *et al.* revealed that the incidence of reoperation in 6 months was greatest with percutaneous transforaminal endoscopic discectomy, followed by microdiscectomy, and lowest with open surgery (P < .01); however, the incidence over 1 to 5 years was greatest with open surgery, followed by microdiscectomy, and lowest with percutaneous transforaminal endoscopic discectomy (P < .01) [70]. The authors concluded that the long-term incidence of reoperation following endoscopy was relatively low. These observations were corroborated by Yeung [24] and Lewandrowski [71] independently and jointly [38]. Yao *et al.* showed that the percutaneous transforaminal endoscopic discectomy, microdiscectomy and minimally invasive transforaminal interbody fusion share similar long-term surgical efficacy [72]. Moreover, these authors concluded that endoscopy has the advantage of short operation time, hospital stay, and low expense, when compared to these other three forms of minimally invasive spine surgery but the risk of recurrence- and reoperation rates were lower with endoscopy. Yeung and Lewandrowski published their five-year reoperation rates for the purpose of comparing outcomes with the outside-in *versus* the inside-out technique [38]. Excellent MacNab outcomes were obtained in 52.8% of their 176 patients whom they treated with transforaminal endoscopic decompression for foraminal stenosis and herniated disc. Good Macnab results were obtained in 35.8%, fair in 9.7%, and poor in 1.7%. The mean preoperative VAS was 6.87+/-1.96. The vast majority of their patients (63.6%) did not require any additional surgery [38]. The reoperation rate was higher in the outside-in patients (35.6%) than the inside-out patients (8.1%) [38]. The subsequent fusion rate was also higher with the outside-in (8.9%) than with the inside-out technique (2.3%). Both authors concluded that patients with symptomatic foraminal stenosis may be treated successfully with either the inside-out or the outside-in endoscopic method. Their long-term outcomes were favorable, with a 3.2x decreased need for secondary fusion at 5-year follow-up compared to recently reported reoperation rates for traditional decompression/fusion [38].

Instrument Breakage

Endoscopic instruments are fragile and may break during surgery. While this occurs rarely, it may be challenging to retrieve parts of broken instruments [73, 74]. A cross-pin from the hinge of a grasper or rongeur may often break if it is stressed beyond its failure point [73]. Typically, this occurs when the surgeon pushes too hard on the instruments' handle. Early-generation instruments did not have a fail-safe mechanism within the rongeur or grasper's handle, which is supposed to break before the cross pin of the hinge within the patient, thus minimizing the risk of loose metallic parts of the rongeur in the patient. Therefore, surgeons should be familiar with their endoscopic instrumentation and only use higher quality products developed later that incorporated these fail-safe mechanisms. Metallic portions of endoscopic instruments may be rapidly flushed away from the surgical site, mainly if the surgeon works in the epidural space because of the constant irrigation. During intradiscal endoscopic decompression work, the broken part may be contained within the disc space. However, finding it may not be simple if the part is entrapped between degenerative fissured disc tissues.

The guidewires commonly used during serial dilation can be another source of intraoperative instrumentation related problems [75]. Steel wires may bend if the surgeon ignores the trajectory of the instruments he advances towards the spine. The guidewire may get stuck to a dilator and inadvertently be advanced beyond the safe confines of the disc space. Advancing the guidewire anterior to the spine may cause vascular, neural, or bowel injury. Fracture of the guidewire in two endoscopic cases was published by Guan *et al.* [75]. The authors were able to retrieve the broken guidewire tip during the same endoscopic operations which they completed. Ultimately, their patients had good clinical outcomes because these surgeons were able to complete the endoscopic operation despite the guidewire complication [75]. Open surgery should only be considered if endoscopic removal does not succeed during the same surgery. However, a shared decision should be made with the patient depending on the broken instrument's size and location and symptomatic. No consensus does exist on this subject.

DISCUSSION

As with every innovation, the risks *versus* benefits have to be carefully weighed. Nowadays, consensus exists that minimally invasive surgery has several advantages over traditional open spinal surgery. Endoscopic spinal surgery, in particular, is characterized by much shorter operation time as the surgeon does not have to spend as much time exposing the target area and closing the wound afterwards. Moreover, lower blood loss, minimal damage to the muscle, and stabilizing ligamentous spine structures are other advantages of endoscopic spinal surgery. Postoperatively, return to work data appear also more favorable when compared to open spinal surgery [76]. To realize these advantages in day-to-day clinical practice, most surgeons face a steep learning curve, especially if they are not exposed or taught the minimally invasive technique in their training period [24, 62, 77]. There is no question that sequelae and complications are less common in experienced and skilled hands [10]. The novice surgeon should expect some initial difficulty in realizing the same clinical outcomes as their traditional well-versed translaminar open and minimally invasive surgical procedures [62]. While there may not be necessarily more complications when the endoscopic procedure is carefully executed, at a minimum, a higher rate of sequelae should be expected initially. Foremost, irritation of the dorsal root ganglion of the exiting nerve root at the surgical level should be expected. As shown by a recent study by the authors, skill level plays an essential role in diminishing the incidence of this problem postoperatively [10]. Therefore, surgeons should not initially target the most complex problems often encountered in spinal stenosis cases. Beginning with straightforward herniated disc surgeries will help master the learning curve and becoming familiar with endoscopic instrumentation, its capabilities, and limitations. The cited study also showed that complications and sequelae are more common in the endoscopic treatment of lumbar motion segment with advanced degenerative changes which may entail severe stenosis due to hypertrophy of the facet joint complex, thickening of the yellow ligament, overt instability, epidural fibrosis, and tethering of the nerve roots [10].

The use of local anesthesia under monitored anesthesia care has been advocated by some key opinion leaders and is widely utilized by many surgeons. The expectation is that nerve root damage and dorsal root ganglion irritations can be minimized since the patient may verbalize complaints to the surgeon during surgery. Some authors apply spinal anesthesia as an adjunct, and others prefer to perform their endoscopic spinal surgeries under general anesthesia with or without neuromonitoring [8]. General balanced anesthesia protocols with propofol, fentanyl, and minimal inhalation anesthesia afford better pain control during surgery and overall higher patient satisfaction with the entire outpatient experience [78]. Severe intraoperative surgical pain may expose the patient to undue cardiovascular stress and, in extreme cases, even acute myocardial infarction [79, 80]. Most established, well-versed endoscopic spine surgeons will admit that their patients' awake state is less and less important to them with increasing experience when pressed hard on the issue. However, a universally accepted standard of care does not exist in this regard. Establishing it may be difficult since the spinal endoscopy's overall complication rate is approximately one magnitude lower than with the established gold standard surgery – the microsurgical discectomy [6]. To lower the incidence of complications and sequelae with spinal endoscopy, every surgeon should determine the most appropriate anesthesia protocol in the context of skill level, patient factors, and vendor support.

Other aspects of the operation need to be carefully planned for understanding the patient's painful pathology's anatomy and how to approach and treat it endoscopically [81]. Therefore, the access planning should be done with attention to detail to ensure the rigid spinal endoscope can reach it with the planned access trajectories. The available decompression equipment and instrumentation are capable of accomplishing the desired bony and soft tissue decompression. Regarding reoperation for incomplete decompression, surgeons should carefully select patients for the procedure [82]. Lateral canal and foraminal stenosis and foraminal or extraforaminal disc herniations are clinical indications with a high probability of favorable clinical outcome when treated with the endoscopic decompression surgery carried out with the transforaminal or interlaminar approach, the inside-out or outside-in technique. Far-migrated disc herniations may be hard to retrieve. Hence, every surgeon should carefully assess where the procedure's limits are in his or her hands.

Of the actual complications, dural tear, foot drop, and infection are the more serious ones [25]. Thankfully, they are not common. However, the increased use of power burrs and drills, particularly with the interlaminar approach, has led to increased reported durotomies with the endoscopic surgery in the lumbar spine. The first and senior authors of this chapter have independently reported very low durotomy rates with the transforaminal approach [6, 24, 38]. There may be several reasons for that observation, even though they are experienced, veteran endoscopic spine surgeons. The dura mater of the nerve root sleeve is somewhat more resilient than the dura mater in the posterior spinal canal. The translaminar decompression with power burrs and drills via the interlaminar approach has been associated with higher durotomy rates [25]. Another potential explanation may be the expansile foraminoplasty that most surgeons perform with the transforaminal approach and the surgical trajectories aiming away from the posterior dural sac and not towards it as with the interlaminar approach [83 - 89]. There is no clear consensus on how to treat dural tears [25]. However, most surgeons do not do much else beyond the application of dural patches, 24 to 48 hours of bed rest, pain killers for spinal headaches, fluid resuscitation, and supportive care measures. Conversion to open surgery is not a commonly applied exit strategy from this intraoperative complication [25]. One risk in endoscopic extraction of extruded, sequestered, herniated nucleus pulposus and severe stenosis, while rare, but has been demonstrated by the senior author in his presentations.

CONCLUSION

Complications after spinal endoscopy are uncommon and can usually be managed without the need for open revision surgery. Dural tears rarely require additional surgery. Foot drop is an infrequent complication that typically improves with supportive and conservative care measures. Reoperations for recurrent herniations or incomplete decompression are also uncommon scenarios but are not difficult to manage with additional endoscopic surgeries. Sequelae are much more common than complications. Implementing preoperative patient education programs may help maintain high patient satisfaction with the endoscopic spinal surgery program even if patients experience possibly annoying problems such as dysesthesia, spinal headaches, or incisional bruising.

CONSENT FOR PUBLICATION

Not applicable.

CONFLICT OF INTEREST

The authors declare no conflict of interest, financial or otherwise.

ACKNOWLEDGEMENT

Declared none.

REFERENCES

[1]   Hernandez-Perez PA, Prinzo-Yamurri H. Analysis of the lumbar discectomy complications. Neurocirugia (Astur) 2005; 16(5): 419-26.
[PMID: 16276450]

[2]   Ramirez LF, Thisted R. Complications and demographic characteristics of patients undergoing lumbar discectomy in community hospitals. Neurosurgery 1989; 25(2): 226-30.
[http://dx.doi.org/10.1227/00006123-198908000-00012] [PMID: 2770987]

[3]   Tafazal SI, Sell PJ. Incidental durotomy in lumbar spine surgery: incidence and management. Eur Spine J 2005; 14(3): 287-90.
[http://dx.doi.org/10.1007/s00586-004-0821-2] [PMID: 15821921]

[4]   Kraemer R, Wild A, Haak H, Herdmann J, Krauspe R, Kraemer J. Classification and management of early complications in open lumbar microdiscectomy. Eur Spine J 2003; 12(3): 239-46.
[http://dx.doi.org/10.1007/s00586-002-0466-y] [PMID: 12799998]

[5]   Lawton MT, Porter RW, Heiserman JE, Jacobowitz R, Sonntag VK, Dickman CA. Surgical management of spinal epidural hematoma: relationship between surgical timing and neurological outcome. J Neurosurg 1995; 83(1): 1-7.
[http://dx.doi.org/10.3171/jns.1995.83.1.0001] [PMID: 7782824]

[6]   Lewandrowski KU. Incidence, management, and cost of complications after transforaminal endoscopic decompression surgery for lumbar foraminal and lateral recess stenosis: a value proposition for outpatient ambulatory surgery. Int J Spine Surg 2019; 13(1): 53-67.
[http://dx.doi.org/10.14444/6008] [PMID: 30805287]

[7]   Silav G, Arslan M, Comert A, *et al.* Relationship of dorsal root ganglion to intervertebral foramen in lumbar region: an anatomical study and review of literature. J Neurosurg Sci 2016; 60(3): 339-44.
[PMID: 27402404]

[8]   de Carvalho PST, Ramos MRF, da Silva Meireles AC, *et al.* Feasibility of using intraoperative neuromonitoring in the prophylaxis of dysesthesia in transforaminal endoscopic discectomies of the lumbar spine. Brain Sci 2020; 10(8): E522.
[http://dx.doi.org/10.3390/brainsci10080522] [PMID: 32764525]

[9]   Cho JY, Lee SH, Lee HY. Prevention of development of postoperative dysesthesia in transforaminal percutaneous endoscopic lumbar discectomy for intracanalicular lumbar disc herniation: floating retraction technique. Minim Invasive Neurosurg 2011; 54(5-6): 214-8.
[http://dx.doi.org/10.1055/s-0031-1287774] [PMID: 22287030]

[10]   Lewandrowski KU, Dowling Á, Calderaro AL, *et al.* Dysethesia due to irritation of the dorsal root ganglion following lumbar transforaminal endoscopy: Analysis of frequency and contributing factors. Clin Neurol Neurosurg 2020; 197: 106073.
[http://dx.doi.org/10.1016/j.clineuro.2020.106073] [PMID: 32683194]

[11]   Dindo D, Demartines N, Clavien PA. Classification of surgical complications: a new proposal with evaluation in a cohort of 6336 patients and results of a survey. Ann Surg 2004; 240(2): 205-13.
[http://dx.doi.org/10.1097/01.sla.0000133083.54934.ae] [PMID: 15273542]

[12]   Lewandrowski KU. Retrospective analysis of accuracy and positive predictive value of preoperative lumbar MRI grading after successful outcome following outpatient endoscopic decompression for lumbar foraminal and lateral recess stenosis. Clin Neurol Neurosurg 2019; 179: 74-80.
[http://dx.doi.org/10.1016/j.clineuro.2019.02.019] [PMID: 30870712]

[13]   Yeung AT, Lewandrowski KU. Retrospective analysis of accuracy and positive predictive value of preoperative lumbar MRI grading after successful outcome following outpatient endoscopic decompression for lumbar foraminal and lateral recess stenosis. Clin Neurol Neurosurg 2019; 181: 52.
[http://dx.doi.org/10.1016/j.clineuro.2019.03.011] [PMID: 30986727]

[14]   Lewandrowski KU. Successful outcome after outpatient transforaminal decompression for lumbar

foraminal and lateral recess stenosis: The positive predictive value of diagnostic epidural steroid injection. Clin Neurol Neurosurg 2018; 173: 38-45.
[http://dx.doi.org/10.1016/j.clineuro.2018.07.015] [PMID: 30075346]

[15]   Lewandrowski KU. Readmissions after outpatient transforaminal decompression for lumbar foraminal and lateral recess stenosis. Int J Spine Surg 2018; 12(3): 342-51.
[http://dx.doi.org/10.14444/5040] [PMID: 30276091]

[16]   Pan M, Li Q, Li S, *et al.* Percutaneous endoscopic lumbar discectomy: indications and complications. Pain Physician 2020; 23(1): 49-56.
[PMID: 32013278]

[17]   Tsou PM, Alan Yeung C, Yeung AT. Posterolateral transforaminal selective endoscopic discectomy and thermal annuloplasty for chronic lumbar discogenic pain: a minimal access visualized intradiscal surgical procedure. Spine J 2004; 4(5): 564-73.
[http://dx.doi.org/10.1016/j.spinee.2004.01.014] [PMID: 15363430]

[18]   Yeung AT, Yeung CA. Advances in endoscopic disc and spine surgery: foraminal approach. Surg Technol Int 2003; 11: 255-63.
[PMID: 12931309]

[19]   Yeung AT, Tsou PM. Posterolateral endoscopic excision for lumbar disc herniation: Surgical technique, outcome, and complications in 307 consecutive cases. Spine 2002; 27(7): 722-31.
[http://dx.doi.org/10.1097/00007632-200204010-00009] [PMID: 11923665]

[20]   Tsou PM, Yeung AT. Transforaminal endoscopic decompression for radiculopathy secondary to intracanal noncontained lumbar disc herniations: outcome and technique. Spine J 2002; 2(1): 41-8.
[http://dx.doi.org/10.1016/S1529-9430(01)00153-X] [PMID: 14588287]

[21]   Bini W, Yeung AT, Calatayud V, Chaaban A, Seferlis T. The role of provocative discography in minimally invasive selective endoscopic discectomy. Neurocirugia (Astur) 2002; 13(1): 27-31.
[http://dx.doi.org/10.1016/S1130-1473(02)70646-5] [PMID: 11939090]

[22]   Yeung AT. The evolution of percutaneous spinal endoscopy and discectomy: state of the art. Mt Sinai J Med 2000; 67(4): 327-32.
[PMID: 11021785]

[23]   Yeung AT. Minimally Invasive Disc Surgery with the Yeung Endoscopic Spine System (YESS). Surg Technol Int 1999; 8: 267-77.
[PMID: 12451541]

[24]   Yeung A, Roberts A, Zhu L, Qi L, Zhang J, Lewandrowski KU. Treatment of soft tissue and bony spinal stenosis by a visualized endoscopic transforaminal technique under local anesthesia. Neurospine 2019; 16(1): 52-62.
[http://dx.doi.org/10.14245/ns.1938038.019] [PMID: 30943707]

[25]   Lewandrowski KU, Hellinger S, De Carvalho PST, *et al.* Dural tears during lumbar spinal endoscopy: surgeon skill, training, incidence, risk factors, and management. Int J Spine Surg 2021; 15(2): 280-94.
[http://dx.doi.org/10.14444/8038] [PMID: 33900986]

[26]   Shin JK, Youn MS, Seong YJ, Goh TS, Lee JS. Iatrogenic dural tear in endoscopic lumbar spinal surgery: full endoscopic dural suture repair (Youn's technique). Eur Spine J 2018; 27 (Suppl. 3): 544-8.
[http://dx.doi.org/10.1007/s00586-018-5637-6] [PMID: 29789920]

[27]   Tamaki Y, Sakai T, Miyagi R, *et al.* Intradural lumbar disc herniation after percutaneous endoscopic lumbar discectomy: case report. J Neurosurg Spine 2015; 23(3): 336-9.
[http://dx.doi.org/10.3171/2014.12.SPINE14682] [PMID: 26068274]

[28]   Ahn Y, Lee HY, Lee SH, Lee JH. Dural tears in percutaneous endoscopic lumbar discectomy. Eur Spine J 2011; 20(1): 58-64.
[http://dx.doi.org/10.1007/s00586-010-1493-8] [PMID: 20582555]

[29]   Deng H, Chan AK, Ammanuel S, *et al*. Risk factors for deep surgical site infection following thoracolumbar spinal surgery. J Neurosurg Spine 2019; 32(2): 292-301.
[http://dx.doi.org/10.3171/2019.8.SPINE19479] [PMID: 32011834]

[30]   Shoji H, Hirano T, Watanabe K, Ohashi M, Mizouchi T, Endo N. Risk factors for surgical site infection following spinal instrumentation surgery. J Orthop Sci 2018; 23(3): 449-54.
[http://dx.doi.org/10.1016/j.jos.2018.02.008] [PMID: 29506769]

[31]   Liu JM, Deng HL, Chen XY, *et al*. Risk factors for surgical site infection after posterior lumbar spinal surgery. Spine 2018; 43(10): 732-7.
[http://dx.doi.org/10.1097/BRS.0000000000002419] [PMID: 28922276]

[32]   Yusuf M, Finucane L, Selfe J. Red flags for the early detection of spinal infection in back pain patients. BMC Musculoskelet Disord 2019; 20(1): 606.
[http://dx.doi.org/10.1186/s12891-019-2949-6] [PMID: 31836000]

[33]   Fei Q, Li J, Lin J, *et al*. Risk factors for surgical site infection after spinal surgery: a meta-analysis. World Neurosurg 2016; 95: 507-15.
[http://dx.doi.org/10.1016/j.wneu.2015.05.059] [PMID: 26054871]

[34]   Gu YT, Cui Z, Shao HW, Ye Y, Gu AQ. Percutaneous transforaminal endoscopic surgery (PTES) for symptomatic lumbar disc herniation: a surgical technique, outcome, and complications in 209 consecutive cases. J Orthop Surg Res 2017; 12(1): 25.
[http://dx.doi.org/10.1186/s13018-017-0524-0] [PMID: 28178992]

[35]   Choi KC, Lee JH, Kim JS, *et al*. Unsuccessful percutaneous endoscopic lumbar discectomy: a single-center experience of 10,228 cases. Neurosurgery 2015; 76(4): 372-80.

[36]   Lee SH, Kang BU, Ahn Y, *et al*. Operative failure of percutaneous endoscopic lumbar discectomy: a radiologic analysis of 55 cases. Spine 2006; 31(10): E285-90.
[http://dx.doi.org/10.1097/01. brs.0000216446.13205.7a] [PMID: 16648734]

[37]   Lewandrowski KU, Yeung A. Lumbar endoscopic bony and soft tissue decompression with the hybridized inside-out approach: a review and technical note. Neurospine 2020; 17 (Suppl. 1): S34-43.
[http://dx.doi.org/10.14245/ns.2040160.080] [PMID: 32746516]

[38]   Yeung A, Lewandrowski KU. Five-year clinical outcomes with endoscopic transforaminal foraminoplasty for symptomatic degenerative conditions of the lumbar spine: a comparative study of inside-out *versus* outside-in techniques. J Spine Surg 2020; 6 (Suppl. 1): S66-83.
[http://dx.doi.org/10.21037/jss.2019.06.08] [PMID: 32195417]

[39]   Ahn Y. Transforaminal percutaneous endoscopic lumbar discectomy: technical tips to prevent complications. Expert Rev Med Devices 2012; 9(4): 361-6.
[http://dx.doi.org/10.1586/erd.12.23] [PMID: 22905840]

[40]   Yao Y, Liu H, Zhang H, *et al*. Risk factors for recurrent herniation after percutaneous endoscopic lumbar discectomy. World Neurosurg 2017; 100: 1-6.
[http://dx.doi.org/10.1016/j.wneu.2016.12.089] [PMID: 28043884]

[41]   Yeung AT. The evolution and advancement of endoscopic foraminal surgery: one surgeon's experience incorporating adjunctive techologies. SAS J 2007; 1(3): 108-17.
[http://dx.doi.org/10.1016/S1935-9810(07)70055-5] [PMID: 25802587]

[42]   Epstein NE. Spine surgery in geriatric patients: Sometimes unnecessary, too much, or too little. Surg Neurol Int 2011; 2: 188.
[http://dx.doi.org/10.4103/2152-7806.91408] [PMID: 22276241]

[43]   Lewandrowski KU, Zhang X, Ramírez León JF, de Carvalho PST, Hellinger S, Yeung A. Lumbar vacuum disc, vertical instability, standalone endoscopic interbody fusion, and other treatments: an opinion based survey among minimally invasive spinal surgeons. J Spine Surg 2020; 6 (Suppl. 1): S165-78.
[http://dx.doi.org/10.21037/jss.2019.11.02] [PMID: 32195425]

[44] Raines JR. Intervertebral disc fissures (vacuum intervertebral disc). Am J Roentgenol Radium Ther Nucl Med 1953; 70(6): 964-6.
[PMID: 13104729]

[45] Ford LT, Gilula LA, Murphy WA, Gado M. Analysis of gas in vacuum lumbar disc. AJR Am J Roentgenol 1977; 128(6): 1056-7.
[http://dx.doi.org/10.2214/ajr.128.6.1056] [PMID: 414544]

[46] Chevrot A, Pillon B, Revel M, Moutounet J, Pallardy G. The radiological phenomenon of lumbar vacuum-disc (author's transl). J Radiol Electrol Med Nucl 1978; 59(4): 267-70.
[PMID: 660575]

[47] Anda S, Støvring J, Rø M. CT of extraforaminal disc herniation with associated vacuum phenomenon. Neuroradiology 1988; 30(1): 76-7.
[http://dx.doi.org/10.1007/BF00341949] [PMID: 3357572]

[48] Latif AB. Vacuum phenomenon in the intervertebral disc. Magy Traumatol Orthop Helyreallito Seb 1991; 34(4): 297-300.
[PMID: 1685543]

[49] Schweitzer ME, el-Noueam KI. Vacuum disc: frequency of high signal intensity on T2-weighted MR images. Skeletal Radiol 1998; 27(2): 83-6.
[http://dx.doi.org/10.1007/s002560050342] [PMID: 9526773]

[50] Lee CH, Cho JH, Hyun SJ, Yoon SH, Kim KJ, Kim HJ. Symptomatic gas-containing herniated disc with the vacuum phenomenon: mechanism and treatment. Case report. Neurol Med Chir (Tokyo) 2012; 52(2): 106-8.
[http://dx.doi.org/10.2176/nmc.52.106] [PMID: 22362295]

[51] Abdu RW, Abdu WA, Pearson AM, Zhao W, Lurie JD, Weinstein JN. Reoperation for Recurrent Intervertebral Disc Herniation in the Spine Patient Outcomes Research Trial: Analysis of Rate, Risk Factors, and Outcome. Spine 2017; 42(14): 1106-14.
[http://dx.doi.org/10.1097/BRS.0000000000002088] [PMID: 28146015]

[52] Wong AYL, Karppinen J, Samartzis D. Low back pain in older adults: risk factors, management options and future directions. Scoliosis Spinal Disord 2017; 12: 14.
[http://dx.doi.org/10.1186/s13013-017-0121-3] [PMID: 28435906]

[53] Akça B, Erdil N, Colak MC, Disli OM, Battaloglu B, Colak C. Is there any difference in risk factors between male and female patients in new-onset atrial fibrillation after coronary artery bypass grafting? Thorac Cardiovasc Surg 2018; 66(6): 483-90.
[http://dx.doi.org/10.1055/s-0038-1629921] [PMID: 29510430]

[54] Katzell JL. Risk factors predicting less favorable outcomes in endoscopic lumbar discectomies. J Spine Surg 2020; 6 (Suppl. 1): S155-64.
[http://dx.doi.org/10.21037/jss.2019.11.04] [PMID: 32195424]

[55] Huang W, Han Z, Liu J, Yu L, Yu X. Risk factors for recurrent lumbar disc herniation: a systematic review and meta-analysis. Medicine (Baltimore) 2016; 95(2): e2378.
[http://dx.doi.org/10.1097/MD.0000000000002378] [PMID: 26765413]

[56] Staartjes VE, de Wispelaere MP, Miedema J, Schröder ML. Recurrent lumbar disc herniation after tubular microdiscectomy: analysis of learning curve progression. World Neurosurg 2017; 107: 28-34.
[http://dx.doi.org/10.1016/j.wneu.2017.07.121] [PMID: 28765022]

[57] Yaman ME, Kazancı A, Yaman ND, Baş F, Ayberk G. Factors that influence recurrent lumbar disc herniation. Hong Kong Med J 2017; 23(3): 258-63.
[http://dx.doi.org/10.12809/hkmj164852] [PMID: 28253483]

[58] Yin S, Du H, Yang W, Duan C, Feng C, Tao H. Prevalence of recurrent herniation following percutaneous endoscopic lumbar discectomy: a meta-analysis. Pain Physician 2018; 21(4): 337-50.
[PMID: 30045591]

[59]   Shin EH, Cho KJ, Kim YT, Park MH. Risk factors for recurrent lumbar disc herniation after discectomy. Int Orthop 2019; 43(4): 963-7.
[http://dx.doi.org/10.1007/s00264-018-4201-7] [PMID: 30327934]

[60]   Yu C, Zhan X, Liu C, *et al.* Risk factors for recurrent l5-s1 disc herniation after percutaneous endoscopic transforaminal discectomy: a retrospective study. Med Sci Monit 2020; 26: e919888.
[http://dx.doi.org/10.12659/MSM.919888] [PMID: 32210223]

[61]   Wang H, Zhou Y, Li C, Liu J, Xiang L. Risk factors for failure of single-level percutaneous endoscopic lumbar discectomy. J Neurosurg Spine 2015; 23(3): 320-5.
[http://dx.doi.org/10.3171/2014.10.SPINE1442] [PMID: 26068272]

[62]   Ransom NA, Gollogly S, Lewandrowski KU, Yeung A. Navigating the learning curve of spinal endoscopy as an established traditionally trained spine surgeon. J Spine Surg 2020; 6 (Suppl. 1): S197-207.
[http://dx.doi.org/10.21037/jss.2019.10.03] [PMID: 32195428]

[63]   Oosterhuis T, Costa LO, Maher CG, de Vet HC, van Tulder MW, Ostelo RW. Rehabilitation after lumbar disc surgery. Cochrane Database Syst Rev 2014; 2014(3): CD003007.
[PMID: 24627325]

[64]   Zhang R, Zhang SJ, Wang XJ. Postoperative functional exercise for patients who underwent percutaneous transforaminal endoscopic discectomy for lumbar disc herniation. Eur Rev Med Pharmacol Sci 2018; 22(1) (Suppl.): 15-22.
[PMID: 30004565]

[65]   Santana-Ríos JS, Chívez-Arias DD, Coronado-Zarco R, Cruz-Medina E, Nava-Bringas T. Postoperative treatment for lumbar disc herniation during rehabilitation. Systematic review. Acta Ortop Mex 2014; 28(2): 113-24.
[PMID: 26040154]

[66]   Telfeian AE, Oyelese A, Fridley J, Gokaslan ZL. Transforaminal endoscopic decompression for foot drop 12 years after lumbar total disk replacement. World Neurosurg 2018; 116: 136-9.
[http://dx.doi.org/10.1016/j.wneu.2018.05.089] [PMID: 29787873]

[67]   Adsul N, Kim HS, Choi SH, Jang JS, Jang IT, Oh SH. Acute bilateral isolated foot drop: changing the paradigm in management of degenerative spine surgery with percutaneous endoscopy. World Neurosurg 2018; 110: 319-22.
[http://dx.doi.org/10.1016/j.wneu.2017.11.128] [PMID: 29191530]

[68]   Chun EH, Park HS. A modified approach of percutaneous endoscopic lumbar discectomy (PELD) for far lateral disc herniation at L5-S1 with foot drop. Korean J Pain 2016; 29(1): 57-61.
[http://dx.doi.org/10.3344/kjp.2016.29.1.57] [PMID: 26839673]

[69]   Kim MJ, Lee SH, Jung ES, *et al.* Targeted percutaneous transforaminal endoscopic diskectomy in 295 patients: comparison with results of microscopic diskectomy. Surg Neurol 2007; 68(6): 623-31.
[http://dx.doi.org/10.1016/j.surneu.2006.12.051] [PMID: 18053857]

[70]   Cheng J, Wang H, Zheng W, *et al.* Reoperation after lumbar disc surgery in two hundred and seven patients. Int Orthop 2013; 37(8): 1511-7.
[http://dx.doi.org/10.1007/s00264-013-1925-2] [PMID: 23695881]

[71]   Lewandrowski KU, Ransom NA. Five-year clinical outcomes with endoscopic transforaminal outside-in foraminoplasty techniques for symptomatic degenerative conditions of the lumbar spine. J Spine Surg 2020; 6 (Suppl. 1): S54-65.
[http://dx.doi.org/10.21037/jss.2019.07.03] [PMID: 32195416]

[72]   Yao Y, Zhang H, Wu J, *et al.* Comparison of three minimally invasive spine surgery methods for revision surgery for recurrent herniation after percutaneous endoscopic lumbar discectomy. World Neurosurg 2017; 100: 641-647.e1.
[http://dx.doi.org/10.1016/j.wneu.2017.01.089] [PMID: 28153616]

[73]   Sureisen M, Tan BB, Teo YY, Wong CC. A rare incidence of breakage of tip of micropituitary forceps during percutaneous discectomy - how to remove it: a case report. Malays Orthop J 2015; 9(3): 58-60.
[http://dx.doi.org/10.5704/MOJ.1511.009] [PMID: 28611913]

[74]   Manabe H, Tezuka F, Yamashita K, *et al.* Operating costs of full-endoscopic lumbar spine surgery in japan. Neurol Med Chir (Tokyo) 2020; 60(1): 26-9.
[http://dx.doi.org/10.2176/nmc.oa.2019-0139] [PMID: 31619601]

[75]   Guan X, Wu X, Fan G, *et al.* Endoscopic retrieval of a broken guidewire during spinal surgery. Pain Physician 2016; 19(2): E339-42.
[PMID: 26815261]

[76]   Lewandrowski KU, Ransom NA, Yeung A. Return to work and recovery time analysis after outpatient endoscopic lumbar transforaminal decompression surgery. J Spine Surg 2020; 6 (Suppl. 1): S100-15.
[http://dx.doi.org/10.21037/jss.2019.10.01] [PMID: 32195419]

[77]   Yeung A, Roberts A, Shin P, Rivera E, Paterson A. Suggestions for a practical and progressive approach to endoscopic spine surgery training and privileges. J Spine 2018; 7: 2.
[http://dx.doi.org/10.4172/2165-7939.1000414]

[78]   Abrão Jo. Dowling Al, León JFRr, Lewandrowski K-U. Anesthesia For Endoscopic Spine Surgery Of The Spine In An Ambulatory Surgery Center. Glob j anesth pain med 2020; 3(5): 326-36.

[79]   Badner NH, Knill RL, Brown JE, Novick TV, Gelb AW. Myocardial infarction after noncardiac surgery. Anesthesiology 1998; 88(3): 572-8.
[http://dx.doi.org/10.1097/00000542-199803000-00005] [PMID: 9523798]

[80]   Charlson ME, MacKenzie CR, Gold JP, *et al.* The preoperative and intraoperative hemodynamic predictors of postoperative myocardial infarction or ischemia in patients undergoing noncardiac surgery. Ann Surg 1989; 210(5): 637-48.
[http://dx.doi.org/10.1097/00000658-198911000-00012] [PMID: 2530940]

[81]   Lewandrowski KU. "Outside-in" technique, clinical results, and indications with transforaminal lumbar endoscopic surgery: a retrospective study on 220 patients on applied radiographic classification of foraminal spinal stenosis. Int J Spine Surg 2014; 8: 8.
[http://dx.doi.org/10.14444/1026] [PMID: 25694915]

[82]   Dowling Á, Lewandrowski KU, da Silva FHP, Parra JAA, Portillo DM, Giménez YCP. Patient selection protocols for endoscopic transforaminal, interlaminar, and translaminar decompression of lumbar spinal stenosis. J Spine Surg 2020; 6 (Suppl. 1): S120-32.
[http://dx.doi.org/10.21037/jss.2019.11.07] [PMID: 32195421]

[83]   Chung J, Kong C, Sun W, Kim D, Kim H, Jeong H. Percutaneous endoscopic lumbar foraminoplasty for lumbar foraminal stenosis of elderly patients with unilateral radiculopathy: radiographic changes in magnetic resonance images. J Neurol Surg A Cent Eur Neurosurg 2019; 80(4): 302-11.
[http://dx.doi.org/10.1055/s-0038-1677052] [PMID: 30887488]

[84]   Hua W, Zhang Y, Wu X, *et al.* Full-endoscopic visualized foraminoplasty and discectomy under general anesthesia in the treatment of l4-l5 and l5-s1 disc herniation. Spine 2019; 44(16): E984-91.
[http://dx.doi.org/10.1097/BRS.0000000000003014] [PMID: 31374002]

[85]   Jasper GP, Francisco GM, Telfeian AE. Transforaminal endoscopic discectomy with foraminoplasty for the treatment of spondylolisthesis. Pain Physician 2014; 17(6): E703-8.
[PMID: 25415785]

[86]   Li ZZ, Hou SX, Shang WL, Cao Z, Zhao HL. Percutaneous lumbar foraminoplasty and percutaneous endoscopic lumbar decompression for lateral recess stenosis through transforaminal approach: Technique notes and 2 years follow-up. Clin Neurol Neurosurg 2016; 143: 90-4.
[http://dx.doi.org/10.1016/j.clineuro.2016.02.008] [PMID: 26907998]

[87]   Lin YP, Wang SL, Hu WX, *et al.* Percutaneous full-endoscopic lumbar foraminoplasty and decompression by using a visualization reamer for lumbar lateral recess and foraminal stenosis in

elderly patients. World Neurosurg 2020; 136: e83-9.
[http://dx.doi.org/10.1016/j.wneu.2019.10.123] [PMID: 31866456]

[88]   Wu JJ, Chen HZ, Zheng C. Transforaminal percutaneous endoscopic discectomy and foraminoplasty after lumbar spinal fusion surgery. Pain Physician 2017; 20(5): E647-51.
[PMID: 28727709]

[89]   Yang JS, Chu L, Chen CM, *et al.* Foraminoplasty at the tip or base of the superior articular process for lateral recess stenosis in percutaneous endoscopic lumbar discectomy: a multicenter, retrospective, controlled study with 2-year follow-up. BioMed Res Int 2018; 2018: 7692794.
[http://dx.doi.org/10.1155/2018/7692794] [PMID: 30662915]

CHAPTER 6

Laser Applications in Full Endoscopy of the Spine

Stefan Hellinger[1,*], Anthony Yeung[2,*], Friedrich Tieber[3], Paulo Sérgio Teixeira de Carvalho[4], André Luiz Calderaro[5] and Kai-Uwe Lewandrowski[6,7,8]

[1] *Department of Orthopedic Surgery, Arabellaklinik, Munich, Germany*

[2] *Clinical Professor, University of New Mexico School of Medicine, Albuquerque, New Mexico Desert Institute for Spine Care, Phoenix, AZ, USA*

[3] *Medical Technologies Consulting, Augsburg, Germany*

[4] *Department of Neurosurgery, Universidade Federal do Estado do Rio de Janeiro, Rio de Janeiro, Brazil*

[5] *Centro Ortopedico Valqueire, Departamento de Full Endoscopia da Coluna Vertebral, Rio de Janeiro, Brazil*

[6] *Center for Advanced Spine Care of Southern Arizona and Surgical Institute of Tucson, Tucson AZ, USA*

[7] *Associate Professor of Orthopaedic Surgery, Universidad Colsanitas, Bogota, Colombia, USA*

[8] *Visiting Professor, Department Orthopaedic Surgery, UNIRIO, Rio de Janeiro, Brazil*

Abstract: Lasers have been popular in spine surgery for decades. Patients frequently ask about laser spine surgery when looking for simplified ways to treat spine pain related to a herniated disc. Percutaneous interventional non-visualized needle-based laser treatments have been replaced with visualized endoscopic decompressions. This chapter reviews the fundamental physics of laser technology applications in spine surgery. Guidelines for safe laser use in the operating room and avoidance of complications are discussed in detail. Lasers suitable for spinal decompressions and their respective tissue interactions are described. The clinical evidence of percutaneous *versus* the hybridized use with the visualized endoscopic decompression is examined in detail.

Keywords: Clinical evidence, Endoscopic discectomy, Hybrid laser endoscopic surgery, Laser decompression.

* **Corresponding authors Stefan Hellinger and Anthony Yeung:** Department of Orthopedic Surgery, Arabellaklinik, Munich, Germany and Clinical Professor, University of New Mexico School of Medicine, Albuquerque, New Mexico Desert Institute for Spine Care, Phoenix, AZ, USA; Tel: +1 602 944 2900; E-mails: hellinger@gmx.de, ayeung@sciatica.com

INTRODUCTION

Albert Einstein, in 1917, first postulated that controlled radiation could be obtained from an atom under certain conditions [1]. The term laser is an acronym. Spelled out, it stands for Light Amplification by the Stimulated Emission of Radiation, which describes the process by which photonic energy is harnessed for useful applications. Lasers may be classified by the material - called the medium - used to produce the laser light. Solid-state, gas, liquid, and semiconductor are all common types of lasers. The medium undergoes an excitation process resulting in a population inversion of photons necessary to produce laser light. The majority of surgical lasers fall in the invisible portion of the electromagnetic radiation spectrum. A coaxial aligned, non-therapeutic aiming beam, typically Helium-Neon (532nm), indicates where the laser energy will impact tissue upon activation. The absorption characteristic of the medium largely determines the extent of penetration in particular tissue types. The application of any laser requires the surgeon to thoroughly understand the specific laser's characteristics for safe and effective use. Lasers have always been very attractive with an overall favorable public perception (Fig. **1**). The public's interest in laser spine care far exceeds its interest in minimally invasive-, endoscopic or laser spine surgery (Fig. **2**). Patients and surgeons are seemingly fascinated with the idea of laser care for common painful spinal conditions. However, there may be a gap between perception and understanding of actual laser protocols.

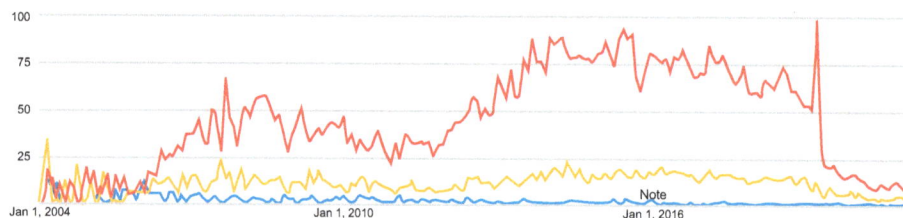

Fig. (1). Graphic depiction of worldwide monthly Google search popularity rating on on "laser discectomy" (blue), "laser spine surgery" (yellow), and "laser spine" (red) from 2004 to the present (data extracted on 12 15 2020). The highest popularity rating of monthly google searches is 100. Therefore, the numbers do not represent actual searches. The public interest in any type of laser treatment is much higher than in laser surgery or discectomy.

Surgeons have long shown an interest in incorporating lasers into minimally invasive spinal surgery procedures. This was first demonstrated by Peter Ascher, who employed neodymium:yttrium-aluminum-garnet (Nd: YAG) laser through an 18 gauge needle introduced fluoroscopically into the intervertebral disc [2]. He ablated the intervertebral disc in a short burst to minimize the heat spread to other adjacent tissues. He vaporized tissue that was allowed to escape through the needle. This procedure was ideally suitable for an outpatient setting as the patient was discharged once the needle is withdrawn in the puncture wound was covered with a small Band-Aid.

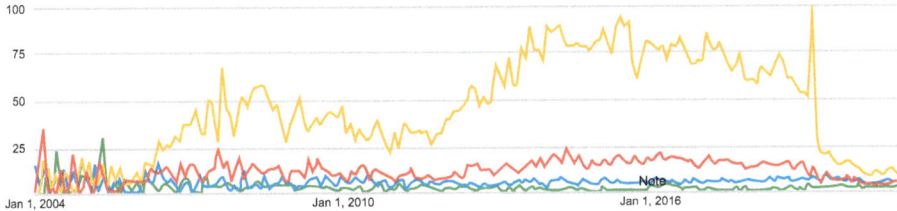

Fig. (2). Graphic depiction of worldwide monthly Google search popularity rating on "minimally invasive spinal surgery" (blue), "laser spine surgery" (red), endoscopic spine surgery (green) and "laser spine" (yellow) from 2004 to the present (data extracted on 12 15 2020). The highest popularity rating of monthly google searches is 100. Therefore, the numbers do not represent actual searches. However, it is evident that the public interest in any type of laser treatment is much higher than in minimally invasive, endoscopic-, and laser spine surgery again illustrating the laser's appeal to the public.

BASIC PHYSICS OF LASERS

The laser was invented in 1958 by Charles H. Townes and Arthur L. Schawlow [1]. They were attempting to create a device for studying molecular structure. They extended research from microwaves to the infrared region of the spectrum and utilized a series of mirrors to focus these shorter wavelengths. In 1960, a patent was granted for the laser. Townes won a Nobel Prize in Physics in 1964 and Schawlow in 1981. Light can be amplified and focused into a very intense beam. The light can be of different wavelengths and is classified as ultraviolet (UV) (150–400 nm), visible (390–700 nm), or infrared (greater than 700 nm) as part of the electromagnetic spectrum.

Atoms at their resting or ground state can be excited to a higher energy level when they absorb electrical, optical, or thermal energy. When the atom returns to its preexcitation state, it releases energy as a photon. This occurs naturally and spontaneously. Emission of two photons of the same frequency occurs if the atom is hit with another photon while on its descent from the excited state to the ground state. This happens in phase (coherence) with and in the same direction as the bombarding photon. This process is called stimulated emission. When these photons stimulate enough atoms to create a population inversion where there are more atoms in the excited stage than the ground state, a powerful coherent beam of energy is produced and emitted radiation (Fig. **3**).

KTP   Nd:YAG Hol:YAG Er:YAG CO_2
532   1,064   2,100   2,940   10,600

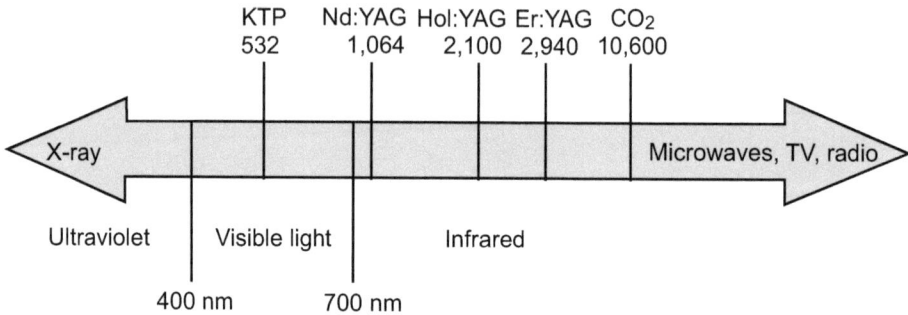

X-ray   Microwaves, TV, radio

Ultraviolet   Visible light   Infrared

400 nm   700 nm

Fig. (3). Wavelengths of the common lasers in the electromagnetic spectrum. The holmium: yttrium-aluminum-garnet (Hol:YAG), neodymium: yttrium-aluminum-garnet (Nd:YAG), erbium: yttrium-aluminu--garnet (Er:YAG), potassium-titanyl-phosphate (KTP) lasers, and carbon dioxide (CO_2) lasers in nanometers (nm).

Lasers consist of three components: (1) an active medium or lasing medium, (2) an optical cavity or resonator, and (3) an energizing source or pump. The energy source activates the atoms of the active medium within the resonator. The active medium can be a gas, solid, or liquid. Different media produce light at different wavelengths or energies. The resonator contains the active media and is fitted with two parallel mirrors facing each other. The back mirror is 100% reflective, while the output mirror is only partially reflective. The stimulated photons are reflected within the resonator and hit atoms in the excited state, producing more photons. The energy builds and is amplified by the reflected photons. This energy is released through the output mirror in the form of an intense beam of monochromatic (same wavelength), collimated (parallel, non-diverging), and coherent (same direction) light. This light beam can be focused with precision to a minute focal point (higher power density). This focused energy can cut or vaporize tissue. The beam can also be diffused and spread over a larger surface area to lessen penetration depth and produce more tissue coagulation (lower power density).

TYPES OF MEDICAL LASERS

Holmium YAG Laser (Ho: YAG Laser)

The Ho: YAG laser is a solid-state laser that emits light with a wavelength of 2,100 nm (2.1 μm). The active medium is the chemical element holmium. The yttrium-aluminum garnet serves as the host crystal. The laser rod is pumped with flash lamps, and the output power is up to 60 watts of laser power. The typical pulse lengths are in the range of 150-3,000 μs. While many wavelengths have been explored for spine applications [3, 4], the 2100nm Holmium: YAG laser remains the most popular laser employed in minimally invasive spine procedures requiring calcific or bone interaction [5, 6]. Yeung [7], Casper [8, 9], Chiu [10,

11] and Knight [12 - 16] further reported Holmium laser's utility to remodel extra-discal boney architecture during endoscopic spine surgery [8, 14, 17]. The combination of the laser beam's non-contact delivery, optical system (endoscope) quality, and surgeon comfort with endoscopic techniques, anatomical considerations, and skill play a critical role in the safe and effective use of the Holmium laser for bony decompression while avoiding damage to the dorsal root ganglion. Rongeurs and reamer systems entering the market for extra discal bone work may be alternatives to lasers for safer, effective, and economical decompression.

Alexandrite Laser

Alexandrite is an artificially produced crystal used as a laser medium in flashlamp-pumped solid-state lasers - usually with a xenon lamp (in pulsed operation) with intensive UV light. It emits in the wavelength range of 720-800 nm (close to the infrared range). Its main emission line is at 755 nm. A laser with Q-switch is characterized by the fact that the laser beam is switched with long pulses. The pulse duration is in the ns range (around 20 ns, and pulse energy of 1 J). Q-switch = Q-switching in principle emits extremely short laser pulses in the nanosecond range ns (10-9 s).

Argon Ion Laser (Argon Laser)

Argon ions are used as the laser medium in the argon laser. The excitation takes place by gas discharge in a glass or ceramic tube. The argon laser (continuous wave laser = CW) emits visible blue and green spectral ranges at 488 and 514 nm. In a particular design, other lines up to the ultraviolet (UV) range are also possible.

Diode Laser

The diode laser with a wavelength of 680 nm, 980nm, or 1470 nm is also known as a semiconductor laser or laser diode. Here the laser source consists of a unique arrangement of individual, special light-emitting diodes that emit laser radiation. The advantage of the diode laser over other laser systems is its compact design and portability. Systems with low laser power (up to 30 watts) usually have water-free cooling. They are easy to install and require less maintenance than others. Another advantage resulting from the technology is the low power consumption. A diode laser with a power of 60 watts is used in dermatology, ophthalmology, lithotripsy, photo-disruption, and epilation.

Erbium YAG Laser (Er: YAG Laser)

The Er: YAG laser has found several medical applications. This solid-state laser belongs to the group of "YAG lasers." It is a flash-lamp-pumped solid-state laser, which emits infrared light with a wavelength of 2,940 nm (2.94 μm). This wavelength corresponds to the maximum absorption of water. The effect of the Erbium-YAG laser is comparable to that of the CO_2 laser. An erbium laser is used in the field of dermatology and aesthetic surgery (wavelength 2,940 nm). Other areas of application are surgery, neurosurgery, dermatology, ophthalmology, plastic surgery, and dentistry.

Excimer Laser

Excimer lasers emit electromagnetic radiation in the ultraviolet wavelength range between 157 and 351 nm. Excimer is an artificial word and is formed from the words "excited state dimer" d. Here, molecules (dimers) are formed from two atoms, particularly from a noble gas and halogen, ArF. If a noble gas (neon, argon, krypton, xenon) is mixed with aggressive molecules such as chlorine, fluorine, or bromine in a tube and applies an electrical voltage, a gas discharge occurs. This process means that the molecule only exists in the excited state. In the basic state, it is unstable. Different wavelengths can be set by different mixing ratios of noble gas and a halogen such as chlorine (Cl), fluorine (F), bromine (Br). With a short pulse duration and very high peak energies, the process of photoablation occurs (material is removed from the surface). Typically, excimer lasers operating at 2-3 bar gas pressure of the laser medium and pulse repetition rates of up to 1,000 Hz. The pulse width ranges from 10 to a few 100 ns (10-9 s). Today's systems, which can only be operated in a pulsed manner, have an output power of up to 200 watts. A filling with xenon chloride (XeCl) can be used for approximately 107 pulses corresponding to an operating time of 10–20 days if the laser is operated four hours a day at a repetition rate of 30 Hz. This laser is primarily employed in ophthalmology.

Dye Laser (FDL)

The functional principle of the dye laser (FDL = flashlamp-pumped dye laser) is based on the excitation (optically pumped) of an organic dye solution for fluorescence, which occurs either through high-energy flashes of light from a flash lamp or with the aid of a second laser (usually argon laser). A relatively broad spectrum of light is emitted here. The main difference between this and other lasers is that a dye laser can emit a single wavelength or several wavelengths. It is tunable over a limited spectral range. The highest efficiency is achieved with the dye rhodamine 6G in the orange-red spectral range. The dye laser can work as a CW or pulsed laser, depending on the pump source.

Employing wavelength-selective filters, only a particular wavelength - defined or selectable depending on the laser device - is amplified and transmitted via the fiber system.

Helium-Neon Laser (Hene Laser)

Red helium-neon laser (632 nm) may serve as pilot lasers for the invisible surgical lasers such as CO_2 and Nd: YAG lasers.

Frequency-Doubled Neodymium Laser (KTP Laser)

With the KTP laser, the laser light from an Nd: YAG laser is passed through a KTP crystal (potassium titanyl phosphate). The Nd's wavelength: YAG laser light (1,064 nm) is halved when passing through this crystal. In this way, the green laser light with a wavelength of 532 nm is generated. Monochromatism, collimation, and coherence are retained as properties of laser light.

Carbon Dioxide Laser (CO₂ Laser)

With the CO_2 laser, carbon dioxide gas is used as the laser medium, excited in a glass tube by an electrical discharge. The CO_2 laser emits invisible, infrared radiation with a wavelength of 10,600 nm (10.6 μm). In continuous operation (CW), this laser is an exact cutting instrument because of its high water absorption and thus low penetration depth into the tissue. The limited applicability in a gas medium and with a mirror system is disadvantageous.

Neodymium YAG Laser (Nd: YAG laser)

The Nd: YAG laser (Nd3+: Y3Al5O12) uses neodymium ions as the laser medium embedded in a yttrium-aluminum-garnet crystal (active crystal). One or more high-performance discharge lamps (*e.g.*, krypton lamp), whose light excites the Nd ions, are arranged parallel to the Nd: YAG crystal rod. The Nd: YAG laser emits infrared, invisible light with a wavelength of 1,064 nm. A typical Nd: YAG laser (100 watts) is mobile with integrated air and water cooling circuit. An Nd: YAG is used in all surgical specialties, in urology, endoscopy, gynecology, pediatric surgery, and orthopedics.

Ruby Laser

The ruby laser is operating at a wavelength of 694 nm. Like other solid-state lasers, it can be used in the following operating modes: regular operation, Q-switch, and mode-locking. In its design as a Q-switched laser device (Q-switch ruby laser (QSRL)), this laser delivers high-energy light with a 20–40 ns pulse duration. Ruby laser devices have recently become available that enable a pulse duration of (0.3-5 ms). With a solid-state laser switched in mode-locked operation, the laser achieves a pulse duration of 1 ps = 1*10-12 s). Compared to a solid-state laser with a pulsed flash lamp, the pulse duration is 10 μs = 1*10-6 s. A ruby laser with 694 nm (10-60 J / cm²) is primarily used in dermatology.

LASER TISSUE INTERACTIONS

Depending on the medium with which the laser is operated, the radiation has different wavelengths. Besides, a distinction is made between continuously emitting (CW) and pulsed lasers. For medical treatments, three main principles of action can be distinguished:

- The photochemical effect,
- The thermal effects and,
- Photoablation.

In the early days, it was primarily thermal laser effects that were used for spatially limited tissue destruction (coagulation), hemostasis (hemostasis), and surgical tissue removal (ablation). With an increasing understanding of the laser and tissue interaction mechanisms, photochemical effects emerged in photodynamic therapy. The latter mechanisms are of lesser relevance to spinal surgery. Additional distinctions is can be made between various laser applications:

- Contact and non-contact between light guide or applicator and tissue;
- Various tissue reactions including hyperthermia, coagulation, vaporization (Table **1**);
- Different depth effects.

Table 1. Thermal effects of the laser on the tissue.

Temperature [C]	Tissue Effect
37-43	Reversible damage to normal tissue
43-60	The detachment of membranes, irreversible changes in enzymes
60-100	Coagulation (precipitation of protein)
> 100	Evaporation of water
> 150	Carbonization (charring)
> 300	Vaporization ("evaporation" of the tissue), non-linear effects (*e.g.* photo disruption)

In addition to the basic physical properties of monochromaticity, coherence, and collimation of the laser beam. The absorption behavior of matter, fluorescence, and scattering are essential for diagnostics with laser light. These properties are evaluated photometrically and spectroscopically. Depending on the irradiation parameters, different effects can be produced at the point of absorption. These can be chemical, thermal, or be mechanical. The initiation of chemical reactions is used in photodynamic tumor therapy. The thermal effects such as coagulation or vaporization form the basis of "classic laser surgery." Mechanical effects can lead to the fragmentation of gallstones or tear membranes. In the transition area, tissue can be ablated very precisely with minimal damage using thermomechanical ablation. Medical specialties and the various processes used by lasers are general surgery, dermatology, gastroenterology, gynecology, ENT surgery, neurosurgery, ophthalmology, orthopedics, pulmonology, and urology. The specifications of the different laser devices must be selected according to the desired requirements.

LASER ROOM, OPERATING ROOM SETUP

Regulations and requirements set forth by the Occupational Safety and Health Administration (OSHA) may vary from country to country. The authors advise the reader to consult with their applicable national and local safety boards, which regulate how to ensure safe working conditions by setting and enforcing standards and providing training, outreach, education, and assistance. However, the authors recommend the reader employ the following checklist when making modifications to the procedure or operating room where the laser will be used:

- Warning signs (yellow triangles with a black laser symbol and a black border) should be installed;
- Laser warning light must be on the entrance door and must indicate the laser "in operation";
- In the entrance area, laser protection goggles (corresponding to the laser) must be available;
- Emergency lighting should be installed in the laser room;
- Install a safety switch that prevents the laser from being used when the access door is opened the beam exits the laser;
- Install optimal restriction of the laser area (*e.g.*, through protective curtains, foils, talking protective glass);
- Apply an anti-reflective coating of all components in the beam path - this applies to the entire accessible area;
- Secure the laser against tilting, ventilation;
- Cover windows and the room areas that can be reached by reflection (*e.g.*, tiled walls).

RISKS, SIDE EFFECTS & COMPLICATIONS OF CLINICAL LASER USE

Dangers and risks associated with using a laser to the patient and the user or staff are often underestimated. When employing laser during spine surgery, possible side effects such as postoperative erythema, hyperpigmentation, or infections must also be considered. The laser is not a miracle instrument, and it replaces neither operative experience nor anatomical knowledge. One example was the introduction of "skin resurfacing" with CO_2 lasers. Comprehensive clinical studies on the effectiveness, safety, and side effect profile of these methods are said to have not been available when the CO_2 laser was introduced to the market. Often the end-user lacked the basis for a well-founded decision. Observed side effects of clinical laser applications in general include:

- Scar formation, hypopigmentation, and fibrosis were observed with the ruby laser in dermatology, followed by;
- tissue aging, edema, blistering, point bleeding;
- modification of the treated surface turning rough, *e.g.*, during LASIK, and photoablation refractive surgery;
- localized as well as generalized urticarial, pruriginous or eczematous skin reactions developing following Nd: YAG laser application in dermatology.

LASERS SUITABLE FOR SPINE DECOMPRESSION

Although many types of lasers have been reported in the literature for spine applications [18], which includes; KTP at 531 nm [16], Nd: YAG at 1,054 nm [3, 6, 19], and CO_2 at 10,600 nm [20, 21]. Only the Ho: YAG laser at 2100 nm has maintained a role in minimally invasive spine surgery [14]. However, it is associated with disadvantages, including a large "footprint," high cost of capital purchase and maintenance, high voltage requirement, and a steep learning curve since the Holmium laser is a non-tactile system delivering energy to tissue [22]. In general, lasers typically occupy ample space, are costly, and require a controlled environment for safe use, including laser signs on entryways and protective eyewear that often hinder vision and comfort for the surgeon staff in the operating room.

Neodymium YAG Laser (Nd: YAG laser)

A typical volume coagulator is the widespread continuous wave (CW) Nd: YAG laser (wavelength 1,064 and 1,320 or 1,318 nm). Depending on the power density used, deep, unspecific coagulation, vaporization, or tissue cutting is possible with this device. In recent years the Nd: YAG laser has also been increasingly used in contact processes. The Nd: YAG laser radiation is less strongly absorbed in the tissue. The tissue's optical scattering appears strongly at this wavelength and promotes the even distribution of the radiation in the tissue. The low absorption leads to up to 8 mm coagulation depths, for which reason it has been widely used in percutaneous laser discectomy. The volume of tissue irradiated by the laser light is heated, leading to a delayed death of the tissue without any noticeable structural change. If the surface defect is minimal, deep coagulation necrosis may occur. Due to the high power density at the contact point, carbonization and vaporization occur very quickly there. However, this also means that no thermally sufficient power density is achieved at a distance of a few millimeters, especially with a short exposure time, since the energy has already been absorbed or heavily scattered. The coagulation margin can thus be limited. The high depth of the Nd: YAG laser leads to the occlusion of blood and lymph vessels.

The laser light can be transported via flexible fibers. The Nd: YAG laser is ideally suited for endoscopic use or a spinal needle to access the intervertebral disc [19, 23]. There is minimal blood loss when cutting with the laser because the heat from the beam closes the wounds very quickly, leading to faster recovery. For the aim of vaporization with the fiber "bare fiber," a laser power of 25-60 W (depending on the fiber diameter and the desired effect) must be available. Higher laser power is required for coagulation to achieve a wide coagulation seam. The penetration depth on cartilage and bone tissue is up to 6 mm. With a suitable application, laser power between 20 and 40 watts, and a pulse rate of 0.05 to 0.1 seconds, the coagulation zone can be limited to 0.6 mm in experimental situations. The Nd: YAG laser's main advantage is the good coagulation effect with a relatively good penetration depth. The disadvantages of using this laser include:

- The considerable thermal effect does not leave a therapeutically desired large area [24].
- During intervertebral disc surgery, there is a risk of damage to the ring apophysis and endplates.

Erbium: YAG

Due to the very high absorption in water, the Er: YAG radiation penetrates only a few μm into biological tissue, which leads to an excellent cutting effect. The tissue absorption is ten to fifteen times stronger than that of the CO_2 laser; this results in the even faster and thinner explosive ablation of the tissue (associated with noise). When using a short pulse duration (approximately 1 ms), an almost athermal removal of outer skin layers (depending on the energy density used up to 10 μm) is possible. The Er: YAG lasers are primarily used in dermatology, plastic surgery, and dentistry. Due to its wavelength, the Er: YAG laser offers an absorption maximum of water, an optimal prerequisite for an exact superficial ablation of the skin, with minimal thermal tissue damage. Neither a hemostatic effect occurs with minimal thermal shrinkage. The postoperative inflammatory reaction should be less. The Er: YAG laser is excellent for controlled bone cutting and should theoretically be useful during spine surgery but has found moderate clinical application [3].

Holmium YAG Laser

The Ho: YAG laser, with its specific wavelength of 2,100 nm, is used wherever a low penetration depth is crucial (*e.g.*, neurosurgery, orthopedics). Depending on the tissue's water content, the Ho: YAG laser radiation penetration depth is up to 500 μm (0.5 mm). In particular, it is used for processing complex substances such as cartilage and bones and therefore has found broad usage in spinal decompression procedures (Fig. **4**). The "Moses effect" in water is exploited with holmium laser energy delivery on stones. It was first described in 1988 and relied on the vaporization of water by laser energy [25, 26]. The successive portion of the laser pulse transmits through vapor instead of water. In urologic applications, this mechanism allows for enhanced transmission of the laser energy to the target stone [27]. Therefore, the recently developed "Moses technology" uses pulse modulation to deliver a considerable fraction of total pulse energy through the vapor channel for ideal energy delivery [27]. Therefore, the Ho: YAG laser is suitable for bone ablation necessary during spinal decompression.

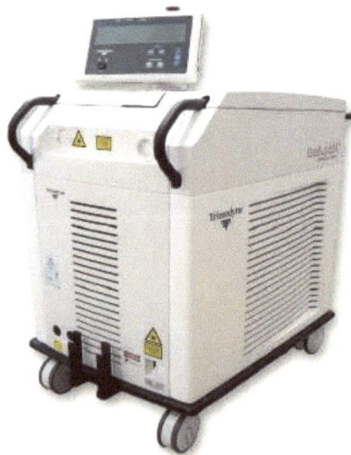

Fig. (4). The holmium: yttrium-aluminum-garnet (Hol:YAG) laser made by Trimedyne. This model is an 80 Watt double pulse laser. The Hol:YAG side-firing laser is one of the most useful tools in posterolateral selective endoscopic discectomy (SED). The small-diameter fiber tip fits down the working channel of the rigid rod-lens endoscope and allows precise tissue removal under direct visualization.

Frequency-Doubled Neodymium Laser (KTP)

Laser light of this wavelength (532 nm) is well absorbed in hemoglobin. The clinical application largely corresponds to the argon-ion laser. Devices with high output power (up to 15 W) allow the use of short-pulse times so that the treatment's painfulness is reduced. The laser light of the KTP laser is more strongly absorbed by the hemoglobin than that of the Nd: YAG laser. However, due to the excellent absorption, the penetration depth is also less. It has found some application in spine surgery because is limited penetration. It is beneficial when employed during endoscopic spine surgery in awake patients because it is not as painful as other lasers [14, 16, 28].

Carbon Dioxide Laser (CO$_2$ Laser)

Due to the wavelength of the CO$_2$ laser, absorption in the tissue is very high, which is why the laser energy is ultimately converted into heat on the tissue surface. Due to the increased tissue absorption, even with a low energy input of approximately 15-25 watts, tremendous heat is generated, leading to the tissue's evaporation in a narrow area. The CO$_2$ laser in continuous wave operation (CW) is an exact cutting instrument because of its high water absorption and low depth of penetration into the tissue. The cutting effect results from rapid vaporization with minimal coagulation necrosis and immediate water absorption by the light of the CO$_2$ laser. The CO$_2$ laser is used wherever microsurgical work or extensive ablation is required. Therefore, it has found significant traction in neurosurgery [29] and intervertebral disc surgery [1 - 3, 20, 21]. Its hemostatic effect is minimal; only capillary bleeding can be prevented. Its disadvantage is the current lack of radiation transmission via the fiber and the resulting articulated mirror arm (waveguide). Thus, hollow light conductors are increasingly being used, which, although they allow flexible beam guidance, have so far offered relatively low focusing capabilities. In the case of the pulsed CO$_2$ laser, instead of a continuous beam, a high-speed sequence of short pulses with high energy density is emitted, which, due to the reduced heat dissipation to the surrounding tissue, enables a cutting or vaporization effect with even less thermal influence on the environment. Pulsed or continuous-wave CO$_2$ lasers with unique scanner systems that will allow the superficial ablation of thin layers of skin are used in dermatology and plastic surgery. The great advantage of the CO$_2$ laser is its particular suitability for cutting with low edema reactions. The high absorption of CO$_2$ radiation in water, which prevents the use of quartz fibers to transport the laser radiation, proves disadvantageous. Therefore, with the CO$_2$ laser, the laser beam is guided to use with joint mirror optics. However, this technique is not suitable for endoscopic use.

PERCUTANEOUS LASER DECOMPRESSION

The percutaneous lumbar laser disc decompression treatment principle is based on the intervertebral disc being a closed hydraulic system. Increased water content may increase intradiscal pressure, shown in in vitro experiments to increase by 312 kPa or 2340 mmHg only by injecting one cc of water [30]. Conversely, reducing the intradiscal pressure by water vaporization within the tissues targeted by the laser may aid in nerve root decompression and reduce symptoms. For example, percutaneous lumbar laser disc decompression (PLDD) this reduction is accomplished by applying laser energy to evaporate water within the nucleus pulposus. The resulting increased water temperature also contributes to the denaturation of proteins changing in the nucleus pulposus, structurally limiting its ability to retain water and permanently reduce intradiscal pressure by more than half [30].

The significant advantages of using a minimally invasive technique for treating degenerative pathology are that the spine's architecture is better preserved, less tissue destruction, and lower risks. Initially, percutaneous interventions used to treat lumbar disc herniation employed chymopapain by way of dissolving the disc. Lasers set themselves apart from other percutaneous ablative techniques such as nucleotomy. They vaporize the intervertebral tissue disc by placing a fiber through a spinal needle into the herniated disc [31]. Often, percutaneous laser disc decompression (PLDD) is done under local anesthesia. The water within the disc tissue is vaporized, and the protein structure is changed so that it causes the intervertebral disc to shrink. As a result, there is a significant reduction of the intervertebral disc volume and the intradiscal pressure that produces an indirect decompression of the compressed nerve root. The first clinical percutaneous lumbar laser disc decompression was performed in Europe by Choy and colleagues in 1986 [30]. The FDA subsequently approved it in 1991 [32].

Despite FDA approval and abundant literature, significant dubiousness continues regarding the PLDD technology. The lack of randomized trials compounds this problem. Several cohort studies demonstrated safety and efficacy, but Brouwer *et al*. were the first to conduct a prospective randomized controlled trial (RCT) comparing PLDD to microsurgical discectomy [32]. Schenk *et al*. brought it on point when they reasoned that despite some 20 years of clinical use of PLDD, the quality of clinical evidence in its support remains weak [31]. Considering the cost-savings PLLD offers compared to the equivalent surgical protocols, discarding it altogether because of low-grade clinical evidence supporting it seems ill-advised. A recent meta-analysis that included 40 randomized controlled trials and two additional quasi-controlled trials comparing surgical and percutaneous forms of treated herniated disc concluded that the indications for

PLDD remain poorly defined and unresolved [33]. Moreover, the authors concluded that trials of percutaneous discectomy and laser discectomy showed inferior outcomes to microdiscectomy. However, good results can be achieved in appropriately selected patients [34]. Then, there remains the concern of the long-term consequences of translaminar microsurgical decompression techniques where iatrogenic instability may accelerate the natural history of the underlying degenerative disease.

While most of the observational studies analyzing percutaneous lumbar laser discectomy showed favorable clinical outcomes, to date, no randomized studies of percutaneous lumbar laser disc decompression were identified [35]. However, when stratifying analyses by design, none of the 33 observational articles had a control group. The authors of a systematic review on PLDD concluded that based on currently available evidence employing the U.S. Preventive Services Task Force (USPSTF) criteria, PLDD should be selectively offered to patients based on the physician's best judgment and the patient preference considering that the net benefit is likely small [35]. Another systematic review assessed the effectiveness of PLDD in comparison to conventional open lumbar discectomy regarding its cost-effectiveness suggesting limited evidence for short- and long-term relief based on 15 included observational studies [36].

In a multicenter, retrospective analysis of 658 cases by Mayer *et al.*, the authors found a 1.1% intraoperative complication rate and a 1.5% postoperative complication rate [37]. Spondylodiscitis - aseptic and septic - is the most common complication. It may occur at a rate of up to 1.2% [30]. Aseptic discitis results from heat damage to either the disc or adjacent vertebral endplates [38]. This heat damage can be minimized by monitoring the patient during the procedure. The laser power, pulse rate, and pulse interval should be adjusted when heat sensations occur. On the other hand, septic discitis is a result of infection during the initial needle placement [39]. Therefore, antibiotic prophylaxis should be given within 1 hour before the procedure [40]. Although it has been stipulated that the laser-induced heat may inhibit infection [41]. Another less-common complication is bleeding and epidural hematoma [42]. Nerve root damage has been reported with the CO_2 laser. In one study, it occurred at an incidence of 8% [31]. Postoperative dysesthesia may occur as well but is typically self-limiting. In a survey on sciatica management due to lumbar disc herniation in the Netherlands, Arts *et al.* showed that recurrent disc herniation was expected to be highest after percutaneous lumbar laser disc decompression [43]. In contrast, it was anticipated to be less after unilateral trans-flaval discectomy and lowest after bilateral discectomy [43].

In the cervical spine, there is a lack of literature on percutaneous PLDD. Siebert *et al.* reported favorable outcomes with cervical PLDD in 1995 [44]. Knight wrote a prospective study to compare the efficacy of the Holmium 2100: YAG with that of the KTP 532 laser in 2000 for symptomatic broad-based cervical disc protrusions [14]. Preoperatively, patients were screened with provocative discography to isolate the painful level. The cervical PLDD was performed on 105 patients at 108 levels under fluoroscopic control employing the anterior approach and side-firing probes. After a minimum follow-up of 12 months, half of the patients had excellent clinical outcomes. Another 25% demonstrated functional improvement on the Vernon-Mior cervical disability and visual analog pain score. There was no difference in outcome between the two types of lasers. The author thought both lasers are helpful in annealing of painful discal tears [14].

THE INITIAL EVOLUTION OF LASERS IN SPINAL ENDOSCOPY

Quigley compared the Ho: YAG to the Nd: YAG laser in a clinical trial conducted in 1991 [6]. They concluded that the Ho: YAG laser was the best compromise between the efficacy of absorption and the convenience of fiber-optic delivery at that time. In 1990, Davis *et al*. reported an 85% favorable outcome in 40 patients who underwent a laser discectomy using the potassium-titanyl-phosphate (KTP 532-nm) laser [28]. Of the 40 patients, six required a traditional open discectomy because the laser discectomy had failed. Casper *et al*. used a side-firing Ho: YAG laser first in 1995 [28]. His observations were later corroborated by Yeung *et al*. [9]. At a one-year follow-up, Casper *et al*. reported an 84% success rate [9]. 5 In the same year, Siebert *et al*. published a 78% success rate on 100 patients with a mean follow-up of 17 months treated with the Nd: YAG laser [44].

Mayer *et al*. were the first to suggest the combined use of an endoscope with laser ablation through an endoscopically introduced fiber. Extensive clinical trials followed and supported the clinical use of lasers for the removal of a herniated disc [37]. Hellinger reported in 1999 on more than 2535 patients he treated with the Ascher technique [22]. The reported success rate was 80%, with a maximum follow-up of 13 years. Also employing the KTP laser, Yeung *et al*. reported an 84% success rate in his patient group of more than 50 [45, 46].

The current state-of-the-art has been summarized by Ahn *et al*. [47] in a recent article by pointing out the three categories of laser application in interventional and minimally invasive spinal surgery: (1) open microscopic laser surgery; (2) percutaneous endoscopic laser surgery; and (3) laser-tissue modulation for spinal pain [47]. However, the lack of evidence with randomized clinical trials regarding clinical indications, safety, and the benefit was of concern [47]. Brouwer *et al*. orchestrated such a multicenter randomized prospective trial employing an intent-to-treat protocol with a non-inferiority design in their study of 115 patients suffering from symptomatic lumbar disc herniation [32]. Only enrolling patients whose disc herniation occupied less than one-third of the spinal canal, the authors randomly assigned 57 patients to conventional microdiscectomy surgery and the remaining 55 patients to percutaneous laser disc decompression (PLDD) [32, 48]. The needle-based (18G) percutaneous PLDD procedure allowed placement of 600-micron glass fiber into the center of the disc where they delivered laser energy employing the Biolitec Diode laser operating at 980 nm, 7 W, 0.6 s pulses, interval 1 s to total energy produced of 1500 J (2000 J per level. The authors could not demonstrate any statistically significant differences in outcome measures between the two treatment groups by analyzing pain reduction postoperatively with the VAS for back and leg pain and the Roland Morris score. However, the laser group's reoperation rate was disproportionally higher in the laser (52%) than in the microdiscectomy (21%) group. Brower's study did not involve the application of a spinal endoscope for direct visualization. Their procedures were done under fluoroscopic guidance. Nonetheless, Brower's study demonstrates tissue interaction with the modern diode lasers where the white intervertebral disc tissue may have limited ability to absorb laser light in any wavelength. Delivery of sufficient energy to achieve the treatment effect may not be possible [48]. Thus, the decompression effect may be minimal when placing the laser fiber inside the intervertebral disc. At 980 nm, laser decompression of white intervertebral disc tissue could be problematic. The laser treatment of bovine intervertebral disc tissue at a 1,470-nm rather than 980 nm wavelength was shown to be beneficial in vitro, but its clinical benefit still has to be demonstrated [48]. In 2012, Cselik *et al.* investigated MRI and histology evaluated the impact of infrared laser light-induced ablation at different wavelengths on bovine intervertebral discs ex vivo [4]. The 1470-nm laser light had affected the entire nucleus pulposus and not just at the tip of the fiber - a problem observed with the 980-nm laser irradiation [4]. The cost-effectiveness of PLDD over standard microdiscectomy has been demonstrated for a simple herniated disc. However, it remains to be seen when integrated with an endoscopic platform and applied in more complex clinical scenarios such as foraminal and lateral recess stenosis [32, 49]. At a minimum, the concern for nerve root injury with laser application in the spine remains [50].

LASER AS AN ADJUNCT TO ENDOSCOPIC EPIDURAL DECOMPRESSION

In 1998, Knight first reported his endoscopic assisted laser for lumbar foraminoplasty, which he saw primarily indicated for patients with unilateral sciatica-type back and leg pain [12]. Through a uniportal transforaminal approach, he employed a side-firing holmium laser to ablate bone from the stenotic neuroforamen of the affected nerve root under direct visualization and constant saline irrigation. The author also used his for debridement of epidural scarring, extruded and sequestrated disc herniations, and bony osteophytes. A total of 219 such laser-assisted endoscopic foraminal decompression surgeries were performed in such a way. The author had favorable minimum one-year follow-up data on 48 cases [12]. Knight found the adjunctive use of his Holmium laser particularly useful when decompressing the lateral recess and stipulated that his technique may delay open spinal decompression with fusion.

Knight followed with a complications analysis of the endoscopic laser foraminoplasty in 2001, analyzing 958 procedures performed on 716 patients [15]. The author found 24 complications in 23 patients. These included discitis (1 infective, 8 aseptic; 0.9%), 1 dural tear (0.1%), 1 deep wound infection (0.1%), 2 patients suffered a foot drop (1 transient) (0.2%), 1 myocardial infarction (0.1%), 1 erectile dysfunction (0.1%), and a final 1 patient who suffered from panic attacks post-operatively (0.1%). Therefore, the overall PLDD complication rate of 1.6%, which the author pointed out, was a magnitude lower than observed with spinal fusion surgery. Failure to cure was observed in 8 patients in whom the postoperative MRI scan showed incomplete decompression with a sizable residual disc herniations (0.8%) [15].

In 2007, Anthony Yeung reported on his first 80 consecutive patients who had undergone endoscopic decompression with adjunctive use of a KTP laser from 1991–1995 before Knight had published his results in 1999 and 2000 [46]. Yeung's initial cohort had a mean age was 41.9 years, ranging from 25 to 69 years. They had surgery at the following levels: L2–L3 (n = 2); L3–L4 (n = 12); L4–L5 (n = 28); L5–S1 (n = 21); and L4–L5 and L5–S1 (n = 17). The inclusion criteria for his study were:

1. symptomatic lumbar disc herniation,

2. an advanced imaging study including MRI or CT scan confirming a lumbar disc herniation corresponding to the patient's symptoms, and

3. failed non-operative care for at least six weeks.

All patients needed to have an associated unilateral or bilateral sciatica. There were no limits on the size or migration distance of extruded fragments within reach of the endoscopic instrumentation. Postoperative MRI scans were available in 28 patients who were used for comparative analysis to preoperative studies. Of those 28 patients with large herniations favorable clinical outcomes, the postoperative MRI scan showed a significant reduction in the symptomatic disc herniation size. Despite excellent results, smaller protrusions of 3 mm at the base or less displayed no noticeable change in size on postoperative MRI scans [46]. Yeung also used chymopapain as an adjunct during the endoscopic removal of extruded herniations if he suspected that he could not remove the disc in its entirety by endoscopic means alone. He also recognized that patients were at increased risk for incomplete discectomy with the YESS "inside-out technique when the disc level's height was greater than the width at the base of the extruded herniation fragments. He found it easier to pull extruded fragments back inside the disc space when chymopapain was injected during surgery [46]. Yeung also used laser disc decompression during the endoscopic microdiscectomy procedures, which later was modified by including unipolar, and bipolar radiofrequency for hemostasis and tissue shrinkage instead of a laser (Fig. **5**).

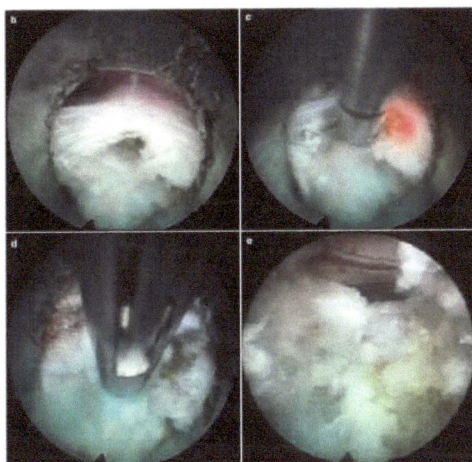

Fig. (5). Illustration of the (**a**) endoscope with the laser fiber (tool) in the working channel and (**b**) intraoperative images of the intact posterior annular fibers, (**c**) laser targeting the posterior annular fibers to free up the extruded herniated disc fragment, (**d**) extracting the herniation with pituitary rongeurs, (**e**) visualization of the decompressed traversing nerve root.

In 1997, Yeung employed a temperature-controlled flexible probe by Oratec Interventions Inc (Menlo Park, California) [46]. Of the 50 patients treated in such a way, two experienced transitory severe dysesthesia, and one patient developed a foot-drop which incompletely resolved. Yeung abandoned the temperature-controlled probe in favor of a steerable, cold temperature bipolar, high-frequency (4.0 MHZ) flexible probe (Ellman International Inc, Baldwin, New York) and the KTP to holmium: yttrium-aluminum-garnet (Ho: YAG) laser (Trimedyne, Irvine, California). The latter he specifically employed for soft tissue and bone ablation. The Ho: YAG laser was used with a side-firing tip and a straight fiber guided with a nitinol curved tube to better direct it (Fig. **6**), ablate osteophytes, and release disc fragments scarred down the annulus and the endplate. Yeung later also employed differently-configured hinged pituitary disc rongeurs for a more efficient discectomy and motorized shavers (Endius Inc, Plainville, Massachusetts) to improve the discectomy.

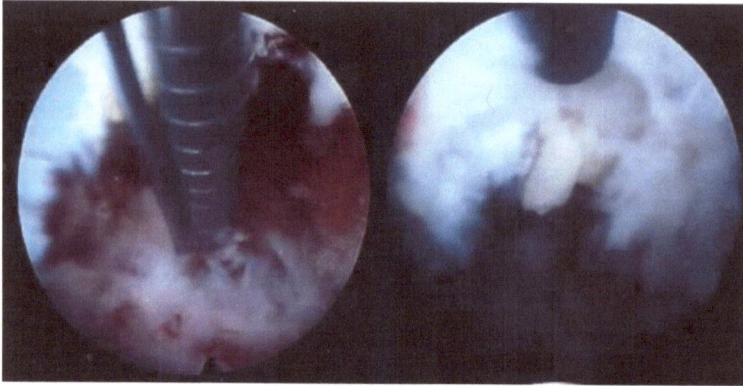

Fig. (6). Intraoperative endoscopic view of holmium: yttrium-aluminum-garnet (Ho: YAG; Dornier) laser ablation employed for ablation of facet joint capsule and bone ablation from the superior articular process during the foraminoplasty (left panel). The fiber was aimed at the target area with a steering wire (Storz). The controlled ablation effect – the Moses effect - by the Ho: YAG Laser is illustrated (right panel.

For the disc ablation, Yeung reported using the KTP laser at 10 watts for 1 second at a time to allow local heat to dissipate. He also paused the lasering if the patient reported discomfort from the heat. The total energy delivery was toped at 1800 joules per disc level. Yeung used indigo carmine dye to preferentially stain the degenerative nuclear material, typically taking on a blue to green color. The pigment also enhanced the effect of the KTP laser on degenerative nuclear disc tissue. Suppose the herniation breaches the annulus in extruded herniations. In that case, the vital dye will stain both the disc material and annular collagen, visually guiding the surgeon on the extent of discectomy and posterior fragmentectomy needed. If the surgeon could not reach the extruded fragment, a biportal approach was established to get the fragment from the opposite foramen. After the herniated fragment was retrieved, the nerve root and epidural space are probed or visualized, and the disc space was further inspected for any loose fragments.

LASER-ASSISTED FORAMINOPLASTY

The Ho: YAG side-firing laser has been used along with high-speed endoscopic burrs to remove boney neuroforaminal stenosis and alleviate radiculopathy. The laser is powerful enough to ablate bone and safe sufficient to operate near the exiting nerve root. Typically, the undersurface of the SAP is removed starting at the base of the caudal pedicle and working cephalad towards the tip of the SAP until the exiting nerve root is decompressed (Figs. **7** and **8**).

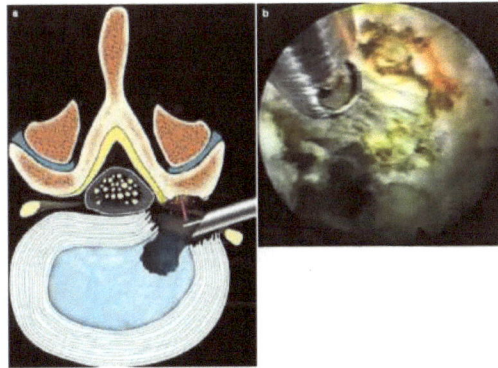

Fig. (7). Illustration of the (**a**) position of the endoscope and laser under the superior articular facet. (**b**) Intraoperative endoscopic view of the side-firing Hol:YAG laser removing bone from the ventral aspect of the superior articular facet.

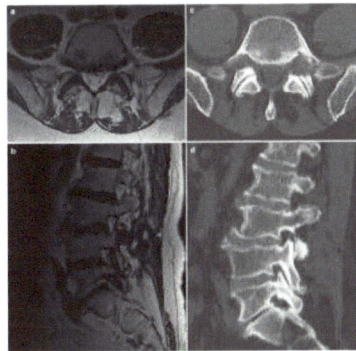

Fig. (8). Preoperative MRI showing symptomatic left foraminal stenosis. (**c, d**) Postoperative CT scan showing the area of foraminal decompression after removal of the undersurface of the superior articular facet (foraminoplasty).

EPIDUROSCOPIC LASER NEURAL DECOMPRESSION

In Asia, epiduroscopic laser discectomy has been applied for neural element decompression, mostly through the sacral hiatus [51]. Additional indications include the epiduroscopic visualization for lysis of adhesions or fibrosis using a laser [52]. The authors advocated epiduroscopic laser neural decompression (ELND) as a means to visualize the epidural space distant from the neuroforamina or lateral recess better. They proposed it as an adjunct to their endoscopic treatment for downward migrated herniated disc where epidural fibrosis is not uncommon. The advocates of ELND built their protocol around the concept of using a Ho: YAG laser operating at a wavelength of 2.1 µm and a limited penetration depth of 0.5 mm to visualize and decompress inflamed neural tissue and release adhesion directly [51]. The authors of this chapter have no clinical experience with the epiduroscopic application of lasers to the spine. However, they felt compelled to mention this technique for completeness sake as it recently has been hybridized with transforaminal full-endoscopy to aid in the complete removal of difficult-to-treat downward migrated lumbar disc herniations.

ENDOSCOPIC *VERSUS* PERCUTANEOUS LASER DECOMPRESSION

PLDD has recently seen a renaissance after nearly have fallen by the wayside for nearly 20 years. The advent of the 1470-nm laser light and more user-friendly clinical applications with tabletop units have simplified the reintegration of lasers into an outpatient spinal surgery or office-based pain management program [53 - 56]. Therefore, PLDD has regained momentum with interventional pain management physicians [57 - 59], and vendors push it as an alternative to microsurgical lumbar discectomy and endoscopic decompression. Recognizing that both the percutaneous laser and the directly visualized endoscopic technologies have advanced, comparing the clinical benefits of these two very different decompression procedures was the focus of a clinical investigation (Fig. 9). Contained lumbar disc herniation causing stenosis-related sciatica symptoms is much more common in the elderly than extruded disc herniations. Age-related bony lateral recess stenosis may cause additional claudication symptoms and limited walking endurance. Employing this clinical vantage point, this comparative clinical outcome analysis between the transforaminal directly visualized endoscopic surgical and the non-visualized percutaneous laser interventional disc decompression by performing Kaplan-Meier survival analysis of the duration of the treatment benefit was recently published.

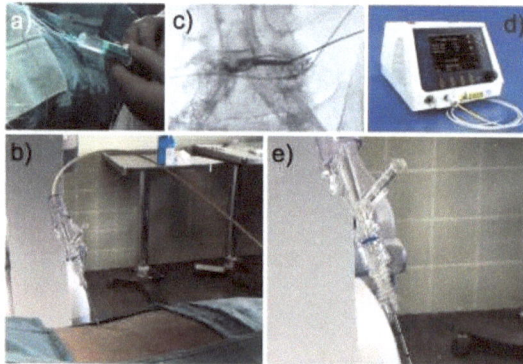

Fig. (9). Leonardo® Dual diode laser platform (biolitec®) deployed into the L5/S1 intervertebral disc space employing a combination of 980 nm and 1470nm set at 7 W, 0.6 s pulses at 1s intervals with total energy delivered of no more than 1500 J **(a-d)**. The flexible laser fiber with a diameter of 360 μm was also introduced into the intervertebral disc via the transforaminal approach. After hydration of the disc space **(e)**, the vaporized disc material is allowed to escape through the proprietary spinal needle (e; Evolve®).

The study population of 248 patients consisted of 162 patients who underwent directly visualized lumbar endoscopic transforaminal microdiscectomy and 86 patients treated with non-visualized interventional percutaneous laser decompression [34]. The mean age was 53.4 ± 14.65 years between the 134 females (54%) and 114 males (46%). Over the mean follow-up period of 43.5 months, the serial time was recorded for the Kaplan-Meier analysis, ranging from 1.5 months to 84 months.

The transforaminal endoscopic decompressions were done using the "outside-in" technique [60, 61]. PLDD was performed using Leonardo® Dual diode laser platform (biolitec®) employing a combination of 980 nm and 1470nm set at 7 W, 0.6 s pulses at 1s intervals with total energy delivered of no more than 1500 J. The flexible laser fiber with a diameter of 360 μm was also introduced into the intervertebral disc via the transforaminal approach [53 - 56]. There were 162 endoscopic decompression patients (65.3%) and 86 percutaneous laser patients (34.7%). Surgery was done for paracentral disc herniations in 180 patients (72.6%) and central herniations in 68 patients (27.4%). There were Excellent Macnab outcomes were achieved in 58.0% of the endoscopically treated patients (p < 0.0001. In the laser group, Excellent Macnab outcomes were reported at 44.2%. Fair and Poor Macnab outcomes were preferentially reported by laser-treated patients (26.7% laser *versus* 8.1% endoscopy; p < 0.0001).

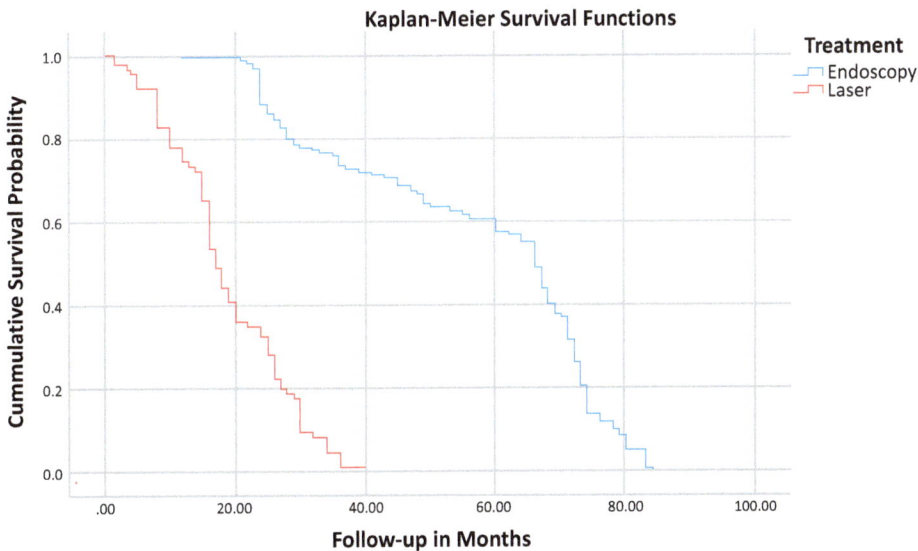

Fig. (10). The 50% percentile median Kaplan-Meier survival for endoscopy patients was 66.0 months with a standard error of 1.515 months, and 95% confidence interval lower boundary of 63.031, and an upper boundary of 68.969 months. For percutaneous laser decompression, the numbers were 17 months with a standard error of .773 months, and 95% confidence interval lower boundary of 15.486 months, and an upper boundary of 18.514 months. This difference was statistically significant (p=0.0001).

Kaplan-Meier (K-M) survival time showed a more prolonged median survival of the treatment benefit of 66 months for patients who underwent visualized endoscopic surgical decompression (Fig. **10**; Table **2**). In the laser-treated patients, the median K-M survival time was 17 months (p = 0.0001).

Table 2. Kaplan-Meier Survival time in patients treated for contained herniated disc (n = 248) with either visualized endoscopic surgical- *versus* **percutaneous laser decompression.**

Treartment	Mean[a]				Median			
-	Estimate	Std. Error	95% Confidence Interval	-	Estimate	Std. Error	95% Confidence Interval	-
-	-	-	Lower Bound	Upper Bound	-	-	Lower Bound	Upper Bound
Endoscopy	56.568	1.613	53.406	59.730	66.000	1.515	63.031	68.969
Laser	18.866	.988	16.931	20.802	17.000	.773	15.486	18.514
Overall	43.494	1.590	40.378	46.610	36.000	4.062	28.039	43.961
[a]Estimation is limited to the largest survival time if it is censored.								
Overall Comparisons								
-	Chi-Square		df		Sig.			
Log Rank (Mantel-Cox)	214.169		1		.< .0001			

While percutaneous non-visualized laser decompression is making a comeback and is promoted as an alternative to aggressive surgery in medically complex patients, endoscopic transforaminal decompression yields better long-term results. What is clear from this study is that a formal visualized transforaminal endoscopic decompression is not interchangeable with the percutaneous laser treatment of herniated disc. Clinical outcomes were better in endoscopy patients, but the duration of the treatment effect demonstrated by the Kaplan-Meier survival analysis was nearly five times as long. Nonetheless, this knowledge gives patients more substantial clinical evidence to make the best choice of spine care in the context of their functional improvement needs at the time when the spine care is needed.

DISCUSSION

Despite the widespread interest in lasers, few high-level clinical studies have been published comparing laser or laser-assisted spine surgery with traditional open or other forms of minimally invasive spinal surgery. Instead, recent systematic reviews including one published by Radcliff *et al.* prompted by the closure of the Laser Spine Institute in 2019 often conflate clinical outcomes with the percutaneous laser disc decompression (PLDD) with other forms of laser applications in spine surgery including endoscopic and open spine surgery [62]. Unfortunately, the obvious lack of attention to detail and the paucity of high-grade evidence in support of PLDD have prompted the North American Spine Society Coverage Recommendations Task Force [63] and the Canadian Agency for Drugs and Technology [64] to have advocated against laser spine surgery even though PLDD is rather an interventional procedure frequently carried out by pain management physicians rather than surgeons. It is a generalization that in the author's opinion does not apply to the current state of the art of lasers in spine surgery. There is no question that the focus on the use of lasers in spine surgery has shifted from PLDD to applications of lasers as an adjunct to other forms of spine surgery. Although the Biolitec™ diode laser system has regained some popularity as a result of its updated dual wavelength application (980 and 1480 nm) coupled with an elegant needle fiber applicator system and a userfriendly interface, our clinical data analysis of the treatment durability of this laser's PLDD treatment benefit *versus* formal visualized endoscopic decompression showed that even modern forms of PLDD cannot replace endoscopic surgery protocols as their median treatment benefit as illustrated by our K-M durability curves outlasted PLDD by a factor of 4. However, Ren *et al.* pointed out that PLDD may be still useful in the elderly in cases where there is predominant anterior compressive pathology below the dural sac thereby contributing foremost to spinal stenosis. The authors reported favorable two-year follow-up data on 21 patients with lumbar claudication due to spinal stenosis that they treated with Nd: YAG laser PLDD [65].

Traditionally, patients have been conditioned by marketing campaigns to consider laser procedures over any surgery because of its perceived cutting-edge technology. However, the short-term benefit and the long-term shortfall of comparing clinical outcomes of PLDD with the surgical outcomes with endoscopy should be discussed preoperatively with the patient. Patient preference and circumstances may favor PLDD even though the transforaminal endoscopic decompression could be more durable in the long-run when considering surgical options for a symptomatic herniated disc. In experienced hands, the median treatment benefit with the full-endoscopic transforaminal discectomy lasted up to six years. Interventional percutaneous non-visualized laser decompression for the same condition may provide favorable outcomes in the short-term with median durability of 17 months.

The endoscopic spine surgery techniques, on the other hand, have been validated with a plethora of peer-reviewed papers that were published in the last five years alone as capable of achieving comparable clinical outcomes as with open or other forms of minimally invasive translaminar spine surgery. The clinical indications and the clinical outcomes that should be expected in terms of recovery and return-to-work time, acceptable readmission-, reoperation- and complication rates are much better understood. The same cannot be said about the non-visualized interventional percutaneous laser decompression procedure (PLDD) [32]. The meta-analysis review of PLDD articles shows a few randomized controlled trials. Most articles are observational studies without a control group, rendering the quality of clinical evidence supporting PLDD weak [49]. Nonetheless, there may be a place for PLDD in medically complex patients or patients that simply reject any surgery. Those patients should be advised that the treatment benefit be short-lived. However, this may be appropriate for some patients. The provided Kaplan-Meier durability analysis for the first time provides clinical evidence that the directly visualized endoscopic procedure provides more durable pain relief than the percutaneous laser discectomy procedure. The Kaplan-Meier (K-M) analysis of the survival times of the treatment benefit for both the endoscopic surgical and the percutaneous interventional laser decompression demonstrates a telling visual demonstration of the laser treatment's rapid deterioration benefit with the 50% percentile median being 17 months. Fifty percent of patients treated with the percutaneous laser procedure had lost the treatment benefit 17 months postoperatively. The same K-M analysis done on endoscopic spine surgery patients revealed a median survival time of 66 months for the directly visualized endoscopic surgery. The K-M curves have some limitations and are certainly not predictions of durability. They are an accurate depiction of the minimum survival until the first patient is censored from a study. At that point, K-M curves become an estimation. Extrapolations on future patient outcomes should be avoided. One could argue that these procedures are not comparable since the endoscopy was primarily carried out in the epidural space and the disc space's laser decompression. Direct endoscopic visualization and treatment of pain generators could improve clinical outcomes more reliably than what can be achieved with the non-visualized PLDD. However, in routine clinical practice, they are being offered for the overlapping clinical indication – herniated disc with or without boney stenosis in the lateral spinal canal or foramina – often by physicians of different subspecialities. Therefore, a side-by-side comparison of outcome data and the respective durability of the treatment benefit is certainly reasonable.

There is, however, no question that lasers are useful as an adjunct to modern spinal surgery techniques [10, 16, 30, 66, 67]. There are clinical applications where lasers are still effective tools in dissecting epidural fibrosis or removing farmigrated extruded disc herniations. Even an epiduroscopic technique has recently been described to illustrate this point exactly [10, 16, 30, 66, 67]. For example, Lee *et al.* analyzed outcomes in 21 patients who underwent laser-assisted conventional microdiscectomy for recurrent disk herniations [68]. Another study by Kim *et al.* reported fewer durotomy with the laser assisted dissection of epidural adhesions than observed with traditional surgical dissection techniques [69]. In one of the few comparative retrospective studies, Ahn *et al.*[31] disclosed posterior cervical laminoforaminotomy and discectomy outcomes with adjunctive use of lasers. Clinical outcomes were no different between the 24 patients who underwent laser-assisted posterior cervical discectomy and the 23 patients who underwent conventional posterior cervical laminoforaminotomy. However, there was less blood loss with the laser-assisted procedure [70]. Hussein *et al.* described the use of a flexible, handpiece-delivered CO_2 laser they employed for ablation of the contralateral ligamentum flavum in 39 patients on whom they had done unilateral hemilaminotomy [71]. The CO_2 was particularly useful in desiccating the ligamentum flavum which the authors thought was then easier to remove. An additional benefit of the CO_2 laser was observed when cauterizing bleeding bony surfaces. Other possible applications of lasers have been demonstrated during discectomy to prepare the interspace for the interbody fusion by employing a CO_2 laser [72]. This study did not find that the use of lasers in such a way did not speed up endplate preparation. Yeung and Hellinger's groundbreaking work demonstrated in this chapter, however, has illustrated how lasers can be a useful adjunct tool during endoscopic spinal surgery.

CONCLUSION

Lasers have had surgical applications for decades. They can be used for disc ablation percutaneously during PLDD or spinal surgery. The Nd: YAG and the Ho: YAG laser has found several applications in endoscopic spine surgery where they can aid in the removal of the disc, bony, or ligamentous tissue to facilitate neural element decompression. Side-firing lasers are useful tools to reach extruded disc fragments that have migrated far from the intervertebral disc space. In those challenging case scenarios, lasers may extend the reach of rigid spinal endoscopes without performing an extensive open decompression only for access reasons. The PLDD procedure has received FDA approval in the 1990ies, and there is a plethora of low-level studies in support of it. PLDD may be of limited therapeutic durability, but its low cost and low burden aspect may be of interest to the elderly with multiple medical comorbidities to whom the lack of long-term benefit is irrelevant. The call of high-level randomized prospective clinical trials to support the use of lasers in spine surgery [62] seems impractical when used as an adjunct to other surgical technologies employed in clinical protocols with their indications and associated validated outcomes. To declare the use of laser in spine surgery unsubstantiated merely based on a lack of high-grade clinical evidence in support of PLDD is, in the authors' opinion, unjustified because the PLDD application is such a small portion of laser application in spine surgery. Lasers have seen a recent renaissance because of the many advantages when used as an adjunct to other spinal surgery techniques, particularly in endoscopic spine surgery. After all, every innovation starts with low-grade level 5 evidence – personal observations – frequently followed by level 3 and 4 observational cohort studies. Lasers will likely remain relevant in spine surgery as innovation in other minimally invasive and endoscopic spinal surgery areas continues.

CONSENT FOR PUBLICATION

Not applicable.

CONFLICT OF INTEREST

The authors declare no conflict of interest, financial or otherwise.

ACKNOWLEDGEMENT

Declared none.

REFERENCES

[1]   Siebert WE. Use of lasers in arthroscopy. Orthopade 1992; 21(4): 273-88.
        [PMID: 1408119]

[2]   Ascher PW. Status quo and new horizons of laser therapy in neurosurgery. Lasers Surg Med 1985; 5(5): 499-506.
        [http://dx.doi.org/10.1002/lsm.1900050509] [PMID: 4068883]

[3]   Choy DS, Altman PA, Case RB, Trokel SL. Laser radiation at various wavelengths for decompression of intervertebral disk. Experimental observations on human autopsy specimens. Clin Orthop Relat Res 1991; (267): 245-50.
        [PMID: 1904334]

[4]   Cselik Z, Aradi M, von Jako RA, *et al.* Impact of infrared laser light-induced ablation at different wavelengths on bovine intervertebral disc ex vivo: evaluation with magnetic resonance imaging and histology. Lasers Surg Med 2012; 44(5): 406-12.
        [http://dx.doi.org/10.1002/lsm.22034] [PMID: 22532099]

[5]   Lee GW, Jang SJ, Kim JD. The efficacy of epiduroscopic neural decompression with Ho:YAG laser ablation in lumbar spinal stenosis. Eur J Orthop Surg Traumatol 2014; 24 (Suppl. 1): S231-7.
        [http://dx.doi.org/10.1007/s00590-013-1407-7] [PMID: 24398702]

[6]   Quigley MR, Maroon JC, Shih T, Elrifai A, Lesiecki ML. Laser discectomy. Comparison of systems. Spine 1994; 19(3): 319-22.
        [http://dx.doi.org/10.1097/00007632-199402000-00011] [PMID: 8171364]

[7]   Yeung AT. The evolution of percutaneous spinal endoscopy and discectomy: state of the art. Mt Sinai J Med 2000; 67(4): 327-32.
        [PMID: 11021785]

[8]   Casper GD, Mullins LL, Hartman VL. Laser-assisted disc decompression: a clinical trial of the holmium:YAG laser with side-firing fiber. J Clin Laser Med Surg 1995; 13(1): 27-32.
        [http://dx.doi.org/10.1089/clm.1995.13.27] [PMID: 10150570]

[9]   Casper GD, Hartman VL, Mullins LL. Percutaneous laser disc decompression with the holmium: YAG laser. J Clin Laser Med Surg 1995; 13(3): 195-203.
        [http://dx.doi.org/10.1089/clm.1995.13.195] [PMID: 10150646]

[10]   Chiu JC, Clifford TJ, Greenspan M, Richley RC, Lohman G, Sison RB. Percutaneous microdecompressive endoscopic cervical discectomy with laser thermodiskoplasty. Mt Sinai J Med 2000; 67(4): 278-82.
       [PMID: 11021777]

[11]   Chiu JC. Endoscopic assisted microdecompression of cervical disc and foramen. Surg Technol Int 2008; 17: 269-79.
       [PMID: 18802913]

[12]   Knight MT, Vajda A, Jakab GV, Awan S. Endoscopic laser foraminoplasty on the lumbar spine--early experience. Minim Invasive Neurosurg 1998; 41(1): 5-9.
       [http://dx.doi.org/10.1055/s-2008-1052006] [PMID: 9565957]

[13]   Knight MT, Goswami A, Patko JT. Cervical percutaneous laser disc decompression: preliminary results of an ongoing prospective outcome study. J Clin Laser Med Surg 2001; 19(1): 3-8.
       [http://dx.doi.org/10.1089/104454701750066875] [PMID: 11547816]

[14]   Knight MT, Goswami A, Patko JT. Comparative outcome of Holmium: YAG and KTP laser disc ablation in degenerative cervical disc disease: results of an ongoing study. Ortop Traumatol Rehabil 2000; 2(2): 39-43.
       [PMID: 18034117]

[15]   Knight MT, Ellison DR, Goswami A, Hillier VF. Review of safety in endoscopic laser foraminoplasty for the management of back pain. J Clin Laser Med Surg 2001; 19(3): 147-57.
       [http://dx.doi.org/10.1089/10445470152927982] [PMID: 11469307]

[16]   Knight M, Goswami A. Lumbar percutaneous KTP532 wavelength laser disc decompression and disc ablation in the management of discogenic pain. J Clin Laser Med Surg 2002; 20(1): 9-13.
       [http://dx.doi.org/10.1089/104454702753474940] [PMID: 11902355]

[17]   Ruetten S, Meyer O, Godolias G. Application of holmium:YAG laser in epiduroscopy: extended practicabilities in the treatment of chronic back pain syndrome. J Clin Laser Med Surg 2002; 20(4): 203-6.
       [http://dx.doi.org/10.1089/104454702760230528] [PMID: 12206722]

[18]   Stith WJ, Judy MM, Hochschuler SH, Guyer RD. Choice of lasers for minimally invasive spinal surgery. Orthop Rev 1991; 20(2): 137-42.
       [PMID: 1901165]

[19]   Hellinger J, Linke R, Heller H. A biophysical explanation for Nd:YAG percutaneous laser disc decompression success. J Clin Laser Med Surg 2001; 19(5): 235-8.
       [http://dx.doi.org/10.1089/10445470152611955] [PMID: 11710617]

[20]   Gropper GR, Robertson JH, McClellan G. Comparative histological and radiographic effects of CO_2 laser *versus* standard surgical anterior cervical discectomy in the dog. Neurosurgery 1984; 14(1): 42-7.
       [http://dx.doi.org/10.1227/00006123-198401000-00009] [PMID: 6420722]

[21]   Jeon HC, Kim CS, Kim SC, *et al.* Posterior cervical microscopic foraminotomy and discectomy with laser for unilateral radiculopathy. Chonnam Med J 2015; 51(3): 129-34.
       [http://dx.doi.org/10.4068/cmj.2015.51.3.129] [PMID: 26730364]

[22]   Hellinger J. Technical aspects of the percutaneous cervical and lumbar laser-disc-decompression and -nucleotomy. Neurol Res 1999; 21(1): 99-102.
       [http://dx.doi.org/10.1080/01616412.1999.11740902] [PMID: 10048065]

[23]   Choy DS. Techniques of percutaneous laser disc decompression with the Nd:YAG laser. J Clin Laser Med Surg 1995; 13(3): 187-93.
       [http://dx.doi.org/10.1089/clm.1995.13.187] [PMID: 10150645]

[24]   Schmolke S, Rühmann O, Lazovic D. The use of lasers in surgical orthopedics. A current review. Orthopade 1997; 26(3): 267-72.
       [PMID: 9198801]

[25] Stern KL, Monga M. The Moses holmium system - time is money. Can J Urol 2018; 25(3): 9313-6.
[PMID: 29900818]

[26] Mullerad M, Aguinaga JRA, Aro T, *et al.* Initial clinical experience with a modulated holmium laser pulse-moses technology: does it enhance laser lithotripsy efficacy? Rambam Maimonides Med J 2017; 8(4)
[http://dx.doi.org/10.5041/RMMJ.10315] [PMID: 28914602]

[27] Leotsakos I, Katafigiotis I, Lorber A, *et al.* Initial experience in combined ultra-mini percutaneous nephrolithotomy with the use of 120-W laser and the anti-retropulsion "Moses effect": the future of percutaneous nephrolithotomy? Lasers Med Sci 2020; 35(9): 1961-6.
[http://dx.doi.org/10.1007/s10103-020-02986-4] [PMID: 32112249]

[28] Davis JK. Percutaneous discectomy improved with KTP laser. Clin Laser Mon 1990; 8(7): 105-6.
[PMID: 10149820]

[29] Büki A, Dóczi T, Vetö F, Horváth Z, Gallyas F. Initial clinical experience with a combined pulsed holmium-neodymium-YAG laser in minimally invasive neurosurgery. Minim Invasive Neurosurg 1999; 42(1): 35-40.
[http://dx.doi.org/10.1055/s-2008-1053366] [PMID: 10228938]

[30] Choy DS, Hellinger J, Tassi GP, Hellinger S. Percutaneous laser disc decompression. Photomed Laser Surg 2007; 25(1): 60.
[PMID: 17352640]

[31] Schenk B, Brouwer PA, van Buchem MA. Experimental basis of percutaneous laser disc decompression (PLDD): a review of literature. Lasers Med Sci 2006; 21(4): 245-9.
[http://dx.doi.org/10.1007/s10103-006-0393-y] [PMID: 16937074]

[32] Brouwer PA, Peul WC, Brand R, *et al.* Effectiveness of percutaneous laser disc decompression *versus* conventional open discectomy in the treatment of lumbar disc herniation; design of a prospective randomized controlled trial. BMC Musculoskelet Disord 2009; 10: 49.
[http://dx.doi.org/10.1186/1471-2474-10-49] [PMID: 19439098]

[33] Gibson JN, Waddell G. Surgical interventions for lumbar disc prolapse: updated Cochrane Review. Spine 2007; 32(16): 1735-47.
[http://dx.doi.org/10.1097/BRS.0b013e3180bc2431] [PMID: 17632394]

[34] Lewandrowski KU, de Carvalho PST, Calderaro AL, *et al.* Outcomes with transforaminal endoscopic *versus* percutaneous laser decompression for contained lumbar herniated disc: a survival analysis of treatment benefit. J Spine Surg 2020; 6 (Suppl. 1): S84-99.
[http://dx.doi.org/10.21037/jss.2019.09.13] [PMID: 32195418]

[35] Singh V, Manchikanti L, Benyamin RM, Helm S, Hirsch JA. Percutaneous lumbar laser disc decompression: a systematic review of current evidence. Pain Physician 2009; 12(3): 573-88.
[http://dx.doi.org/10.36076/ppj.2009/12/573] [PMID: 19461824]

[36] Singh V, Manchikanti L, Calodney AK, *et al.* Percutaneous lumbar laser disc decompression: an update of current evidence. Pain Physician 2013; 16(2) (Suppl.): SE229-60.
[http://dx.doi.org/10.36076/ppj.2013/16/SE229] [PMID: 23615885]

[37] Mayer HM, Brock M, Berlien HP, Weber B. Percutaneous endoscopic laser discectomy (PELD). A new surgical technique for non-sequestrated lumbar discs. Acta Neurochir Suppl (Wien) 1992; 54: 53-8.
[http://dx.doi.org/10.1007/978-3-7091-6687-1_7] [PMID: 1595409]

[38] Turgut M, Onol B, Kiliniç K, Tahta K. Extensive damage to the end-plates as a complication of laser discectomy. An experimental study using an animal model. Acta Neurochir (Wien) 1997; 139(5): 404-9.
[http://dx.doi.org/10.1007/BF01808875] [PMID: 9204108]

[39] Manchikanti L, Malla Y, Wargo BW, Fellows B. Infection control practices (safe injection and

medication vial utilization) for interventional techniques: are they based on relative risk management or evidence? Pain Physician 2011; 14(5): 425-34.
[PMID: 21927046]

[40]   Willems PC, Jacobs W, Duinkerke ES, De Kleuver M. Lumbar discography: should we use prophylactic antibiotics? A study of 435 consecutive discograms and a systematic review of the literature. J Spinal Disord Tech 2004; 17(3): 243-7.
[http://dx.doi.org/10.1097/00024720-200406000-00013] [PMID: 15167342]

[41]   Vescovi P, Conti S, Merigo E, *et al.* In vitro bactericidal effect of Nd:YAG laser on Actinomyces israelii. Lasers Med Sci 2013; 28(4): 1131-5.
[http://dx.doi.org/10.1007/s10103-012-1197-x] [PMID: 23053244]

[42]   Paikin JS, Wright DS, Eikelboom JW. Effectiveness and safety of combined antiplatelet and anticoagulant therapy: a critical review of the evidence from randomized controlled trials. Blood Rev 2011; 25(3): 123-9.
[http://dx.doi.org/10.1016/j.blre.2011.01.007] [PMID: 21354678]

[43]   Arts MP, Peul WC, Koes BW, Thomeer RT. Management of sciatica due to lumbar disc herniation in the Netherlands: a survey among spine surgeons. J Neurosurg Spine 2008; 9(1): 32-9.
[http://dx.doi.org/10.3171/SPI/2008/9/7/032] [PMID: 18590408]

[44]   Siebert W. Percutaneous laser discectomy of cervical discs: preliminary clinical results. J Clin Laser Med Surg 1995; 13(3): 205-7.
[http://dx.doi.org/10.1089/clm.1995.13.205] [PMID: 10150647]

[45]   Yeung AT, Gore S. In-vivo endoscopic visualization of patho-anatomy in symptomatic degenerative conditions of the lumbar spine II: intradiscal, foraminal, and central canal decompression. Surg Technol Int 2011; 21: 299-319.
[PMID: 22505004]

[46]   Yeung AT. The evolution and advancement of endoscopic foraminal surgery: One surgeon's experience incorporating adjunctive techologies. SAS J 2007; 1(3): 108-17.
[http://dx.doi.org/10.1016/S1935-9810(07)70055-5] [PMID: 25802587]

[47]   Ahn Y, Lee U. Use of lasers in minimally invasive spine surgery. Expert Rev Med Devices 2018; 15(6): 423-33.
[http://dx.doi.org/10.1080/17434440.2018.1483236] [PMID: 29855205]

[48]   Brouwer PA, Brand R, van den Akker-van Marle ME, *et al.* Percutaneous laser disc decompression *versus* conventional microdiscectomy in sciatica: a randomized controlled trial. Spine J 2015; 15(5): 857-65.
[http://dx.doi.org/10.1016/j.spinee.2015.01.020] [PMID: 25614151]

[49]   van den Akker-van Marle ME, Brouwer PA, Brand R, *et al.* Percutaneous laser disc decompression *versus* microdiscectomy for sciatica: Cost utility analysis alongside a randomized controlled trial. Interv Neuroradiol 2017; 23(5): 538-45.
[http://dx.doi.org/10.1177/1591019917710297] [PMID: 28679342]

[50]   Kobayashi S, Uchida K, Takeno K, *et al.* A case of nerve root heat injury induced by percutaneous laser disc decompression performed at an outside institution: technical case report. Neurosurgery 2007; 60(2 Suppl 1): ONSE171-2; discussion ONSE2.
[http://dx.doi.org/10.1227/01.NEU.0000249228.82365.D2]

[51]   Epstein JM, Adler R. Laser-assisted percutaneous endoscopic neurolysis. Pain Physician 2000; 3(1): 43-5.
[PMID: 16906206]

[52]   Jo DH, Kim ED, Oh HJ. The comparison of the result of epiduroscopic laser neural decompression between FBSS or not. Korean J Pain 2014; 27(1): 63-7.
[http://dx.doi.org/10.3344/kjp.2014.27.1.63] [PMID: 24478903]

[53]   Soracco JE, D'Ambola JO. New wavelength for the endovascular treatment of lower limb venous insufficiency. Int Angiol 2009; 28(4): 281-8.
        [PMID: 19648871]

[54]   Pannier F, Rabe E, Rits J, Kadiss A, Maurins U. Endovenous laser ablation of great saphenous veins using a 1470 nm diode laser and the radial fibre--follow-up after six months. Phlebology 2011; 26(1): 35-9.
        [http://dx.doi.org/10.1258/phleb.2010.009096] [PMID: 21148467]

[55]   Pannier F, Rabe E, Maurins U. 1470 nm diode laser for endovenous ablation (EVLA) of incompetent saphenous veins - a prospective randomized pilot study comparing warm and cold tumescence anaesthesia. Vasa 2010; 39(3): 249-55.
        [http://dx.doi.org/10.1024/0301-1526/a000037] [PMID: 20737384]

[56]   Pannier F, Rabe E, Maurins U. First results with a new 1470-nm diode laser for endovenous ablation of incompetent saphenous veins. Phlebology 2009; 24(1): 26-30.
        [http://dx.doi.org/10.1258/phleb.2008.008038] [PMID: 19155338]

[57]   Patel N, Singh V. Percutaneous lumbar laser discectomy: literature review and a retrospective analysis of 65 cases. Photomed Laser Surg 2018; 36(10): 518-21.
        [http://dx.doi.org/10.1089/pho.2018.4460] [PMID: 30227091]

[58]   Choi KC, Lee DC, Park CK. A novel combination of percutaneous endoscopic lumbar discectomy and epiduroscopic laser neural decompression for down-migrated disc herniation. Pain Physician 2017; 20(4): E605-9.
        [PMID: 28535570]

[59]   Menchetti PP, Canero G, Bini W. Percutaneous laser discectomy: experience and long term follow-up. Acta Neurochir Suppl (Wien) 2011; 108: 117-21.
        [http://dx.doi.org/10.1007/978-3-211-99370-5_18] [PMID: 21107947]

[60]   Lewandrowski KU. "Outside-in" technique, clinical results, and indications with transforaminal lumbar endoscopic surgery: a retrospective study on 220 patients on applied radiographic classification of foraminal spinal stenosis. Int J Spine Surg 2014; 8: 8.
        [http://dx.doi.org/10.14444/1026] [PMID: 25694915]

[61]   Lewandrowski KU, León JFR, Yeung A. Use of "inside-out" technique for direct visualization of a vacuum vertically unstable intervertebral disc during routine lumbar endoscopic transforaminal decompression-a correlative study of clinical outcomes and the prognostic value of lumbar radiographs. Int J Spine Surg 2019; 13(5): 399-414.
        [http://dx.doi.org/10.14444/6055] [PMID: 31741829]

[62]   Radcliff K, Vaccaro AR, Hilibrand A, Schroeder GD. Lasers in spine surgery. J Am Acad Orthop Surg 2019; 27(17): 621-32.
        [http://dx.doi.org/10.5435/JAAOS-D-18-00001] [PMID: 30628998]

[63]   North American Spine Society. Laser Spine Surgery Coverage Recommendation, NASS Coverage Recommendations eBook. 2014.

[64]   Khangura S. A R. Laser spine surgery for herniated discs and/or nerve root entrapment: a review of clinical effectiveness Cost-Effectiveness and Guidelines. Ottawa, ON, Canada 2017.
        https://www.ncbi.nlm.nih.gov/books/ NBK470816/

[65]   Ren L, Han Z, Zhang J, *et al.* Efficacy of percutaneous laser disc decompression on lumbar spinal stenosis. Lasers Med Sci 2014; 29(3): 921-3.
        [http://dx.doi.org/10.1007/s10103-013-1429-8] [PMID: 23996073]

[66]   Savitz MH, Doughty H, Burns P. Percutaneous lumbar discectomy with a working endoscope and laser assistance. Neurosurg Focus 1998; 4(2): e9.
        [http://dx.doi.org/10.3171/foc.1998.4.2.12] [PMID: 17206772]

[67]   Chiu JC, Negron F, Clifford T, Greenspan M, Princethal RA. Microdecompressive percutaneous

endoscopy: spinal discectomy with new laser thermodiskoplasty for non-extruded herniated nucleosus pulposus. Surg Technol Int 1999; 8: 343-51.
[PMID: 12451548]

[68] Lee DY, Shim CS, Ahn Y, Choi YG, Kim HJ, Lee SH. Comparison of percutaneous endoscopic lumbar discectomy and open lumbar microdiscectomy for recurrent disc herniation. J Korean Neurosurg Soc 2009; 46(6): 515-21.
[http://dx.doi.org/10.3340/jkns.2009.46.6.515] [PMID: 20062565]

[69] Kim CH, Chung CK, Jahng TA, Yang HJ, Son YJ. Surgical outcome of percutaneous endoscopic interlaminar lumbar diskectomy for recurrent disk herniation after open diskectomy. J Spinal Disord Tech 2012; 25(5): E125-33.
[http://dx.doi.org/10.1097/BSD.0b013e31825bd111] [PMID: 22744610]

[70] Ahn Y, Moon KS, Kang BU, Hur SM, Kim JD. Laser-assisted posterior cervical foraminotomy and discectomy for lateral and foraminal cervical disc herniation. Photomed Laser Surg 2012; 30(9): 510-5.
[http://dx.doi.org/10.1089/pho.2012.3246] [PMID: 22793668]

[71] Hussain NS, Perez-Cruet M. Application of the flexible CO_2 laser in minimally invasive laminectomies: technical note. Cureus 2016; 8(6): e628.
[http://dx.doi.org/10.7759/cureus.628] [PMID: 27433407]

[72] Villavicencio AT, Burneikiene S, Babuska JM, Nelson EL, Mason A, Rajpal S. A preliminary report on the CO_2 laser for lumbar fusion: Safety, efficacy and technical considerations. Cureus 2015; 7(4): e262.
[http://dx.doi.org/10.7759/cureus.262] [PMID: 26180686]

CHAPTER 7

High Frequency Surgery for the Treatment of Herniated Discs

Friedrich Tieber[1], Stefan Hellinger[2], Hyeun-Sung Kim[3] and Kai-Uwe Lewandrowski[4,5,6]

[1] *Medical Technologies Consulting, Augsburg, Germany*

[2] *Department of Orthopedic Surgery, Arabellaklinik, Germany*

[3] *Nanoori Hospital, Nonhyeon-dong, Gangnam-gu, Seoul, South Korea*

[4] *Center for Advanced Spine Care of Southern Arizona and Surgical Institute of Tucson, Tucson AZ, USA*

[5] *Department of Orthopaedic Surgery, Universidad Colsanitas, Bogota, Colombia, USA*

[6] *Visiting Professor, Department Orthopaedic Surgery, UNIRIO, Rio de Janeiro, Brazil*

Abstract: High-frequency coagulation, cutting, and coblation technology have long been applied during endoscopic spine surgery. Endoscopic visualization devices and high-frequency surgical devices can be found in almost every surgical subspecialty. During surgical HF applications, electrical energy is converted into heat, used to cut biological tissue and stop bleeding. This technology works with high voltages in cutting and coagulation mode. The difference is in the creation of arcs, which have a cutting effect. In simplified terms, voltages of ≤ 200 Volts are generated during coagulation and > 200 Volts during cutting. The interaction of HF with biological tissue can be explained by the faradic, electrolytic, and thermal effect. A frequency of over 400 kHz has no harmful effect on body tissue. Frequencies over 1MHz have a "cold cutting effect" allowing for safe bipolar applications and minimizing thermal damage. This chapter reviews how modern high-frequency generators work and how to minimize risk during clinical applications, including electrode bonding and burns by applying automatic power metering, two-part neutral electrode, and bipolar techniques. During spinal endoscopy, the effects of HF treatment can be directly assessed under very high magnification factors. This complementary overlap of the videoendoscopic and HF technique in modern endoscopic spine surgery is the key to superior clinical outcomes compared to non-visualized percutaneous procedures performed under fluoroscopic control.

Keywords: Coblation, Cutting, Endoscopic surgery, Herniated disc, High frequency.

---

* **Corresponding author Stefan Hellinger:** Department of Orthopedic Surgery, Arabellaklinik, Germany; Tel: +1 520 204-1495; Fax: +1 623 218-1215; E-mail: hellinger@gmx.de

Kai-Uwe Lewandrowski, Jorge Felipe Ramírez León, Anthony Yeung, Gun Choi, Stefan Hellinger and Álvaro Dowling (Eds.)

INTRODUCTION

The trend in minimally invasive spine treatment of axial discogenic pain non-responsive to conservative treatment methods continues to expand throughout the medical community worldwide. With this minimalist evolution, techniques and technologies have progressed to permit atraumatic access, preserve anatomy, maintain the viability of endplates, and minimize scar tissue formation with overall reduced tissue incision, dissection, and manipulation. Surgeons are faced with an array of accessory devices, primarily energy-based technologies, to facilitate soft tissue access, preparation, and tissue modulation.

The use of thermal energy to modulate and ablate tissue is not new. In one form or another, electrical current has been applied to human tissues as a surgical modality for over 100 years. Modern electrosurgery traces its roots to Doyen's machines in the 1920s and Bovie in the 1930s. Electrosurgical units generally operate from 200 to 500 kHz. Devices operating in this frequency range cause the electrode that comes in contact with the tissue to become hot, therefore acting like true heat cautery. In the 1950s, Malis invented a spark gap machine consisting of a bipolar generator and forceps designed to control lateral heat spread to adjacent tissues.

High frequency (HF) surgery for the treatment of herniated discs and spinal endoscopy are complementary procedures. Galvano- and diathermy surgery are twins of the modern HF treatments and have been used since the middle of the 19th century. It was the beginning of the 20th century when Erbe developed HF surgical devices in Europe and Bowie in the USA. Endoscopic visualization devices and high-frequency surgical devices can be found in almost every operating theater globally, both of which are used in all surgical disciplines, both in a hospital and ambulatory surgery setting. In high-frequency surgery, HF alternating current is passed through the human body to achieve targeted hemostasis and sever through the tissue heating it causes in monopolar applications.

Generators with a maximum power of 400 Watts are usually used for HF electrosurgery. The output voltage can be a high voltage of up to 4 kilovolts (kV) when idling. In dentistry and ophthalmology, weaker devices with maximum outputs of 50 Watts with lower voltages are common. The generators on the market usually allow different operating modes. This includes cutting and coagulation. The difference is in the creation of arcs which have a cutting effect. In simplified terms, it can be said that generator voltages of ≤ 200 Volts are generated during coagulation. In cutting mode, the voltages are greater than 200 Volts.

DIFFERENTIATION BETWEEN RF, HIGH RF AND RADIO WAVES

All these descriptions are synonymous with high-frequency (HF) waves. There is no difference between the radiofrequency (RF) and radio wave (RW). In European literature, they are called high-frequency waves. In the North American literature, the term radiofrequency is preferred. The typical range for medical applications is between 3 and 300 MHZ. Waves above this range are called High RF.

GENERAL ASPECTS OF HF SURGERY

Electrosurgery and Radiofrequency energy occupy a range upon the Electromagnetic Radiation Spectrum. The frequency at which the device operates will determine the absorption characteristics, tissue effects, and surgical utility, much like the medium of a laser. Standard monopolar or bipolar devices emitting frequencies under 500kHz are limitedly applied or avoided by the energy source savvy clinician to prevent unwanted tissue destruction. Control of penetration and target tissue effects have led to an interest in various electrosurgical devices and delivery systems. One must realize that the frequency with which the device operates mainly dictates the unique properties and capabilities or limitations of the technology.

High-frequency or radiofrequency in the frequency range between 1.7MHz and 4.0MHz of the radiation spectrum emits energy that is non-thermal with absorption characteristics of water-rich tissues. Transferred from the long-term use in ocular plastics, reconstructive and neurosurgical fields, the frequencies of 1.7 and 4.0Mhz have been reported to be optimal for controlled absorption with minimal tissue alteration. The spine and neurosurgical communities are widely accepting radio-wave technology for the cell-specific precision it affords which played out favorably in endoscopic spine surgery. The demands of critical-anatomy-based surgery warranting precision make this specific technology attractive and a compliment to the equipment armamentarium.

With electrical energy converted into heat, one can cut biological tissue and stop bleeding. Since this technology works with high voltages, there are certain risks. In order to minimize them, it is crucial to be aware of how the technology works. The higher the current density, the greater the temperature increase and the damaging thermal effect. The current density increases at the tip of the monopolar electrocautery - the active electrode. An arc is formed, leading to a very high temperature locally with which tissue can be cut or obliterated. In contrast, at the neutral electrode's - typically a large surface - the current density and temperature development are so low that no harmful effect occurs. The electric current's interaction with biological tissue can be explained by three effects: faradic, electrolytic, and thermal effect.

The Faradic Effect

Nerve and muscle cells are electrically excitable and are excited by an electric current at approximately 100 Hz. Muscle contractions are potentially dangerous reactions to electric shocks as well as rhythm disturbances of the nerve tracts. This may lead to considerable damage and even death. In higher frequency ranges, this effect creates electromagnetic reactions on tissue and nerve membranes.

The Electrical Effect

Direct current is unsuitable for tissue separation and coagulation applications. When a high-frequency alternating current is used, the charged particles constantly change their direction of movement, generate vibrations and, from a frequency of 400 kHz, do not exert any stimulus on the body tissue and therefore have no damaging effect.

The Thermal Effect

Tissue is heated by applying an electric current. The degree of warming depends on:

- The current density,
- The specific resistance of the tissue,
- From the surface of the inserted electrode,
- The exposure time to electrical energy, and
- Irrigation.

During the procedure, this means the correct setting of the current density and type of current on the device and the selection of the electrode suitable for the application and the application time. The rule to be observed is that the higher the current density, the higher the tissue's heating. The HF current characteristic can be varied in many ways. These variations form the basis of all different surgical procedures using HF current. The manufacturer's variety of devices is based on these characteristics' unique design, a large number of differently designed electrodes for various indications, and specially developed software with assigned device operation.

The power specifications for the variation of current characteristics are:

- Form of the HF voltage may be sinusoidal constant, sinusoidal mixed voltage, or pulse-shaped modulated. It is measured in volts (V).
- The peak voltage is specified as Vp.
- The rated load is given in ohms.
- The frequency is given in Herz (Hz).
- Other descriptors are the frequency modulation per duty circle.
- The energy consumption of a device is given in watts.
- *The ohmic resistances is given in ohm* [Ω]. For example, the output power P [W] as a function of the load resistance R [Ω] with the setting "Bipolar Cutting Standard"may be 100 W.

ELECTROTOMY

The cutting of the tissue (instead of cutting with a scalpel) in HF surgery is called electrotomy. The HF surgical device is operated with a needle or a narrow blade in a monopolar mode when cutting. Recently, bipolar scissors have also been used very successfully for cutting. High-density electricity heats the fluid in the body's cells quickly that the resulting vapor pressure bursts the cell membrane. The tissue is superficially coagulated on both sides of the incision. The depth of the coagulation seam depends on the tissue and the cutting speed. A distinction is made between the smooth and the scabbed cut. For the smooth cut, an unmodulated or 100 Hz modulated current is used. For the scabbed cut, a pulse-modulated current with a significantly higher modulation frequency is used.

COAGULATION

This fast and efficient method of hemostasis is used when there is no spontaneous clotting. In most cases, it replaces a ligature of vessels, or the more costly alternatives such as fibrin glue. During the coagulation HF has the following effects:

- Protein molecules are denatured.
- Tissue is shrunk.
- Vessels are closed.
- Result of these processes is hemostasis.

The term coagulation encompasses two different surgical techniques: deep coagulation and (electrical) hemostasis. With deep coagulation, the tissue is heated to 50 - 80 °C cover a large area. This is done with ball and plate electrodes and is used to remove the tissue later (ablation). A large current density and current without pulse modulation are used. The magnitude of the current strength in relation to the frequency can influence the depth of the coagulation. When the tissue is slowly heated, the liquid evaporates inside and outside the cells without destroying the cell walls. The tissue shrinks and parts capable of coagulation are thermally obliterated. A stoppage of the blood flow, even from larger vessels, is achieved.

ARGON PLASMA COAGULATION

A newer form of HF surgery is argon plasma coagulation, in which electricity is transmitted via ionized argon (argon plasma). The arc ignites without direct contact between the probe and the tissue. APC's main area of application is interventional gastroenterology for the endoscopic therapy of bleeding and devitalization of abnormal tissue structures. The APC is also used in open surgery and interventional bronchoscopy.

COBLATION

The high-energy ions in the plasma can separate human tissue at relatively low temperatures below 70 ° C. This technology is used for surgical measures on intervertebral discs, tonsils, or the nasal turbinates.

RISKS OF HF SURGERY

Electrode Bonding

Suppose the power is too high, a scab (carbonization) forms, which inhibits the further spread of heat into the tissue's depth. Upon removing the electrode, the burnt tissue may also be removed because it sticks to the electrode. If, on the other hand, the HF power is too low and combined with a long exposure time, the tissue around the electrode and a scarcely deeper and beyond the diameter of the electrode will boil off.

Burns

Avoiding burns and other risks to the patient in HF surgery requires that general safety precautions for monopolar electrosurgery are followed:

- The patient must be kept isolated on the operating table (dry cloths, plastic pads, *etc.*). It may come into contact with metal parts and conductive (antistatic) hoses. Otherwise, there is a risk of current leakage and burns.

- Sweat builds up in skin folds, and between extremities may leading the current away from the site of application and cause burns. The body should be covered in such places with dry sheets.
- Ensure that the neutral electrode has a large and firmly adhering surface. Liquids must not get under the neutral electrode as they lead to a high current density at the contact area and, thus, may cause burns.
- So-called two-part neutral electrodes should always be used. These monitor the correct position of the neutral electrode. An additional measuring current is generated and monitored between electrode pairs. If this current is too low, one electrode does not make good contact, and the device switches off.
- For preoperative heart monitoring, only ECG cables with high-resistance inputs or HF chokes may be used.
- When using explosive anesthetic gases, shielding gas is necessary (similar to shielding gas welding in metal construction).
- Before the operation, ensure that the current from the active electrode to the neutral electrode is not, or as little as possible, passed through the heart area.
- Careful handling of flammable disinfectants such as alcohol since they may ignite from electrical sparks.

The surgeon's hand may also be at risk for burns through a small hole in the surgical glove since that creates a high current density between the surgical instrument and the doctor's hand. Heat may be generated quickly. The high temperature released destroys the surgical glove's further and very painful burns on the surgeon's hand may develop. While surgeons may think that they have been electrocuted, the intense local heating can destroy surgical gloves made of natural latex as well as synthetic latex. High-quality surgical gloves can reduce the likelihood of punctures. The surgeon should also change gloves at regular intervals during extended operations and, if possible, should double glove.

ELECTROSURGERY AND HIGH FREQUENCY

In 1999, multiple companies began using the term 'radiofrequency' as a technology reference to high frequency. What continues to be misleading is the frequency range of the particular energy source, which, much like lasers, is the determining factor of resulting tissue effect, control of absorption depth, utility, versatility, and most important, safety. Standard electrosurgical units, including low frequency of less than 500k Hz devices marketed under 'Radiofrequency' or 'RF,' produces greater thermal effects without controlled absorption. Radio-wave technology in the range of 1.7 MHz and 4.0 MHz has proven to offer the most significant degree of absorption control, therapeutic versatility, and effectiveness adding to the confusion when faced with the array of commercially available radiofrequency technologies. Monopolar RF units (IDET™) and Bipolar RF units (ArthroCare™) were marketed for specific percutaneous disc procedures.

However, both these devices emit frequency in the range of standard electrosurgical units such as Valleylab™ or ConMed™.

FREQUENCY & MODULATION - PULSED RADIO FREQUENCY

The electric influence on the neural structures related to the frequency modulation occurs during pulsed RF. When designing HF applicators, the distribution of the electromagnetic field generated is decisive for their characteristics — the distribution of the electrical power density and the heating in the tissue results from the field distribution. The HF Generator produces the waves in the MHZ range and the modulation of a single wave. This individual solution influences together with the shape of the HF applicator the magnetic field. Analyzing all vendors who offer medical HF-devices, one will find out that these are the basic principles of all different HF solutions.

INCREASED SAFETY THROUGH INNOVATION

Automatic Power Metering

The development of HF surgery has led to devices that have automatic power dosing. These enable a homogeneous and reproducible cutting effect, regardless of the influencing variables tissue, electrode shape, and operating mode. The sensors of modern regulated HF surgical devices continuously record current, voltage, and arc intensity parameters and dose them to an optimal performance level as required.

Two-Part Neutral Electrode (Monopolar)

A two-part neutral electrode (NE) checks the correct, full-surface contact with the patient's body and continuously compares the currents that flow through the NE's two surfaces. A different distribution of the currents indicates that the NE is not correctly applied. There is a risk of a partially high current density and tissue heating. The HF voltage source is connected to the body *via* the sizeable neutral electrode. The other pole is connected to the surgical instrument and flows from the active electrode to the neutral electrode *via* the least resistance path. No heat is generated on the neutral electrode due to the low current density; heat is generated on the active electrode due to high current density (Fig. **1**).

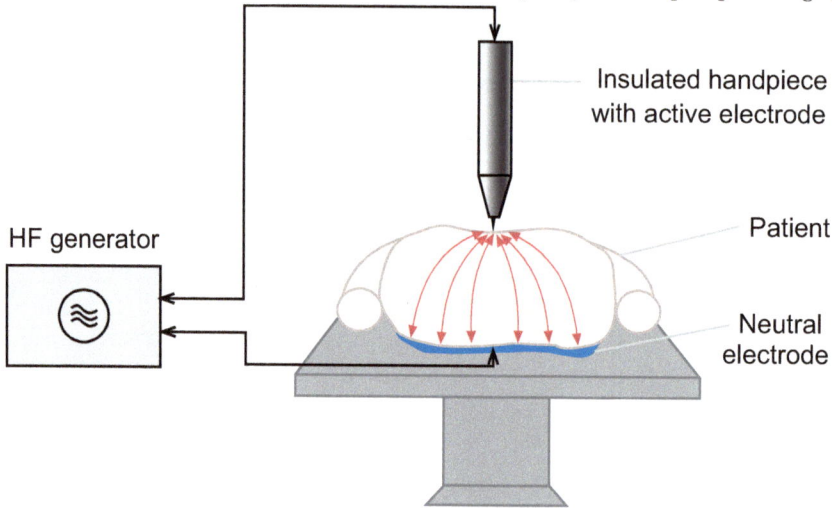

Fig (1). Schematic of monopolar HF electrotomy. The HF voltage source is connected to the body *via* the sizeable neutral electrode. The other pole is connected to the surgical instrument and flows from the active electrode to the neutral electrode *via* the least resistance path.

Bipolar Technique

The bipolar technique is mainly used in microsurgery and neurosurgery and can only be used for coagulation. Work is carried out with a two-pole active electrode (tweezers), whereby both poles are in contact with the surgical field. A neutral electrode is not required. Electrical energy is fed into the forceps, and the thermal effect at the tips causes the tissue to coagulate (Figs. **2** and **3**).

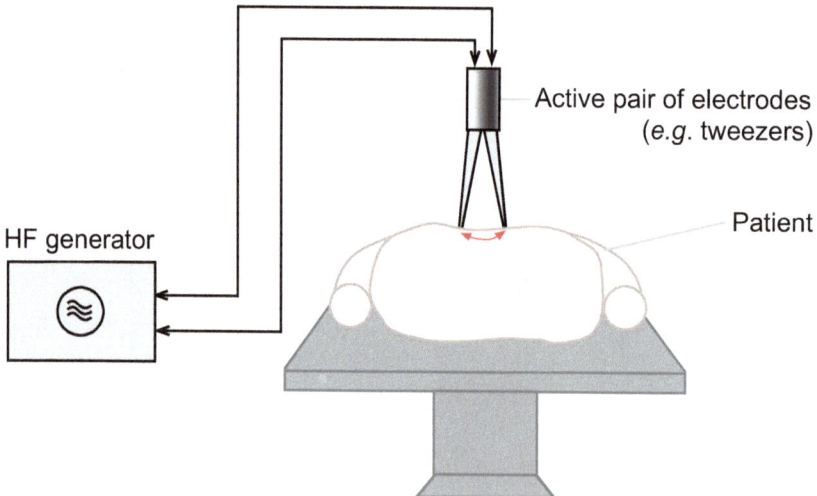

Fig. (2). Schematic of bipolar HF electrotomy. The HF voltage runs through poles that are in contact with the surgical field. A neutral electrode is not required. Electrical energy is fed into the forceps, and the thermal effect at the tips causes the tissue to coagulate.

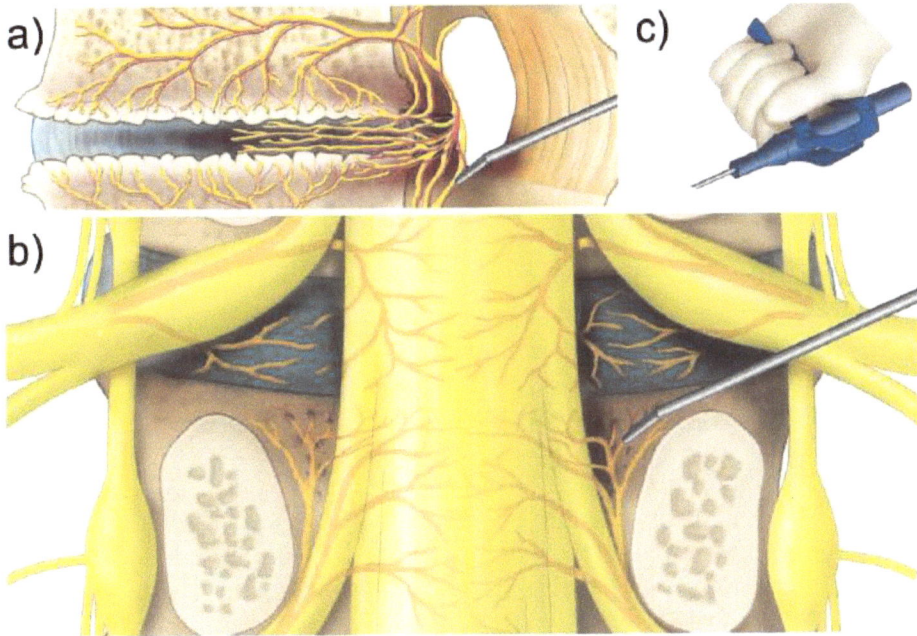

Fig (3). An example of a bipolar high-frequency probe used during basivertebral nerve ablation in the lumbar spine for unrelenting chronic low back pain [1, 2].

The origin of bipolar instruments are bayonet shaped forceps. The current does not flow over the body but between the two tips of the forceps. One of the pointed tweezers acts as an active electrode, the other as a neutral electrode. The energy required is, of course, much lower than with the monopolar technique. When used within neural structures (brain and nerves), the biggest problem is the sticking of tissue to the forceps' tips when too much energy is applied. In spinal endoscopic surgery, approximately 30 cm long electrodes are used that are passed through the channel of the foraminoscope. They consist of an outer tube and an inner electrode or two parallel electrodes on the tip. The outer tube forms the neutral electrode and the inner one the active electrode. Bipolar versions of spinal electrodes can be found in the catalogs of Elliquence™, Joimax™, and Kirwan™.

IMPEDANCE & CAPACITIVE RESISTANCE

The specific resistance of muscle tissue and tissue with an abundant blood supply is relatively low. That of fat is around a factor of 15 higher and that of bones by a factor of 1000. Therefore, the shape and level of the current must be tailored to the type of tissue being operated on. In principle, the lowest possible frequency for the tissue is used (Table **1**).

Table 1. Preferred HF frequency by tissue type.

Tissue Type (Frequency = 1 Mhz)	Specific Resistance (kΩ. cm)
Blood	O.16
Muscle, kidney, heart	0.2
Liver, spleen	0.3
Brain	0.7
Lung	1
Fat	3.3

COLD CUTTING HIGH-FREQUENCY

The first cold cutting device with high-frequency radio wave energy was developed in the 1960s by Ellman [3]. Ellman manipulated standard cautery units operating in the low-frequency range, searching for a more delicate tissue effect. Ellman first introduced the 3.8MHz frequency and was awarded a patent in 1976. Above 1,500kHz (1.5 MHz), high-frequency radiosurgery transmits pure radio-waves to the tissue without heating the electrode. High-frequency radio wave energy has been used extensively in many different medical applications and specialties for its ability to achieve a precise and controlled thermal ablation of soft tissue. The heat for this ablation is generated by a natural resistance of the tissue, which comes in the path of the waves released through the device's electrode tip. The cellular water in the soft tissues gets heated. When the temperature reaches 100 degrees Celsius, it starts boiling and produces steam, which results in the cellular, molecular dissolution of individual tissue cells. The cells exposed to these waves are destroyed while the surrounding tissues remain unaffected. This property of radiofrequency eliminates the possibility of undue damage to healthy tissues while improving surgical precision.

Technology advancement, including high-frequency radio waves and navigational bipolar delivery systems, has resulted in the incidence of dysesthesia dramatically decreasing [4]. Tsou *et al.* identified that nerve root irritation occurred more frequently when a temperature-controlled, low-frequency monopolar device was used [4]. The authors reported less severe or frequent dysesthesia with the use of Ellman's high-frequency radio wave and bipolar delivery system was used [4]. Radio-wave technology presents a modern tool with a multiplicity of applications in every surgical procedure. With tissue sparing as a basis for minimally invasive procedures, Ellman's current technology offers a therapeutic option in precision, preservation, versatility, and safety (Fig. **4**) [5]. Thermal and mechanical artifacts at the tissue margins showed the thermal damage depending on the type of laser and RF use but most consistent cut with the RF technology [6].

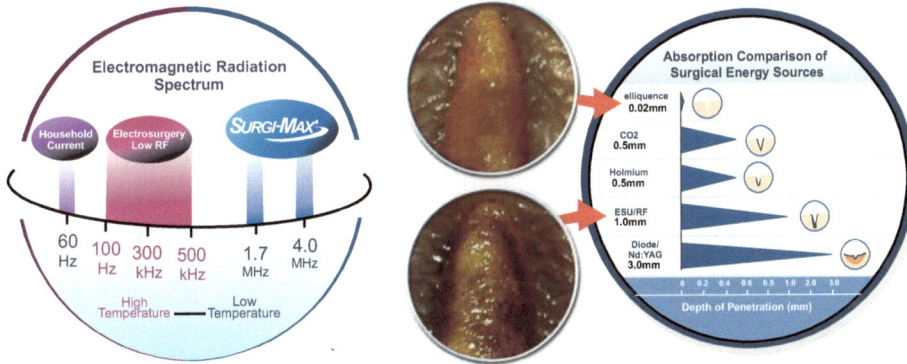

Fig. (4). Comparison of the frequency range employed in electrosurgery with low RF and with the cold cutting technology employed by the Elliquence Surgi-Max Ultra™ HF generator and graphic depiction of the energy absorption and thermal skin penetration in comparison to various lasers and the ESU RF [6].

THERMAL ENERGY IN SPINE APPLICATIONS

The use of thermal energy may play a significant role in reducing radicular symptoms and back pain by depopulating sensitized pain nociceptors in the annulus [7]. Yeung *et al.* reported positive results when applying thermal energy (4.0MHz) to treat debilitating discogenic back pain resulting from annular tears and internal disk disruption [8 - 10]. Percutaneous foraminoplastic lumbar discectomy was reported in a study of 2320 patients with contained, extruded, sequestered herniation with mild migration and lateral recess stenosis [11]. With an evolutionary technique that included Ellman's Surgitron Dual Frequency unit and navigational bipolar Trigger-Flex delivery system for thermal annuloplasty, the success rate was 95% in the leg and low back pain. The indications of a percutaneous discectomy with thermal discoplasty were broadened from small contained through large herniations to lateral spinal stenosis and degenerative disc diseases [11]. Freeman *et al.* concluded that ALADD with thermal modulation is a more fundamental and effective treatment modality than IDET for chronic discogenic low back pain [12].

The steerable high-frequency bipolar Trigger-Flex probe is used to contract and thicken the annular collagen at the herniated site and is also used for hemostasis throughout the endoscopic surgery [13]. Radio-wave energy application for removal of the offending nucleus, modulation of weak collagen fibrils, and sealing of annular tears contribute to depopulating nerve fibers sensitizing the outer annulus allowing for more rapid pain relief compared with traditional techniques [13]. Multiple fusion procedures may be avoided by opting for tissue sparing techniques. Tissue modulation with high radio wave technology can shrink or eliminate defects in the annulus fibrosis [7, 14]. Use of high-frequency radio wave technology is also being used to prepare the intravertebral space or vertebral segment for nucleus implants and artificial disc devices.

HF INTERVERTEBRAL DISC SURGERY

For the intervertebral disc's coagulation, it is desirable to keep a temperature of 60 to 80°C constant over a more extended time ranging from 90 to 180 seconds. This approach is the only way to ensure that the collagen fibers within the annulus and nucleus are transformed through shrinkage. The coagulation result does not only depend on the settings of the HF generator. To a large extent, it is also influenced by the impedance of the intervertebral disc. For an HF generator that has constant voltage regulation, this means the following: Since the generator voltage (U) is constant, the power (P) released in the tissue decreases with increasing intervertebral disc resistance (R). The voltage and the setting of the HF generator must consequently be adapted to the disc impedance to achieve power in the range of 4 to 6W reliably. However, it would be much better to use generators which by themselves guarantee a set output in the tissue. For this purpose, objective criteria would be required that can be continuously analyzed during the operation. Such electrical parameters would assure better the operation's success with lower recurrence- and complication rates.

HF IN PERCUTANEOUS & ENDOSCOPIC SPINE PROCEDURES

The accepted indications for percutaneous and endoscopic spinal surgeries have significantly expanded over the last ten years. Through the endoscopic access route, treatment of common painful degenerative conditions of the spine has gone way beyond the scope of just herniated discs. Compared to open surgery, where direct visualization is often provided *via* an operating microscope during microsurgical dissection, the extent of material removal and effects of HF treatment can be directly assessed during the endoscopic surgery under very high magnification factors. In general, percutaneous surgical procedures achieve better results when they are performed under direct visualization. This complementary overlap of the videoendoscopic and HF technique in modern endoscopic spine surgery is the key to superior clinical outcomes otherwise observed with non-visualized percutaneous procedures performed under fluoroscopic control.

PERCUTANEOUS COBLATION

The details of reaching the spinal canal and the foramina with the spinal endoscope *via* the interlaminar, transforaminal, and other contemporary versions of uni- or multi portal access have been described in several chapters of this text. One of the commercially available HF probes used during spinal endoscopy is connected to a generator that generates an electric plasma field around the probe during the procedure. The HF application to the intervertebral disc causes coagulation of the proteins, and the stiffness of the gel-like nucleus increases resulting HF induced shrinkage. Hence, protrusions may recede and diminish in size. This coblation maneuver is primarily suitable for contained disc herniations. The observed complications with HF coagulation, including tissue traumatization, infection, retroperitoneal bleeding, and allergic reactions, are only too infrequent. The level of impedance shows a significant difference between the nucleus pulposus and the annulus fibrosus. In this performance range, a maximum temperature of 71∘C should ideally be reached after an average of 80 seconds. The temperature should remain constant until the end of the coagulation, not exceeding a total of 180 seconds. The diameter of the devitalization zone should not surpass 20 mm. This protocol ensures that surrounding sensitive tissue, including nerves and vessels, are not unnecessarily destroyed (Fig. **5**).

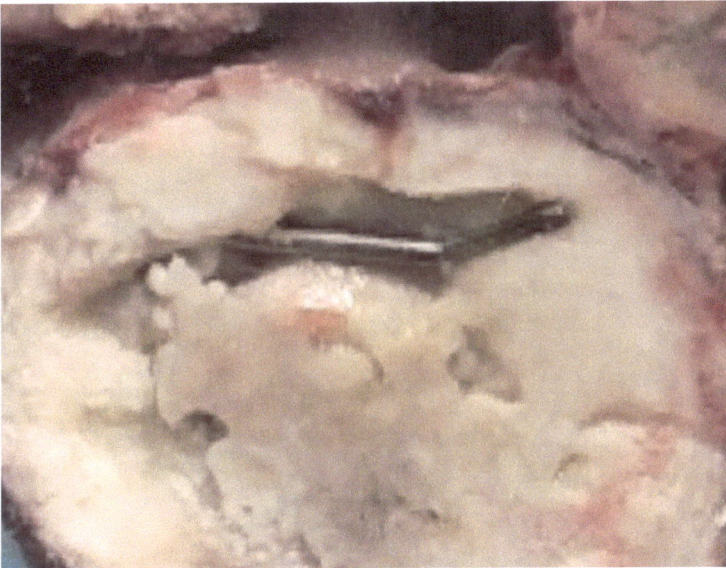

Fig. (5). Intradiscal application of a bipolar steerable Elliquence HF probe for shrinkage and stabilization of the annulus [42].

HF SYSTEMS FOR ENDOSCOPIC DISC SURGERY

Many vendors offer HF generators designed and intended for endoscopic spinal surgery. For discussion purposes, the authors list a few below without suggesting that these products are the only contenders. Percutaneous Intradiscal Thermocoagulation. However, several devices are in the market for the non-visualized treatment of chronic discogenic back pain referred to as intradiscal electrothermal annuloplasty or percutaneous intradiscal radiofrequency thermocoagulation.

Nucleoplasty by ArthroCare™

Nucleoplasty by ArthroCare™ [15] and Intradiscal Disc Electro-Thermal by ORATEC [16 - 18]. Smith and Nephew treatments are delivery system devices geared towards targeting thermal energy to either the nucleus or annulus, respectively. These percutaneous treatments produce varied results as the physician cannot visualize the exact treatment target's anatomy or pathology. Considering the non-visualized nature of these devices and the thermal nature of low frequency (under 500kHz), post-operative results have been difficult to predict [4, 17, 19, 20]. The FDA cleared the ORATEC SpineCATH Intradiscal Catheter system also in 1999 to treat chronic low back pain associated with contained herniated discs [16 - 18]. The SpineCATH is intended for the coagulation and decompression of disc material to treat symptomatic patients with contained herniated discs [16].

Arthrocare DISC Nucleoplasty™

DISC nucleoplasty™ (Arthrocare) [12, 15] is another method of applying heat treatment to the intervertebral disc using low radiofrequency. DISC nucleoplasty is closer in concept to a laser discectomy, in that tissue is removed or ablated to provide decompression of a bulging disc. Arthrocare received Food and Drug Administration (FDA) clearance in 1999 for its spine system. Indications for this system are ablation, coagulation, and disc material decompression to treat symptomatic patients with contained herniated discs.

Intradiscal Electrothermal Annuloplasty (IDET™)

Electrothermal annuloplasty (IDET™) describes explicitly a procedure whereby a thermal catheter is inserted posterolaterally into the disc annulus or nucleus [21 - 30]. The catheter is then passed through the disc circuitously to return posteriorly. Using low radiofrequency energy, electrothermal heat is generated within the thermal resistive coil at 90 degrees centigrade; the disc material is heated for up to 20 minutes. The mechanism of pain relief action is not precisely understood. However, it is thought to be either shrinkage of the collagen fibers within the annulus or destruction of the adjacent nociceptive pain fibers. Subsequently, the IDET™ system fell out of favor because of complications [31 - 36].

Radionics RF Disc Catheter System™

The Radionics RF Disc Catheter System™ is a low radiofrequency probe placed into the disc's center rather than around the annulus [37]. The device is activated for only 90 seconds at a temperature of 70 degrees centigrade. Again, this procedure's mechanism of action is not precisely understood but is thought to reduce the nociceptive pain input from the free nerve ending in the outer annulus fibrosis. Based on the destruction of nociceptive pain fibers, the Radionics Disc Catheter System is similar in concept to IDET™.

Joimax® Karlsruhe, Germany

The Legato® and Vaporflex® bipolar probes are disposable RF electrodes and are designed especially for minimally invasive electro-surgical spinal interventions through the endoscope under constant irrigation [38]. The probes are guided through the endoscope's working channel, and the electrical power is transferred directly to the tissue at the surgical site. They are used to cut, coagulate, shrink and remove soft tissue or for the denervation of the surface and are operated with a proprietary RF generator. Handles, Cables, and shafts are reusable and can be sterilized. More information is available in the appropriate user manuals and instructions for use (IFU).

Kirwan® Rockwell, Massachusetts, USA

This company offers two HF probes: The 14-7018 reusable TRP bipolar nonstick pencil, point Tip, 10° angle, measuring 30 cm in length, and the 14-9030 - 14-9034 disposable bipolar suction coagulator in French diameters of 8, 11, 13, 15, measuring 28 cm in length.

Elliquence® Baldwin, New York 11510, USA

Elliquence offers the Disc-Fix®, or Trigger Fix®, in conjunction with their proprietary RF generator Surgi-max ultra® (Fig. 6). Several clinical applications have been demonstrated [10, 39 - 41].

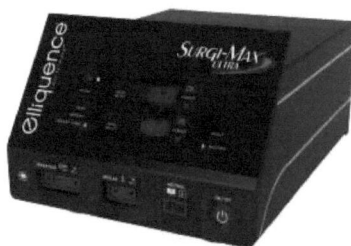

Fig (6). Photo of the Elliquence Surgi-Max Ultra™ HF generator that works in conjunction with a bipolar RF probe typically used during spinal endoscopy procedures.

TARGETING PAIN GENERATORS BY PROBE STEERING

Another factor of the outcome using Surgical HF-Devices is how they are moved by steering the HF-applicator during the endoscopic operation. For this to work well in conjunction with the spinal endoscope, the entire endoscopic spine system has to be integrated to maximize benefits of both surgical decompression and HF coblation and shrinkage of pathologic tissues (Figs. **7 - 9**).

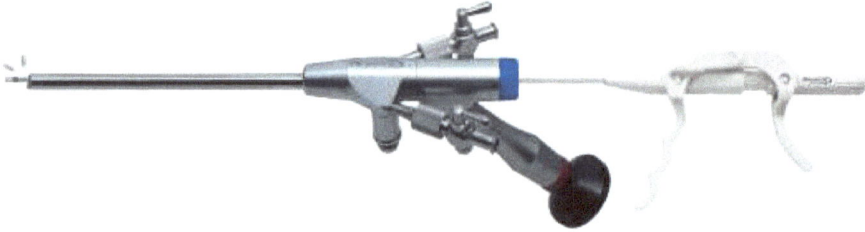

Fig (7). Illustration of the Elliquence lumbar foraminoscope with the HF radiofequency probe introduced through the center working channel of the endoscope.

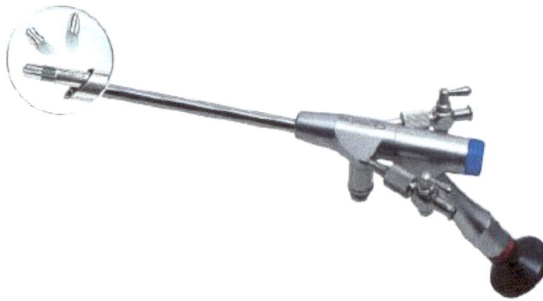

Fig (8). Illustration of the Elliquence lumbar foraminoscope with the HF radiofequency probe than can be easily flexed and directed at the target pain generator by pressing the handle shown in Fig. (**5**).

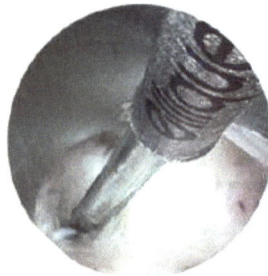

Fig. (9). Illustration of the Elliquence radiofequency Triggerflex ™ probe than can be directed at the target area by pressing the handle shown in Fig. **7**.

INFLUENCE OF IRRIGATION FLUIDS ON THE IMPEDANCE & TISSUE EFFECTS

The benefits of irrigation during endoscopic disc surgery have been overlooked for an extended period. During the development of the Destandau Endospine™ device and the YESS™ system, an irrigation channel was incorporated, improving endoscopic spine surgery in two ways: a) A clear view of the region of interest was finally provided, and b) it aided in hemostasis and diminished bleedings by maintaining a hydrostatic fluid pressure at the surgical site similar to knee arthroscopy. Soon it was recognized that the foraminal space was not contained as during knee arthroscopy and that neural structures were at risk of injury if irrigation pressures would be excessively high. Dr. Destandau, Dr. Leu, and Dr. A. Yeung advised avoiding this problem. Joimax™ and R. Wolf™ offer specialized irrigation equipment for endoscopic disc treatment.

USER FRIENDLY CONFIGURATION

Most HF devices offer the option of creating a personalized start screen. This appears after switching on the device for a selectable duration. For percutaneous endoscopic HF applications, 2 to 3 presets from the multitude of current characteristic variations are often sufficient. The providers of HF products for endoscopic disc surgery offer devices with a software configuration with a myriad of possibilities, some of which are very complex. From the surgeon's point of view, they appear mostly over-engineered. The Elliquence™ HF generator is a device specially manufactured for this frequent use. The company has decades of experience providing HF equipment to surgeons across multiple subspecialties and offers the best possible purchase and maintenance solution. In comparison, Kirwan offers reusable probes with the HF generator for endoscopic disc surgery besides disposables.

DISCUSSION

High-frequency is commonly used during endoscopic spinal surgery in bi-polar probes, which are also named radiofrequency probes. They have found application as a cutting, coagulation, and coblation tool to aid in tissue dissection, shrinkage, and hemostasis. Many surgeons use these high-radiofrequency probes routinely without knowing much about the underlying technology and how to use it to maximize its advantage. Some aspects of the technology can potentially be harmful to the patient and the surgeon end-user. Modern RF generators intended for endoscopic spine surgery have built-in checks and balances, including automatic power metering, and two-part neutral electrodes to avoid burns and electrode bonding.

The primary mechanism of action of endoscopic RF probes is generating an electric plasma field around the probe directed at the disc, ligamentous, and other tissues within the spinal canal. Typically, this energy delivery results in temperature-induced dehydration and coagulation of proteins and other biological building blocks of the tissues making up the spinal motion segment. The gel-like consistency of the nucleus is changed to higher stiffness induced shrinkage. This is the primary mechanism of action applied to the endoscopic and percutaneous treatment of herniated discs. The bipolar RF probes can be applied in the epidural space or intradiscally. The non-visualized percutaneous intradiscal application's clinical application has been studied more thoroughly since the RF probe is the primary decompression tool. An example of such a device is DiscFix™ [42].

In contrast, the RF probe's added benefit during directly visualized endoscopic procedures is less well researched since the clinical benefit is primarily attributed to the mechanical endoscopic decompression tools. However, the authors of this chapter stipulate an added benefit of the RF technology does exist even if used in conjunction with endoscopy. It requires further clinical study as innovation of HF technologies may contribute to simplify minimally invasive spinal surgery techniques further and, thus, contribute to more reliable and durable clinical improvements in patients suffering from sciatica-type low back and leg pain. In short, such HF technologies could further realize future cost-savings despite the added upfront cost.

CONCLUSION

In this chapter, the authors attempted to provide a brief look into the field of high-frequency technology applications in medicine in general and in endoscopic spinal surgery in particular [4, 9, 11 - 13, 36, 37, 41 - 72]. By no means did they attempt to provide an in-depth view of how these technologies are currently applied. Instead, we wanted to brief the spine surgeon on the underlying principles, so they feel enabled to apply them more effectively in their patients' treatment. Moreover, the authors wanted to highlight areas in need of further clinical research in the modern context of recent endoscopic spine surgery – a very fast-moving dynamic subspecialty field of spine surgery as a whole. As indications for endoscopic spine surgery expand and more complex decompression and reconstructive scenarios are attempted, HF applications will require continued innovation.

CONSENT FOR PUBLICATION

Not applicable.

CONFLICT OF INTEREST

The authors declare no conflict of interest, financial or otherwise.

ACKNOWLEDGEMENT

Declared none.

REFERENCES

[1]   Becker S, Hadjipavlou A, Heggeness MH. Ablation of the basivertebral nerve for treatment of back pain: a clinical study. Spine J 2017; 17(2): 218-23.
[http://dx.doi.org/10.1016/j.spinee.2016.08.032] [PMID: 27592808]

[2]   Kim HS, Adsul N, Yudoyono F, *et al.* Transforaminal epiduroscopic basivertebral nerve laser ablation for chronic low back pain associated with modic changes: A preliminary open-label study. Pain Res Manag 2018; 2018: 6857983.
[http://dx.doi.org/10.1155/2018/6857983] [PMID: 30186540]

[3]   Welch WC, Gerszten PC. Alternative strategies for lumbar discectomy: intradiscal electrothermy and nucleoplasty. Neurosurg Focus 2002; 13(2): E7.
[http://dx.doi.org/10.3171/foc.2002.13.2.8] [PMID: 15916404]

[4]   Tsou PM, Alan Yeung C, Yeung AT. Posterolateral transforaminal selective endoscopic discectomy and thermal annuloplasty for chronic lumbar discogenic pain: a minimal access visualized intradiscal surgical procedure. Spine J 2004; 4(5): 564-73.
[http://dx.doi.org/10.1016/j.spinee.2004.01.014] [PMID: 15363430]

[5]   Sperli AE. The use of radiosurgery in plastic surgery and dermatology. Surg Technol Int 1998; 7: 437-42.
[PMID: 12722012]

[6]   Turner RJ, Cohen RA, Voet RL, Stephens SR, Weinstein SA. Analysis of tissue margins of cone biopsy specimens obtained with "cold knife," CO_2 and Nd:YAG lasers and a radiofrequency surgical unit. J Reprod Med 1992; 37(7): 607-10.
[PMID: 1522568]

[7]   Ramírez-León JF, Rugeles-Ortiz JG, Barreto-perea JA, Alonso-cuéllar GO. Intradiscal temperature variation resulting from radiofrequency thermal therapy. Cadaver study. Acta Ortop Mex 2014; 28(1): 12-8.
[PMID: 26031132]

[8]   Yeung AT, Gore S. *In-vivo* endoscopic visualization of patho-anatomy in symptomatic degenerative conditions of the lumbar spine ii: intradiscal, foraminal, and central canal decompression. Surg Technol Int 2011; 21: 299-319.
[PMID: 22505004]

[9]   Yeung AT. The evolution of percutaneous spinal endoscopy and discectomy: state of the art. Mt Sinai J Med 2000; 67(4): 327-32.
[PMID: 11021785]

[10]   Yeung A, Gore S. Endoscopically guided foraminal and dorsal rhizotomy for chronic axial back pain based on cadaver and endoscopically visualized anatomic study. Int J Spine Surg 2014; 8: 8.
[http://dx.doi.org/10.14444/1023] [PMID: 25694936]

[11]   Yeung AT. The evolution and advancement of endoscopic foraminal surgery: one surgeon's experience incorporating adjunctive techologies. SAS J 2007; 1(3): 108-17.
[http://dx.doi.org/10.1016/S1935-9810(07)70055-5] [PMID: 25802587]

[12]   Freeman BJ, Mehdian R. Intradiscal electrothermal therapy, percutaneous discectomy, and nucleoplasty: what is the current evidence? Curr Pain Headache Rep 2008; 12(1): 14-21.
[http://dx.doi.org/10.1007/s11916-008-0004-7] [PMID: 18417018]

[13]   Kapural L, Hayek S, Malak O, Arrigain S, Mekhail N. Intradiscal thermal annuloplasty *versus* intradiscal radiofrequency ablation for the treatment of discogenic pain: a prospective matched control trial. Pain Med 2005; 6(6): 425-31.
[http://dx.doi.org/10.1111/j.1526-4637.2005.00073.x] [PMID: 16336479]

[14]   Zhou H, Yang X, Jiang L, Wei F, Liu X, Liu Z. Radiofrequency ablation in gross total excision of cervical chordoma: ideas and technique. Eur Spine J 2018; 27(12): 3113-7.

[http://dx.doi.org/10.1007/s00586-018-5628-7] [PMID: 29915886]

[15]   Nau WH, Diederich CJ. Evaluation of temperature distributions in cadaveric lumbar spine during nucleoplasty. Phys Med Biol 2004; 49(8): 1583-94.
[http://dx.doi.org/10.1088/0031-9155/49/8/015] [PMID: 15152694]

[16]   Saal JS, Saal JA. Management of chronic discogenic low back pain with a thermal intradiscal catheter. A preliminary report. Spine 2000; 25(3): 382-8.
[http://dx.doi.org/10.1097/00007632-200002010-00021] [PMID: 10703114]

[17]   Kleinstueck FS, Diederich CJ, Nau WH, *et al.* Temperature and thermal dose distributions during intradiscal electrothermal therapy in the cadaveric lumbar spine. Spine 2003; 28(15): 1700-8.
[http://dx.doi.org/10.1097/01.BRS.0000083160.16853.6E] [PMID: 12897495]

[18]   Kleinstueck FS, Diederich CJ, Nau WH, *et al.* Acute biomechanical and histological effects of intradiscal electrothermal therapy on human lumbar discs. Spine 2001; 26(20): 2198-207.
[http://dx.doi.org/10.1097/00007632-200110150-00009] [PMID: 11598508]

[19]   Kaplan LD, Ernsthausen JM, Bradley JP, Fu FH, Farkas DL. The thermal field of radiofrequency probes at chondroplasty settings. Arthroscopy 2003; 19(6): 632-40.
[http://dx.doi.org/10.1016/S0749-8063(03)00128-2] [PMID: 12861202]

[20]   Freeman BJ, Walters RM, Moore RJ, Fraser RD. Does intradiscal electrothermal therapy denervate and repair experimentally induced posterolateral annular tears in an animal model? Spine 2003; 28(23): 2602-8.
[http://dx.doi.org/10.1097/01.BRS.0000097889.01759.05] [PMID: 14652477]

[21]   Spruit M, Jacobs WC. Pain and function after intradiscal electrothermal treatment (IDET) for symptomatic lumbar disc degeneration. Eur Spine J 2002; 11(6): 589-93.
[http://dx.doi.org/10.1007/s00586-002-0450-6] [PMID: 12522718]

[22]   Shah RV, Lutz GE, Lee J, Doty SB, Rodeo S. Intradiskal electrothermal therapy: a preliminary histologic study. Arch Phys Med Rehabil 2001; 82(9): 1230-7.
[http://dx.doi.org/10.1053/apmr.2001.23897] [PMID: 11552196]

[23]   Saal JA, Saal JS. Intradiscal electrothermal therapy for the treatment of chronic discogenic low back pain. Clin Sports Med 2002; 21(1): 167-87.
[http://dx.doi.org/10.1016/S0278-5919(03)00064-4] [PMID: 11877870]

[24]   Saal JA, Saal JS. Intradiscal electrothermal treatment for chronic discogenic low back pain: prospective outcome study with a minimum 2-year follow-up. Spine 2002; 27(9): 966-73.
[http://dx.doi.org/10.1097/00007632-200205010-00017] [PMID: 11979172]

[25]   Saal JA, Saal JS. Intradiscal electrothermal treatment for chronic discogenic low back pain: a prospective outcome study with minimum 1-year follow-up. Spine 2000; 25(20): 2622-7.
[http://dx.doi.org/10.1097/00007632-200010150-00013] [PMID: 11034647]

[26]   Mayer HM. [Discogenic low back pain and degenerative lumbar spinal stenosis - how appropriate is surgical treatment?]. Schmerz 2001; 15(6): 484-91.
[http://dx.doi.org/10.1007/s004820100036] [PMID: 11793155]

[27]   Lee J, Lutz GE, Campbell D, Rodeo SA, Wright T. Stability of the lumbar spine after intradiscal electrothermal therapy. Arch Phys Med Rehabil 2001; 82(1): 120-2.
[http://dx.doi.org/10.1053/apmr.2001.19021] [PMID: 11239297]

[28]   Heary RF. Intradiscal electrothermal annuloplasty: the IDET procedure. J Spinal Disord 2001; 14(4): 353-60.
[http://dx.doi.org/10.1097/00002517-200108000-00013] [PMID: 11481560]

[29]   Endres SM, Fiedler GA, Larson KL. Effectiveness of intradiscal electrothermal therapy in increasing function and reducing chronic low back pain in selected patients. WMJ 2002; 101(1): 31-4.
[PMID: 12025752]

[30]   Derby R, Eek B, Chen Y, O'neill C, Ryan D. Intradiscal Electrothermal Annuloplasty (IDET): A Novel Approach for Treating Chronic Discogenic Back Pain. Neuromodulation 2000; 3(2): 82-8.
[http://dx.doi.org/10.1046/j.1525-1403.2000.00082.x] [PMID: 22151403]

[31]   Wegener B, Rieskamp K, Büttner A, *et al.* Experimental evaluation of the risk of extradiscal thermal damage in intradiscal electrothermal therapy (IDET). Pain Physician 2012; 15(1): E99-E106.
[http://dx.doi.org/10.36076/ppj.2012/15/E99] [PMID: 22270753]

[32]   Stamuli E, Kesornsak W, Grevitt MP, Posnett J, Claxton K. A cost-effectiveness analysis of intradiscal electrothermal therapy compared with circumferential lumbar fusion. Pain Pract 2018; 18(4): 515-22.
[http://dx.doi.org/10.1111/papr.12641] [PMID: 28898530]

[33]   Kircelli A, Coven I, Cansever T, Sonmez E, Yilmaz C. Patient selection and efficacy of intradiscal electrothermal therapy with respect to the dallas discogram score. Turk Neurosurg 2017; 27(4): 623-30.
[PMID: 27593796]

[34]   Helm Ii S, Simopoulos TT, Stojanovic M, Abdi S, El Terany MA. Effectiveness of thermal annular procedures in treating discogenic low back pain. Pain Physician 2017; 20(6): 447-70.
[http://dx.doi.org/10.36076/ppj/447] [PMID: 28934777]

[35]   Helm Ii S, Deer TR, Manchikanti L, *et al.* Effectiveness of thermal annular procedures in treating discogenic low back pain. Pain Physician 2012; 15(3): E279-304.
[http://dx.doi.org/10.36076/ppj.2012/15/E279] [PMID: 22622914]

[36]   Gelalis I, Gkiatas I, Spiliotis A, *et al.* Current concepts in intradiscal percutaneous minimally invasive procedures for chronic low back pain. Asian J Neurosurg 2019; 14(3): 657-69.
[http://dx.doi.org/10.4103/ajns.AJNS_119_17] [PMID: 31497082]

[37]   Rosen S, Falco F. Radiofrequency stimulation of intervertebral discs. Pain Physician 2003; 6(4): 435-8.
[http://dx.doi.org/10.36076/ppj.2003/6/435] [PMID: 16871294]

[38]   Jones PD, Moskalyuk A, Barthold C, *et al.* Low-Impedance 3D PEDOT:PSS Ultramicroelectrodes. Front Neurosci 2020; 14: 405.
[http://dx.doi.org/10.3389/fnins.2020.00405] [PMID: 32508562]

[39]   Chen KT, Jabri H, Lokanath YK, Song MS, Kim JS. The evolution of interlaminar endoscopic spine surgery. J Spine Surg 2020; 6(2): 502-12.
[http://dx.doi.org/10.21037/jss.2019.10.06] [PMID: 32656388]

[40]   Palea O, Granville M, Jacobson RE. Selection of tubular and endoscopic transforaminal disc procedures based on disc size, location, and characteristics. Cureus 2018; 10(1): e2091.
[http://dx.doi.org/10.7759/cureus.2091] [PMID: 29564196]

[41]   Beyaz SG, İnanmaz ME, Zengin ES, Ülgen AM. Combined use of high radiofrequency disk ablation, annulus modulation, and manual nucleotomy in a patient with extruded disk herniation. Pain Pract 2016; 16(5): E74-80.
[http://dx.doi.org/10.1111/papr.12426] [PMID: 26991910]

[42]   Hellinger S. Treatment of contained lumbar disc herniations using radiofrequency assisted micro-tubular decompression and nucleotomy: four year prospective study results. Int J Spine Surg 2014; 8: 8.
[http://dx.doi.org/10.14444/1024] [PMID: 25694932]

[43]   Kanpolat Y, Savas A, Bekar A, Berk C. Percutaneous controlled radiofrequency trigeminal rhizotomy for the treatment of idiopathic trigeminal neuralgia: 25-year experience with 1,600 patients. Neurosurgery 2001; 48(3): 524-32.
[http://dx.doi.org/10.1097/00006123-200103000-00013] [PMID: 11270542]

[44]   Mathews ES, Scrivani SJ. Percutaneous stereotactic radiofrequency thermal rhizotomy for the treatment of trigeminal neuralgia. Mt Sinai J Med 2000; 67(4): 288-99.

[PMID: 11021779]

[45]   Dreyfuss P, Halbrook B, Pauza K, Joshi A, McLarty J, Bogduk N. Efficacy and validity of radiofrequency neurotomy for chronic lumbar zygapophysial joint pain. Spine 2000; 25(10): 1270-7.
       [http://dx.doi.org/10.1097/00007632-200005150-00012] [PMID: 10806505]

[46]   van Kleef M, Barendse GA, Kessels A, Voets HM, Weber WE, de Lange S. Randomized trial of radiofrequency lumbar facet denervation for chronic low back pain. Spine 1999; 24(18): 1937-42.
       [http://dx.doi.org/10.1097/00007632-199909150-00013] [PMID: 10515020]

[47]   Göçer AI, Cetinalp E, Tuna M, Ildan F, Bağdatoğlu H, Haciyakupoğlu S. Percutaneous radiofrequency rhizotomy of lumbar spinal facets: the results of 46 cases. Neurosurg Rev 1997; 20(2): 114-6.
       [http://dx.doi.org/10.1007/BF01138194] [PMID: 9226670]

[48]   Rocco AG. Radiofrequency lumbar sympatholysis. The evolution of a technique for managing sympathetically maintained pain. Reg Anesth 1995; 20(1): 3-12.
       [PMID: 7727325]

[49]   Andersen KH, Mosdal C, Vaernet K. Percutaneous radiofrequency facet denervation in low-back and extremity pain. Acta Neurochir (Wien) 1987; 87(1-2): 48-51.
       [http://dx.doi.org/10.1007/BF02076015] [PMID: 2960131]

[50]   Shealy CN. Percutaneous radiofrequency denervation of spinal facets. Treatment for chronic back pain and sciatica. J Neurosurg 1975; 43(4): 448-51.
       [http://dx.doi.org/10.3171/jns.1975.43.4.0448] [PMID: 125787]

[51]   Adakli B, Cakar Turhan KS, Asik I. The comparison of the efficacy of radiofrequency nucleoplasty and targeted disc decompression in lumbar radiculopathy. Bosn J Basic Med Sci 2015; 15(2): 57-61.
       [http://dx.doi.org/10.17305/bjbms.2015.427] [PMID: 26042514]

[52]   Blume HG. Cervicogenic headaches: radiofrequency neurotomy and the cervical disc and fusion. Clin Exp Rheumatol 2000; 18(2) (Suppl. 19): S53-8.
       [PMID: 10824288]

[53]   Cohen SP, Bhaskar A, Bhatia A, *et al.* Consensus practice guidelines on interventions for lumbar facet joint pain from a multispecialty, international working group. Reg Anesth Pain Med 2020; 45(6): 424-67.
       [http://dx.doi.org/10.1136/rapm-2019-101243] [PMID: 32245841]

[54]   Engel A, King W, Schneider BJ, Duszynski B, Bogduk N. The effectiveness of cervical medial branch thermal radiofrequency neurotomy stratified by selection criteria: A systematic review of the literature. Pain Med 2020; 21(11): 2726-37.
       [http://dx.doi.org/10.1093/pm/pnaa219] [PMID: 32935126]

[55]   Ji K, Wang S, Miao W, Yu J, Wang Z. Application of esophageal radiography technique in the treatment of herniation of cervical disc with radiofrequency thermocoagulation and target ablation. J Neurosurg Sci 2019; 63(5): 615-7.
       [http://dx.doi.org/10.23736/S0390-5616.17.04165-0] [PMID: 28869374]

[56]   Kanpolat Y, Berk C, Savas A, Bekar A. Percutaneous controlled radiofrequency rhizotomy in the management of patients with trigeminal neuralgia due to multiple sclerosis. Acta Neurochir (Wien) 2000; 142(6): 685-9.
       [http://dx.doi.org/10.1007/s007010070113] [PMID: 10949444]

[57]   Khalil JG, Smuck M, Koreckij T, *et al.* A prospective, randomized, multicenter study of intraosseous basivertebral nerve ablation for the treatment of chronic low back pain. Spine J 2019; 19(10): 1620-32.
       [http://dx.doi.org/10.1016/j.spinee.2019.05.598] [PMID: 31229663]

[58]   Kvarstein G, Måwe L, Indahl A, *et al.* A randomized double-blind controlled trial of intra-annular radiofrequency thermal disc therapy--a 12-month follow-up. Pain 2009; 145(3): 279-86.
       [http://dx.doi.org/10.1016/j.pain.2009.05.001] [PMID: 19647940]

[59]   Kwak SG, Lee DG, Chang MC. Effectiveness of pulsed radiofrequency treatment on cervical radicular

pain: A meta-analysis. Medicine (Baltimore) 2018; 97(31): e11761.
[http://dx.doi.org/10.1097/MD.0000000000011761] [PMID: 30075599]

[60]   Lee DG, Ahn SH, Lee J. Comparative effectivenesses of pulsed radiofrequency and transforaminal steroid injection for radicular pain due to disc herniation: a prospective randomized trial. J Korean Med Sci 2016; 31(8): 1324-30.
[http://dx.doi.org/10.3346/jkms.2016.31.8.1324] [PMID: 27478346]

[61]   Mamlouk MD, Vansonnenberg E, Schraml F, Theodore N. Radiofrequency ablation of an unusual vertebral body osteoid osteoma contiguous with the intervertebral disc. J Vasc Interv Radiol 2013; 24(11): 1756-8.
[http://dx.doi.org/10.1016/j.jvir.2013.05.029] [PMID: 24160834]

[62]   Mehta M, Sluijter ME. The treatment of chronic back pain. A preliminary survey of the effect of radiofrequency denervation of the posterior vertebral joints. Anaesthesia 1979; 34(8): 768-75.
[http://dx.doi.org/10.1111/j.1365-2044.1979.tb06410.x] [PMID: 160757]

[63]   Niemisto L, Kalso E, Malmivaara A, Seitsalo S, Hurri H. Radiofrequency denervation for neck and back pain. A systematic review of randomized controlled trials. Cochrane Database Syst Rev 2003; (1): CD004058.
[PMID: 12535508]

[64]   O'Gara A, Leahy A, McCrory C, Das B. Dorsal root ganglion pulsed radiofrequency treatment for chronic cervical radicular pain: a retrospective review of outcomes in fifty-nine cases. Ir J Med Sci 2020; 189(1): 299-303.
[http://dx.doi.org/10.1007/s11845-019-02087-4] [PMID: 31441007]

[65]   Pan F, Shen B, Chy SK, et al. Transforaminal endoscopic system technique for discogenic low back pain: A prospective Cohort study. Int J Surg 2016; 35: 134-8.
[http://dx.doi.org/10.1016/j.ijsu.2016.09.091] [PMID: 27693825]

[66]   Rohof O. Intradiscal pulsed radiofrequency application following provocative discography for the management of degenerative disc disease and concordant pain: a pilot study. Pain Pract 2012; 12(5): 342-9.
[http://dx.doi.org/10.1111/j.1533-2500.2011.00512.x] [PMID: 22008239]

[67]   Teixeira A, Grandinson M, Sluijter ME. Pulsed radiofrequency for radicular pain due to a herniated intervertebral disc--an initial report. Pain Pract 2005; 5(2): 111-5.
[http://dx.doi.org/10.1111/j.1533-2500.2005.05207.x] [PMID: 17177757]

[68]   Vallejo R, Benyamin RM, Kramer J, Stanton G, Joseph NJ. Pulsed radiofrequency denervation for the treatment of sacroiliac joint syndrome. Pain Med 2006; 7(5): 429-34.
[http://dx.doi.org/10.1111/j.1526-4637.2006.00143.x] [PMID: 17014602]

[69]   van Tilburg CW, Stronks DL, Groeneweg JG, Huygen FJ. Randomized sham-controlled, double-blind, multicenter clinical trial on the effect of percutaneous radiofrequency at the ramus communicans for lumbar disc pain. Eur J Pain 2017; 21(3): 520-9.
[http://dx.doi.org/10.1002/ejp.945] [PMID: 27734550]

[70]   Walter SG, Schildberg FA, Rommelspacher Y. Endoscopic Sacrolumbar Facet Joint Denervation in Osteoarthritic and Degenerated Zygapophyseal Joints. Arthrosc Tech 2018; 7(12): e1275-9.
[http://dx.doi.org/10.1016/j.eats.2018.08.014] [PMID: 30591874]

[71]   Wang ZJ, Zhu MY, Liu XJ, Zhang XX, Zhang DY, Wei JM. Cervical intervertebral disc herniation treatment *via* radiofrequency combined with low-dose collagenase injection into the disc interior using an anterior cervical approach. Medicine (Baltimore) 2016; 95(25): e3953.
[http://dx.doi.org/10.1097/MD.0000000000003953] [PMID: 27336892]

[72]   Zeng Z, Yan M, Dai Y, Qiu W, Deng S, Gu X. Percutaneous bipolar radiofrequency thermocoagulation for the treatment of lumbar disc herniation. J Clin Neurosci 2016; 30: 39-43.
[http://dx.doi.org/10.1016/j.jocn.2015.10.050] [PMID: 27234606]

CHAPTER 8

Lumbar MRI– How Useful is It in Surgical Decision Making for Spinal Endoscopy?

Kai-Uwe Lewandrowski[1,2,3], Stefan Hellinger[4], Paulo de Carvalho[5], Max Rogério Freitas Ramos[6,7] and Jorge Felipe Ramírez León[8]

[1] *Center for Advanced Spine Care of Southern Arizona and Surgical Institute of Tucson, Tucson AZ, USA*

[2] *Associate Professor of Orthopaedic Surgery, Universidad Colsanitas, Bogota, Colombia, USA*

[3] *Visiting Professor, Department Orthopaedic Surgery, UNIRIO, Rio de Janeiro, Brazil*

[4] *Department of Orthopedic Surgery, Arabellaklinik,, Munich, Germany*

[5] *Department of Neurosurgery, Universidade Federal do Estado do Rio de Janeiro, Rio de Janeiro, Brazil*

[6] *Associate Professor of Orthopedics and Traumatology, Federal University of the Rio de Janeiro State UNIRIO, Rio de Janeiro - RJ, Brazil*

[7] *Head of Orthopedic Clinics at Gaffrée Guinle University Hospital HUGG, Rio de Janeiro - RJ, Brazil*

[8] *Orthopedic and Minimally Invasive Spine Surgeon; Reina Sofía Clinic and Center of Minimally Invasive Spine Surgery – Bogotá Colombia. Chairman, Spine Surgery Program, Universidad Sanitas, Bogotá, D.C., Colombia, USA*

Abstract: The commonly used preoperative lumbar MRI grading lags behind modern patient selection criteria to prognosticate favorable outcomes with the endoscopic decompression for lumbar herniated disc and foraminal and lateral recess stenosis. Since its utilization has evolved into a primary medical necessity criterion for surgical intervention, surgeons often find themselves with clinical symptoms whose treatment is not supported by the MRI report. Therefore, this chapter's authors established the need to determine the MRI's accuracy and positive predictive value for successful postoperative pain relief after endoscopic transforaminal decompression. Using the transforaminal endoscopic technique, the authors performed a critical retrospective analysis of 1839 patients who had surgery for herniated disc and stenosis in the foramina or lateral spinal canal. They calculated the sensitivity, specificity, accuracy, and positive predictive value of preoperative MRI grading, correctly identifying the

* **Corresponding author Kai-Uwe Lewandrowski:** Center for Advanced Spine Care of Southern Arizona and Surgical Institute of Tucson, Tucson, AZ, USA, Department of Orthopaedic Surgery, UNIRIO, Rio de Janeiro, Brazil and Department of Orthoapedic Surgery, Fundación Universitaria Sanitas, Bogotá, D.C., Colombia, USA; Tel: +1 520 204-1495; Fax: +1 623 218-1215; E-mail: business@tucsonspine.com

symptomatic surgical level by correlating it with the directly visualized pathology during surgery and clinical improvements. The lumbar MRI verbal report's sensitivity was calculated at 68.34%, the specificity at 68.29%, the accuracy at 68.24%, and the positive predictive value at 97.38%. The use of surgical MRI criteria for nerve compression detailed within this manuscript improved the calculated sensitivity to 87.2%, specificity to 73.03%, and accuracy to 86.51%. The likely explanation lies in the lack of consensus between radiologists and spine surgeons when grading compression syndromes of the exiting and traversing nerve root. The grading of a preoperative MRI scan for lumbar foraminal and lateral recess stenosis may significantly differ between radiologists and surgeons. The authors conclude that the endoscopic spine surgeon should read and grade the lumbar MRI scan independently.

Keywords: Lumbar endoscopic transforaminal decompression, Preoperative MRI scan.

INTRODUCTION

Magnetic resonance imaging (MRI) is commonly used to evaluate patients with sciatica-type low back and leg pain [1]. Frequently, MRI suggests multilevel degeneration with disc herniations, facet hypertrophy, and stenosis but should they be interpreted as causes of sciatica-type back and leg pain? What is the predictive value of MRI findings in prompting interventional or surgical care? Unfortunately, the answer is unclear. MRI is integral to the preoperative workup, and its reporting is sometimes the only means insurance companies use to determine the medical necessity of surgical decompression of spinal stenosis. MRI reporting has also become the primary means of communicating the severity of the patient's lumbar degenerative disease among the stakeholders involved in patient care to document the location and extent of lumbar spinal decompression needed to treat the patient's symptoms.

THE PROGNOSTIC VALUE OF THE MRI SCAN

The predictive value of MRI in therapeutic decision-making has been debated [1 - 3]. More than half of the asymptomatic volunteers may have abnormal findings. This number increased between 57% to 80% for those older than 60 years of age [4, 5]. Such MRI abnormalities have been correlated with self-reported pain and appear to have a negligible effect on patient care or outcome [6]. The ultimate gold standard to assess the accuracy of a diagnostic study such as MRI is not another imaging study but direct visualization of pathology during surgery and response to treatment evaluated with clinical outcome studies. Some studies have used surgery as the gold standard to assess lumbar MRI scan accuracy, with some analyses correlating the imaged neural impingement with directly intraoperatively visualized pathology [7 - 13]. Outcome has been employed as another gold standard in assessing lumbar MRI accuracy [14 - 18]. This chapter's focus is simple: What is the predictive value of MRI image-based diagnostic criteria in routine preoperative planning for endoscopic decompression for lumbar spinal stenosis and herniated disc? The authors aimed to analyze the accuracy and positive predictive value (PPV) of a preoperative lumbar MRI grading concerning intraoperatively visualized pathology. They wanted to correlate the visualized pathology with the findings on the preoperative MRI scan, and these MRI findings predicted pain relief with the transforaminal endoscopic lumbar decompression surgery. The accuracy and PPV of MRI reporting in the author's community were calculated and compared to surgeon grading of spinal stenosis using clinical outcome measures and what painful pathology was visualized during the endoscopic surgery.

THE VALUE-BASED SOLUTION

Nowadays, minimally invasive spinal procedures are commonplace [19 - 25]. The volume of these procedures in outpatient surgery centers has disproportionally increased compared to outpatient departments in a hospital setting [26 - 28]. Patients prefer the procedure over open surgery because of much lower complication rates, blood loss, fewer pain killer requirements postoperatively, and faster return to work [29, 30]. The latter problem is significant considering the narcotic epidemic in the United States [31 - 33]. Payors have implemented more front-end scrutiny on the vetting of the medical necessity of spine surgery in general. Some consider endoscopic spine surgery experimental and excluded from coverage as they consider it outside value-based purchasing health care measures. In comparison, some other forms of translaminar minimally invasive spinal surgery have been accepted to serve the aging baby-boomer population [34, 35]. The medical necessity is best explained with a definitive diagnostic workup to make a case for endoscopic spine surgery.

SURGICAL DECISION MAKING

The patients' workup included history, physical examination, plain films, and MRI imaging. Diagnostic transforaminal epidural injections with lidocaine were done preoperatively to validate pain generators amenable to transforaminal endoscopic decompression [36 - 42]. A lidocaine-containing transforaminal diagnostic injection is employed to determine the location of foraminal pain generators. It is confirmed when the patient reports 50% pain relief within 15 minutes of the injection. In conjunction with corroborating findings on the physical examination and the advanced imaging studies, the location of the surgical intervention is most reliably identified [43].

RADIOLOGIC CLASSIFICATIONS

Foraminal and lateral recess stenosis causing traversing nerve root compression was evaluated employing Lee's classification system that focuses on recording the location of the compressive pathology within the neuroforamen by dividing it from medial to lateral into the entry (dura to pedicle; zone 1), middle (medial pedicle wall to center pedicle; zone 2), and exit zone (center pedicle to the lateral border of the facet joint; zone 3) [44]. The offending pathology was stratified as an extruded herniated disc or a disc bulge with or without associated stenosis from osteophytosis or ligament hypertrophy [45]. The location of the disc herniation and its migration wherever applicable was graded according to Lee's four-zone classification. This system classifies a lumbar disc herniation according to its size and direction of migration - upward, downward, or centered around this disc space [46]. Hypertrophy of the facet joint's superior articular process was reported as the predominant pathology in the foraminal exit zone [45]. An osteophyte underneath the pars interarticularis was considered a mid-zone problem. In contrast, subluxation of the inferior articular process often leads to entry-zone stenosis. [45, 19] Hasegawa's numbers obtained from cadaver dissections were used to analyze the foraminal and posterior disc height [47]. fifteen mm was considered the cutoff number below which the neuroforamen was deemed to be stenotic (Fig. **1**).

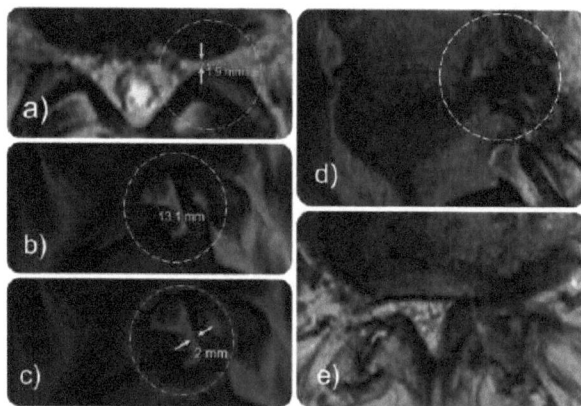

Fig. (1). Several axial MRI cuts at L5/S1 illustrating foraminal stenosis in the foraminal entry and mid zone. The width of the neuroforamen was diminished at 1.9 mm **(a)**. Sagittal imaging **(b-c)** of the symptomatic left side revealed diminished neuroforaminal height of 13.1 mm and **c)** width of 2 mm. According to Lee *et al.* [45] and Hasegawa *et al.* [47] these MRI images were graded by the treating surgeon as MRI Positive. The radiologist's grading was "mild foraminal narrowing" [49] *i.e.*, MRI Negative. Another patient's MRI was grade MRI Positive by both the radiologist and surgeon **(d-e)**. Both patients had excellent outcomes with the endoscopic transforaminal decompression.

The patients' advanced imaging studies were assessed to grade the foraminal stenosis's location and extent. The stenosis criteria were neuroforaminal width of

3 mm or less on sagittal MRI scans, or lateral recess height of 3 mm or less on axial MRI scans. Only one category was chosen at the time, considering the most predominant location of the compressive pathology from lateral to medial consistent with the transforaminal outside-in lateral to medial approach to the neuroforamen.

Table 1. Representative lumbar MRI report of a patient graded as MRI-Negative by the radiologist and MRI Positive by surgeon.

MRI-L TECHNIQUE: Inversion-recovery, T1-, and T2-weighted images of the lumbar spine were obtained in multiple imaging planes without intravenous contrast
FINDINGS: ANATOMY/ALIGNMENT: No significant anterior or posterior subluxation. Slight leftward convexity lower lumbar levels. VERTEBRAE: Degenerative endplate marrow signal changes at L5-S1. Negative for acute compression fractures. VISUALIZED SPINAL CORD/CAUDA EQUINA: Conus terminates at L1. Negative for cord signal abnormality. VISUALIZED LOWER THORACIC DISC LEVELS: Unremarkable. L1-2: No significant canal or foraminal stenosis. L2-3: No significant canal or foraminal stenosis. L3-4: No significant canal or foraminal stenosis. L4-5: No significant central or foraminal stenosis. Facet hypertrophic changes bilaterally. L5-S1: Mild facet hypertrophic changes. Loss of disc space height. Slight disc bulging/ridging. No significant canal stenosis. Mild bilateral foraminal narrowing. OTHER: No abnormal edema in the visualized sacral ala. IMPRESSION: 1. At L5-S1, loss of disc space height with degenerative endplate marrow signal changes. Shallow disc bulging/ridging. Mild bilateral foraminal narrowing. 2. At L4-5, facet hypertrophic changes bilaterally. 3. No significant central canal stenoses.
SURGICAL LEVEL: L5-S1: Mild facet hypertrophic changes. Loss of disc space height. Slight disc bulging/ridging. No significant canal stenosis. Mild bilateral foraminal narrowing.

The Pfirrmann classification was used to analyze the MRI appearance of disc degeneration [48]. The radiologists' MRI reporting of the clinically relevant symptomatic stenotic process was recorded utilizing the grading categories of the Lee classification's exiting nerve root compression [49]. Essentially, Lee's classification assigns increasing grades from 0 to 5 with more severe neuroforaminal stenosis using the perineural fat obliteration in two, three, or all four opposing directions in addition to morphologic changes in the nerve root [49]. For this analysis, patients were classified as MRI stenosis positive if graded by the radiologist with a grade 2 or greater. One representative case of MRI Positive and MRI Negative each are illustrated in Fig. (1). Their respective MRI reports are summarized in Tables 1 and 2.

Table 2. Representative lumbar MRI report of a patient graded as MRI-Positive by both radiologist and surgeon.

MRI-L TECHNIQUE: Inversion-recovery, T1-, and T2-weighted images of the lumbar spine were obtained in multiple imaging planes without intravenous contrast.

FINDINGS:

ANATOMY/ALIGNMENT: Scoliosis convex to left with apex at 3. Left lateral subluxation of L3 on L4. Grade 1 anterolisthesis again noted of L4 on L5.

VERTEBRAE: Degenerative endplate marrow signal changes. Negative for acute compression fractures.

VISUALIZED SPINAL CORD: Conus terminates at L1. Negative for cord signal abnormality.

VISUALIZED LOWER THORACIC DISC LEVELS: Unremarkable.

L1-2: Loss of disc space height. Posterior osseous ridging with mild canal narrowing. Mild bilateral foraminal narrowing.

L2-3: Slight disc bulging. No significant central or foraminal stenosis.

L3-4: Loss of disc space height. Facet hypertrophic changes bilaterally. Mild to moderate canal stenosis. Moderate to severe right foraminal narrowing.

L4-5: Facet hypertrophic changes bilaterally. Anterolisthesis. Left central disc extrusion with cranial extension posterior to L4 again noted. Superior component in the left L4 lateral recess appears smaller. Hypointense regions may reflect calcification. Moderate central canal stenosis. 3 mm cystic focus medial to the left facets on image 29 axially and 9 sagittally likely a synovial cyst. Severe left foraminal stenosis.

L5-S1: Disc bulging. Mild facet hypertrophic changes. No significant central canal stenosis. No significant foraminal narrowing.

OTHER: No abnormal signal in the sacral ala. Probable bilateral peripelvic renal cysts again noted but incompletely characterized.

IMPRESSION:

1. At L1-2, mild canal narrowing.

2. At L3-4, mild to moderate canal stenosis. Moderate to severe right foraminal narrowing.

3. At L4-5, anterolisthesis with left central disc extrusion again noted. Component in the left L4 lateral recess appears slightly smaller but could be due to differences in slice selection. Moderate canal stenosis. Small left synovial cyst. Severe high-grade left foraminal stenosis again noted.

4. Scoliosis.

5. Probable bilateral peripelvic renal cysts but incompletely characterized.

(Table 2) cont.....

> SURGICAL LEVEL: L4-5: Facet hypertrophic changes bilaterally. Anterolisthesis. Left central disc extrusion with cranial extension posterior to L4 again noted. Superior component in the left L4 lateral recess appears smaller. Hypointense regions may reflect calcification. Moderate central canal stenosis. 3 mm cystic focus medial to the left facets on image 29 axially and 9 sagittally likely a synovial cyst. Severe left foraminal stenosis.

SURGICAL TECHNIQUES AND VVISUALIZED PATHOLOGY

The "outside-in" technique was employed during the foraminal endoscopic decompression [50 - 53]. The superior- and inferior articular process was drilled out to accomplish a foraminoplasty to increase both the neuroforaminal height and width. The endoscopic observations of the location and type of the painful offending pathology were recorded either as 1) herniated disc or 2) spinal stenosis due to a ligament or bony overgrowth in relation to its location in the neuroforamen according to Lee [45]. Before initiation of the foraminoplasty, Intraoperatively, the stenosis was graded under direct videoendoscopic visualization by attempting to pass a 2-mm diameter flexible neural probe into the lateral recess [52, 53].

The stenotic lesion location was documented on the MRI by location, *i.e.* the entry-, mid-, or exit zone of the neuroforamen (Fig. **2**). Only one category of stenosis location was assigned both on the preoperative MRI scan and during the intraoperative assessment of the compressive pathology location assessing from lateral to medial. The lateral recess was graded intraoperatively during the endoscopic surgery as stenotic if a 2-mm diameter probe could not be passed into the lateral recess stenosis (Fig. **3**). Hasegawa described this finding to be associated with symptomatic spinal stenosis 80% of the time [47]

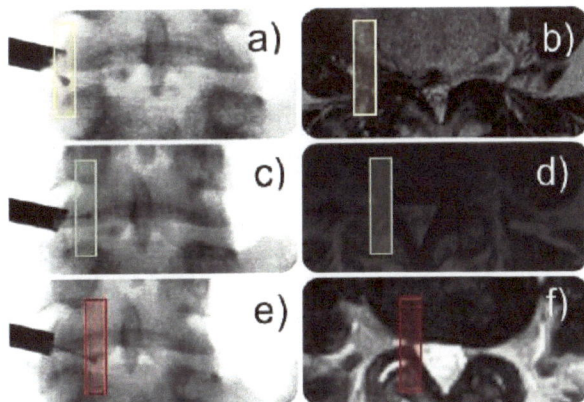

Fig. (2). Intraoperative determination of the location of the foraminal stenosis on AP fluoroscopic views (**a, c, and e**) at the L4/5 level. These findings were compared to preoperative axial lumbar T2-weighted lumbar spine MRI scan. Foraminal entry zone stenosis (**a, b**), foraminal mid zone (**c, d**), and entry zone (**e, f**).

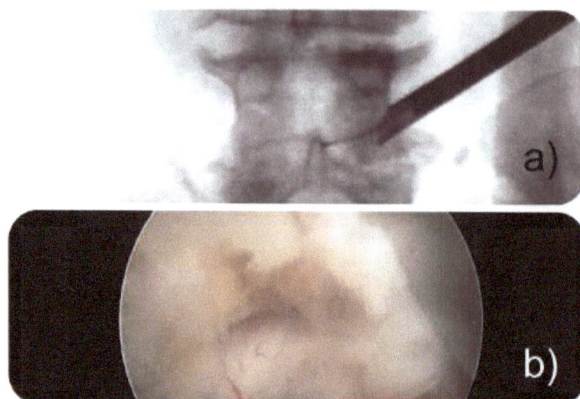

Fig. (3). The completion of the decompression was demonstrated fluoroscopically by being able to pass the probe underneath the dural sac (**a**) and visualized videoendoscopically (**b**).

CORRELATION OF MRI, VISUALIZED PATHOLOGY AND SURGICAL OUTCOMES

Statistical measures of association between preoperative MRI grading, patient functioning, intraoperatively visualized pathology and clinical outcomes were calculated using IBM SPSS Statistics software, Version 25.0. Such correlation matrixes were essentially two-by-two tables to calculate the Pearson χ^2. Differences in pre- and postoperative numerical outcome measures including the VAS score were tested for statisitical significance using the paired T-test. The surgeon grading of the preoperative MRI stenosis zone classification was recorded by converting the categorical zone variable into a numerical variable by assigning the following numbers: entry zone - 1, mid zone - 2, exit zone - 3. The intraclass coefficient (ICC) was calculated using the two-way mixed test option since the subject effect was assumed to be random, but the reader effect was fixed. Besides, the absolute agreement option was used to get an accurate assessment of the agreement of the two scores between MRI and videoendoscopically visualized location of the painful pathology by the surgeon. The single measure ICC option was used to measure reliability since all assessments were by the same rater (surgeon). ICC can test the same rater's reliability by grading the same data set more than once and testing the reliability of the assessment of a data set using two methods. As an additional measure of intraobserver reliability, the agreement between the radiologist's and surgeon MRI grading Cohen's kappa, κ, was calculated. The MRI sensitivity of predicting painful nerve root compression responsive to surgery with excellent, good, and fair Macnab outcomes (true positive rate; TP) was calculated for both gradings by the radiologist and surgeon as the percentage of patients (MRI Positives) whose endoscopic visualization confirmed painful pathology either due to spinal stenosis, or herniated disc. Those patients with intraoperatively visualized neural compression where the MRI grading missed its presence were deemed false negatives (FN). The MRI sensitivity was calculated as follows:

$$\frac{\text{MRI Positives with visualized pathology responsive to decompression (TP)}}{\text{TP + MRI Negatives with visualized pathology responsive to decompression (FN)}}$$

Conversely, the MRI specificity (true negative rate; TN) was calculated as the percentage of patients correctly identified without painful neural compression and without surgical benefit and poor Macnab outcome. False-positive (FP) were MRI Positives without endoscopically visualized pain generators unresponsive to surgery and with the poor clinical outcomes as defined by Macnab criteria. Therefore, the MRI specificity of predicting benefit from the endoscopic decompression procedure was calculated as follows:

$$\frac{\textit{MRI Negatives} \text{ without visualized pathology unresponsive to decompression (TN)}}{\text{TN + } \textit{MRI Positives} \text{ without visualized pathology unresponsive to decompression (FP)}}$$

The MRI diagnostic accuracy (ACC) to prognosticate benefit with endoscopic surgery of the painful pathology was calculated as follows [54, 55]:

$$\text{ACC} = \frac{\text{TP+TN}}{\text{TP+FN+FP+TN}}$$

CLINICAL SERIES

Over ten years between 2006 and 2015, we recruited 1839 patients for this retrospective study, all of whom underwent endoscopic surgery at 2076 levels. The follow-up averaged 33 months, and the patients' age 50.7 ± 18.8 years. Primary clinical outcome tools were the VAS for leg pain and the modified Macnab criteria [44]. Patients were also asked to select a VAS score and rate functioning using the Glasgow Pain Questionnaire [42]. These validated outcome tools were used to determine the accuracy of preoperative lumbar MRI scan reporting by the radiologist with MRI grading by the surgeon of the same scan.

OUTCOMES CORRELATION TO PREOP MRI GRADING

Excellent and good results were reported by 82.2% of patients who underwent transforaminal endoscopic discectomy surgery for an extruded disc fragment (331/1839). These patients reported a significant reduction of the VAS leg score from a mean preoperative value of 5.9 ± 2.5 to 2.4 ± 1.8 at the final follow-up (P < 0.01). More commonly, though, patients carried a preoperative diagnosis of a contained herniated disc (648/1839). Of those, 69.7% reported excellent and good results. Their mean VAS leg score lowered from 7.2 ± 1.6 preoperatively to $3.1 \pm$

1.5 at the final follow-up (P < 0.01). The largest group of study patients suffered from spinal stenosis-related symptoms (860/1839). Seventy-five percent of these patients had excellent to good results, and their mean preoperative VAS score reduced from 6.5 ± 1.8 to 2.3 ± 1.4 at final follow-up (P < 0.001). Nine of the 331 patients with disc extrusions had recurrent disc herniation. Therefore, the recurrence rate was 2.7%. Thirty-nine (4.5%) of the 860 stenosis patients failed to improve. Of the 648 patients with contained disc bulges, 41 (6.3%) also failed to improve.

There were 1196 true positive, 554 false negatives, 30 false positive, and 59 true negative patients. Therefore, the MRI's sensitivity using the radiologist's report was 68.34%, and the specificity was 66.29%. The radiologist's MRI report accuracy of predicting patients' benefit with the endoscopic decompression surgery was determined to be 68.24%. These calculations based on surgeons' grading of the preoperative MRI scan images revealed 1526 true positive, 224 false negative, 24 false positive, and 65 true negative patients. Surgeons' grading of the preoperative MRI improved the calculated sensitivity to 87.2%, specificity to 73.03%, and the MRI accuracy of prognosticating successful clinical outcome of the subsequent endoscopic surgery to 86.51%. The intraclass coefficient (ICC) was 0.514 with a Cronbach's alpha of 0.758. The surgeon MRI grading of the preoperative lumbar MRI scan by zone classification is summarized in Table **3**.

Table 3. Crosstabulation of intraoperatively observed zone location of foraminal stenosis *versus* zone classification on preoperative MRI grading of stenosis by surgeon.

-	-	-	MRI Zone Classification by Surgeon			Total
-	-	-	**Entry Zone**	**Exit Zone**	**Mid Zone**	-
Intraoperatively observed Zone of Foraminal Stenosis	Entry Zone	Count	437	22	89	548
		% within MRI	81.1%	5.3%	10.1%	29.8%
	Exit Zone	Count	18	347	29	394
		% within MRI	3.3%	82.8%	3.3%	21.4%
	Mid Zone	Count	84	50	763	897
		% within MRI	15.6%	11.9%	86.6%	48.8%
Total		Count	539	419	881	1839
		% within MRI	100.0%	100.0%	100.0%	100.0%

Pearson Chi-Square = 2126.437, df = 4, p < .000, Likelihood Ratio =1912.289, df = 4, P < .000, N of Valid Cases = 1839, 0 cells (.0%) have expected count less than 5. The Pearson correlation coefficient = 0.628, p < .000, correlation is significant at the 0.01 level (2-tailed). Intraobserver reliability single measure = 0.514 (absolute agreement definition), p < .000, average measure (computed without interaction effect) = 0.679, p < .000, Cronbach's Alpha = 0.758.

Considering that radiologist reporting is primarily based on exiting nerve root compression [49] compared to surgeon grading of the traversing nerve root compression [45], Kappa agreement analysis showed different degrees of concordance rates for extruded herniated disc ($\kappa = 0.42$; 331/1839 patients), contained disc herniation ($\kappa = -0.01$; 648/1839 patients), and stenosis ($\kappa = 0.25$; 860/1939 patients). The overall measurement of the agreement for the total group of 1839 patients was calculated as $\kappa = 0.216$ and was statistically significant ($p < 0.000$; Tables **4** and **5**).

Table 4. Crosstabulation of preoperative MRI Grading of Stenosis by Radiology reporting *versus* Surgeon by Diagnosis.

Crosstabulation MRI Grading Radiologist Stenois [YES/NO] vs. MRI Grading Surgeon Stenosis [YES/NO] by						
Diagnosis	-	-	-	**MRI Grading Surgeon**		**Total**
-	-	-	-	no	yes	-
Contained Disc	MRI Grading Radiologist	no	Count	28	**178**	206
-	-	-	Expected Count	29.2	**176.8**	206.0
-	-	yes	Count	64	378	442
-	-	-	Expected Count	62.8	379.2	442.0
-	Total	-	Count	92	556	648
-	-	-	Expected Count	92.0	556.0	648.0
Extruded Disc	MRI Grading Radiologist	no	Count	82	**62**	144
-	-	-	Expected Count	48.7	**95.3**	144.0
-	-	yes	Count	30	157	187
-	-	-	Expected Count	63.3	123.7	187.0
-	Total	-	Count	112	219	331
-	-	-	Expected Count	112.0	219.0	331.0
Stenosis	MRI Grading Radiologist	no	Count	63	**200**	263
-	-	-	Expected Count	26.0	**237.0**	263.0
-	-	yes	Count	22	575	597
-	-	-	Expected Count	59.0	538.0	597.0
-	Total	-	Count	85	775	860
-	-	-	Expected Count	85.0	775.0	860.0
Total	MRI Grading Radiologist	no	Count	173	**440**	613

(Table 4) cont.....

Crosstabulation MRI Grading Radiologist Stenois [YES/NO] vs. MRI Grading Surgeon Stenosis [YES/NO] by						
Diagnosis	-	-	-	**MRI Grading Surgeon**		**Total**
-	-	-	Expected Count	96.3	**516.7**	613.0
-	-	yes	Count	116	1110	1226
-	-	-	Expected Count	192.7	1033.3	1226.0
-	Total	-	Count	289	1550	1839
-	-	-	Expected Count	289.0	1550.0	1839.0
Symmetric Measures of Agreement						
Diagnosis	-	-	**Value**	**Asymptotic Standard Error[a]**	**Approximate T[b]**	**Approximate Significance**
Contained Disc	Measure of Agreement	Kappa	-.010	.034	-.301	.763
-	N of Valid Cases	-	648	-	-	-
Extruded Disc	Measure of Agreement	Kappa	.420	.050	7.797	.000
-	N of Valid Cases	-	331	-	-	-
Stenosis	Measure of Agreement	Kappa	.250	.032	9.177	.000
-	N of Valid Cases	-	860	-	-	-
Total	Measure of Agreement	Kappa	.216	.023	10.421	.000
-	N of Valid Cases	-	1839	-	-	-
[a]Not assuming the null hypothesis. [b]Using the asymptotic standard error assuming the null hypothesis.						

The areas of largest disagreement are mentioned in bold.

Table 5. Crosstabulation of preoperative MRI Grading of Stenosis by Radiologist *versus* Surgeon by Foraminal Zone Classification.

Crosstabulation MRI Grading Radiologist Stenosis [YES/NO] vs. MRI Grading Surgeon Stenosis [YES/NO] by Foraminal Zone Classification by Surgeon						
-	-	-	-	**MRI Grading Surgeon**		**Total**
Zone	-	-	-	**no**	**yes**	-
Entry Zone	MRI Grading Radiologist	no	Count	162	**278**	440
-	-	-	Expected Count	159.2	**280.8**	440.0
-	-	yes	Count	33	66	99
-	-	-	Expected Count	35.8	63.2	99.0

(Table 5) cont.....

Crosstabulation MRI Grading Radiologist Stenosis [YES/NO] vs. MRI Grading Surgeon Stenosis [YES/NO] by Foraminal Zone Classification by Surgeon

-	-	-	-	MRI Grading Surgeon		Total
Zone	-	-	-	**no**	**yes**	-
-	Total	-	Count	195	344	539
-	-	-	Expected Count	195.0	344.0	539.0
Exit Zone	MRI Grading Radiologist	no	Count	6	**41**	47
-	-	-	Expected Count	4.3	**42.7**	47.0
-	-	yes	Count	32	340	372
-	-	-	Expected Count	33.7	338.3	372.0
-	Total	-	Count	38	381	419
-	-	-	Expected Count	38.0	381.0	419.0
Mid Zone	MRI Grading Radiologist	no	Count	5	**121**	126
-	-	-	Expected Count	8.0	**118.0**	126.0
-	-	yes	Count	51	704	755
-	-	-	Expected Count	48.0	707.0	755.0
-	Total	-	Count	56	825	881
-	-	-	Expected Count	56.0	825.0	881.0
Total	MRI Grading Radiologist	no	Count	173	**440**	613
-	-	-	Expected Count	96.3	**516.7**	613.0
-	-	yes	Count	116	1110	1226
-	-	-	Expected Count	192.7	1033.3	1226.0
-	Total	-	Count	289	1550	1839
-	-	-	Expected Count	289.0	1550.0	1839.0

Symmetric Measures of Disagreement

Foraminal Zone	-	-	Value	Asymptotic Standard Error[a]	Approximate T[b]	Approximate Significance
Entry Zone	**Measure of Agreement**	**Kappa**	**.018**	**.027**	**.652**	**.514**
-	N of Valid Cases	-	539	-	-	-
Exit Zone	Measure of Agreement	Kappa	.045	.055	.937	.349
-	N of Valid Cases	-	419	-	-	-

(Table 5) cont.....

Symmetric Measures of Disagreement						
Foraminal Zone	-	-	Value	Asymptotic Standard Error[a]	Approximate T[b]	Approximate Significance
Entry Zone	**Measure of Agreement**	**Kappa**	**.018**	**.027**	**.652**	**.514**
Mid Zone	Measure of Agreement	Kappa	-.036	.025	-1.187	.235
-	N of Valid Cases	-	881	-	-	-
Total	Measure of Agreement	Kappa	.216	.023	10.421	.000
-	N of Valid Cases	-	1839	-	-	-
[a]Not assuming the null hypothesis. [b]Using the asymptotic standard error assuming the null hypothesis.						

The areas of largest disagreement are mentioned in bold.

DISCUSSION

This study shows that a preoperative lumbar MRI scan has a high predictive diagnostic value regardless of whether a radiologist or the treating surgeon reads it. It is integral to a conclusive preoperative workup of spinal stenosis patients to arrive at a sound surgical plan to treat their sciatic-type low back and leg pain symptoms with a lumbar endoscopic transforaminal decompression. Since the endoscopic decompression is typically carried out in a tiny area of a degenerative spine that often displays multilevel involvement, the surgeon has to rely on accurate preoperative prognosticators for the lumbar endoscopic decompression procedures to relieve pain effectively. The lumbar MRI scan is an essential tool to identify potential pain generators. Unfortunately, it suffers from low accuracy and positive predictive value of clinical success with surgical decompression. Examples of poor MRI include assessing spinal stenosis [56], integrity of the posterior longitudinal ligament [57], and facet joint complex [58]. Its poor predictive value of low back pain has been demonstrated in asymptomatic volunteers [59]. It is also an inadequate predictor of the duration of low back pain [60]. While endoscopic lumbar surgery is widely popular with patients because of less exposure-related pain and dramatically reduces the surgery's overall burden to the patient by performing it in an outpatient setting where recovery and return to work are faster than with traditional inpatient lumbar decompressions done under general anesthesia, the simplified endoscopic decompression procedure relies on a highly accurate preoperative diagnostic workup to identify the pain generator responsible for the patient's symptoms.

This study on 1839 patients carried out over nearly ten years demonstrates a small, targeted endoscopic transforaminal foraminoplasty and discectomy procedure. The overall readmission rate of 0.87% over the nine-year study period observed was low [61] compared to readmission rates reported with traditional microdiscectomy (4.1% to 5.8%) [24]. Our observed clinical success rates were comparable to success rates reported by patients undergoing laminectomy for spinal stenosis [61 - 67]. There were stark differences in the surgeon and radiologist grading of MRI Positives with a lower sensitivity (68.34%) and specificity (66.29%) of the MRI report compared to the surgeon image-read sensitivity of 87.2% and a specificity of 73.03%. This lower accuracy with routine radiologist reporting of lumbar MRI scan may create over-, but more likely, under-treatment of symptomatic patients. The additional 330 patients negatively graded (FN) by the radiology report would have never received their endoscopic surgery had their surgeons not read and graded their MRI images themselves. Clinical outcome analysis showed that these 330 patients benefited from the endoscopic transforaminal decompression.

Employing a foraminal zone classification system to treat traversing nerve root compression pain syndromes improved the value of the statistical MRI prognosticators of a successful clinical outcome. Sensitivity (87.2%) and specificity (73.03%) were higher when the treating surgeon read the actual MRI images and graded the stenotic process both by location and severity while attempting to arrive at a surgical strategy to reduce the patient's traversing nerve root compression pain syndrome and improve function. When the preoperative lumbar MRI scan is graded by the surgeon its clinical utility and accuracy in predicting successful postoperative improvement of patients' clinical functioning is improved from 68.24% (radiology report) to 86.5% using the clinical result as the gold standard.

A large number of FN patients were incorrectly graded as MRI Negative at different rates by the radiologist (554/1839 patients) and surgeon (224/1839 patients). The difference in FN patients between grading based on the radiology report and grading by the treating surgeon was 330 patients (Tables 2 and 3). These 330 patients underwent successful endoscopic transforaminal decompression to resolve their sciatica-type low back and leg pain despite the lumbar MRI report (radiology) being graded as not providing evidence of foraminal stenosis. This large difference in FN patients between the radiology report and surgeon grading of the lumbar MRI is likely explained by the use of different clinical grading protocols employed when reading the same scan. The neuroforaminal stenosis classification used in the author's area was published by Lee *et al.* [49] is purely based on the description of the compressive pathology of the exiting nerve root rather than the traversing nerve root. However, traversing nerve root compression pain syndromes are more common than those stemming from the exiting nerve root [19 - 22].

Reporting seemingly minor details of the foraminal anatomy and using them when communicating the need for surgical decompression is crucially essential for the transforaminal spinal endoscopy considering the small surgical decompression area and the small amount of bone and soft tissue removed during the foraminoplasty and discectomy. Many musculoskeletal radiologists may be unaware of this newer minimally invasive endoscopic transforaminal lumbar decompression technique and may be accustomed to describing the spinal anatomy on MRI imaging in much broader terms lumbar level concerning central and foraminal stenosis ranging from mild, to moderate, to severe [49]. Although this seems appropriate and sufficient for planning more aggressive, open lumbar laminectomy and fusion surgeries, more detail of the foraminal anatomy is required to select symptomatic patients for the endoscopic transforaminal surgery adequately. Otherwise, lack of detail could leave too many patients falsely classi-fied as MRI Negative (FN) and may result in non-coverage of endoscopic treatment.

The authors' retrospective study may have suffered from cognitive-, outcome-, or hindsight biases in the clinical diagnostic and surgical decision-making process [68, 69], which are virtually unavoidable in retrospective review as knowledge of the clinical outcome has been recognized to inflate the predictability of an event after it happened [70 - 73]. Nevertheless, the findings of the authors' study highlight the need for better utilization of the lumbar MRI scan during patient selection for lumbar endoscopic surgery. When the care is delivered, the context of lumbar spine care is critical to identifying pain generators with diagnostic injections in conjunction with the history and physical examination and careful analysis of the advanced imaging studies. The authors expect that additional research and application of artificial intelligence application – as demonstrated in one chapter of this Bentham book series – will likely produce further insight into the most efficient and appropriate use of the preoperative lumbar MRI scan to improve its positive predictive value with intervention in patients with refractory symptomatic lumbar herniated disc and spinal stenosis.

CONCLUSION

Radiologists and surgeons may grade the preoperative MRI scan for lumbar foraminal and lateral recess stenosis differently. Surgical translational research on the intraoperatively visualized spinal pathology should analyze the effectiveness of endoscopic surgery interventions in the lumbar spine using advanced MRI criteria of central, lateral recess, and neural foraminal stenosis to determine how they impact the prognosis of surgical treatment for neurogenic claudication and lumbar radiculopathy. This research may aid in the identification of more reliable predictors of favorable clinical outcomes.

CONSENT FOR PUBLICATION

Not applicable.

CONFLICT OF INTEREST

The authors declare no conflict of interest, financial or otherwise.

ACKNOWLEDGEMENT

Declared none.

REFERENCES

[1]   Boos N, Rieder R, Schade V, Spratt KF, Semmer N, Aebi M. 1995 Volvo Award in clinical sciences. The diagnostic accuracy of magnetic resonance imaging, work perception, and psychosocial factors in identifying symptomatic disc herniations. Spine 1995; 20(24): 2613-25.
      [http://dx.doi.org/10.1097/00007632-199512150-00002] [PMID: 8747239]

[2]   Buirski G, Silberstein M. The symptomatic lumbar disc in patients with low-back pain. Magnetic resonance imaging appearances in both a symptomatic and control population. Spine 1993; 18(13): 1808-11.
      [http://dx.doi.org/10.1097/00007632-199310000-00016] [PMID: 8235866]

[3]   Modic MT, Ross JS. Lumbar degenerative disk disease. Radiology 2007; 245(1): 43-61.
      [http://dx.doi.org/10.1148/radiol.2451051706] [PMID: 17885180]

[4]   Jensen MC, Brant-Zawadzki MN, Obuchowski N, Modic MT, Malkasian D, Ross JS. Magnetic resonance imaging of the lumbar spine in people without back pain. N Engl J Med 1994; 331(2): 69-73.
      [http://dx.doi.org/10.1056/NEJM199407143310201] [PMID: 8208267]

[5]   Boden SD, Davis DO, Dina TS, Patronas NJ, Wiesel SW. Abnormal magnetic-resonance scans of the lumbar spine in asymptomatic subjects. A prospective investigation. J Bone Joint Surg Am 1990; 72(3): 403-8.
      [http://dx.doi.org/10.2106/00004623-199072030-00013] [PMID: 2312537]

[6]   Beattie PF, Meyers SP, Stratford P, Millard RW, Hollenberg GM. Associations between patient report of symptoms and anatomic impairment visible on lumbar magnetic resonance imaging. Spine 2000; 25(7): 819-28.
      [http://dx.doi.org/10.1097/00007632-200004010-00010] [PMID: 10751293]

[7]   Dutta S, Bhave A, Patil S. Correlation of 1.5 Tesla Magnetic Resonance Imaging with Clinical and Intraoperative Findings for Lumbar Disc Herniation. Asian Spine J 2016; 10(6): 1115-21.
      [http://dx.doi.org/10.4184/asj.2016.10.6.1115] [PMID: 27994789]

[8]   Kulkarni AG, Patel R, Dutta S, Patil V. Stand-alone Lateral Recess Decompression Without Discectomy in Patients Presenting With Claudicant Radicular Pain and MRI Evidence of Lumbar Disc Herniation: A Prospective Study. Spine 2017; 42(13): 984-91.
      [http://dx.doi.org/10.1097/BRS.0000000000001944] [PMID: 27792115]

[9]   Crosby CG, Even JL, Song Y, Block JJ, Devin CJ. Diagnostic abilities of magnetic resonance imaging in traumatic injury to the posterior ligamentous complex: the effect of years in training. Spine J 2011;

11(8): 747-53.
[http://dx.doi.org/10.1016/j.spinee.2011.07.005] [PMID: 21840264]

[10]   Jia LS, Shi ZR. MRI and myelography in the diagnosis of lumbar canal stenosis and disc herniation. A comparative study. Chin Med J (Engl) 1991; 104(4): 303-6.
[PMID: 2065548]

[11]   Lurie JD, Moses RA, Tosteson AN, *et al.* Magnetic resonance imaging predictors of surgical outcome in patients with lumbar intervertebral disc herniation. Spine 2013; 38(14): 1216-25.
[http://dx.doi.org/10.1097/BRS.0b013e31828ce66d] [PMID: 23429684]

[12]   Mannion AF, Fekete TF, Pacifico D, *et al.* Dural sac cross-sectional area and morphological grade show significant associations with patient-rated outcome of surgery for lumbar central spinal stenosis. Eur Spine J 2017; 26(10): 2552-64.
[http://dx.doi.org/10.1007/s00586-017-5280-7] [PMID: 28856447]

[13]   Watanabe K, Yamazaki A, Morita O, Sano A, Katsumi K, Ohashi M. Clinical outcomes of posterior lumbar interbody fusion for lumbar foraminal stenosis: preoperative diagnosis and surgical strategy. J Spinal Disord Tech 2011; 24(3): 137-41.
[http://dx.doi.org/10.1097/BSD.0b013e3181e1cd99] [PMID: 20634730]

[14]   Diagnosis   and   Treatment   of   Lumbar   Disc   Herniation   with   Radiculopathy 2012.https://www.spine.org/Documents/ResearchClinicalCare/Guidelines/ LumbarDiscHerniation.pdf

[15]   Diagnosis   and   Treatment   of   Degenerative   Lumbar   Spinal   Stenosis 2011.https://www.spine.org/Documents/ResearchClinicalCare/ Guidelines/ LumbarStenosis.pdf

[16]   Kent DL, Haynor DR, Larson EB, Deyo RA. Diagnosis of lumbar spinal stenosis in adults: a metaanalysis of the accuracy of CT, MR, and myelography. AJR Am J Roentgenol 1992; 158(5): 1135-44.
[http://dx.doi.org/10.2214/ajr.158.5.1533084] [PMID: 1533084]

[17]   Bischoff RJ, Rodriguez RP, Gupta K, Righi A, Dalton JE, Whitecloud TS. A comparison of computed tomography-myelography, magnetic resonance imaging, and myelography in the diagnosis of herniated nucleus pulposus and spinal stenosis. J Spinal Disord 1993; 6(4): 289-95.
[http://dx.doi.org/10.1097/00002517-199306040-00002] [PMID: 8219542]

[18]   Modic MT, Masaryk T, Boumphrey F, Goormastic M, Bell G. Lumbar herniated disk disease and canal stenosis: prospective evaluation by surface coil MR, CT, and myelography. AJR Am J Roentgenol 1986; 147(4): 757-65.
[http://dx.doi.org/10.2214/ajr.147.4.757] [PMID: 3489378]

[19]   Lewandrowski KU. "Outside-in" technique, clinical results, and indications with transforaminal lumbar endoscopic surgery: a retrospective study on 220 patients on applied radiographic classification of foraminal spinal stenosis. Int J Spine Surg 2014; 8: 8.
[http://dx.doi.org/10.14444/1026] [PMID: 25694915]

[20]   Yeung AT, Yeung CA. Minimally invasive techniques for the management of lumbar disc herniation. Orthop Clin North Am 2007; 38(3): 363-72.
[http://dx.doi.org/10.1016/j.ocl.2007.04.005] [PMID: 17629984]

[21]   Tsou PM, Alan Yeung C, Yeung AT. Posterolateral transforaminal selective endoscopic discectomy and thermal annuloplasty for chronic lumbar discogenic pain: a minimal access visualized intradiscal surgical procedure. Spine J 2004; 4(5): 564-73.
[http://dx.doi.org/10.1016/j.spinee.2004.01.014] [PMID: 15363430]

[22]   Tsou PM, Yeung AT. Transforaminal endoscopic decompression for radiculopathy secondary to intracanal noncontained lumbar disc herniations: outcome and technique. Spine J 2002; 2(1): 41-8.
[http://dx.doi.org/10.1016/S1529-9430(01)00153-X] [PMID: 14588287]

[23]   Clark AJ, Safaee MM, Khan NR, Brown MT, Foley KT. Tubular microdiscectomy: techniques, complication avoidance, and review of the literature. Neurosurg Focus 2017; 43(2): E7.

[http://dx.doi.org/10.3171/2017.5.FOCUS17202] [PMID: 28760036]

[24] Overdevest GM, Peul WC, Brand R, *et al.* Tubular discectomy *versus* conventional microdiscectomy for the treatment of lumbar disc herniation: long-term results of a randomised controlled trial. J Neurol Neurosurg Psychiatry 2017; 88(12): 1008-16.
[http://dx.doi.org/10.1136/jnnp-2016-315306] [PMID: 28550071]

[25] Soriano-Sánchez JA, Quillo-Olvera J, Soriano-Solis S, *et al.* Microscopy-assisted interspinous tubular approach for lumbar spinal stenosis. J Spine Surg 2017; 3(1): 64-70.
[http://dx.doi.org/10.21037/jss.2017.02.07] [PMID: 28435920]

[26] Yeung AT, Yeung CA. Advances in endoscopic disc and spine surgery: foraminal approach. Surg Technol Int 2003; 11: 255-63.
[PMID: 12931309]

[27] Debono B, Sabatier P, Garnault V, *et al.* Outpatient Lumbar Microdiscectomy in France: From an Economic Imperative to a Clinical Standard-An Observational Study of 201 Cases. World Neurosurg 2017; 106: 891-7.
[http://dx.doi.org/10.1016/j.wneu.2017.07.065] [PMID: 28735120]

[28] Hersht M, Massicotte EM, Bernstein M. Patient satisfaction with outpatient lumbar microsurgical discectomy: a qualitative study. Can J Surg 2007; 50(6): 445-9.
[PMID: 18053372]

[29] Zolot J. A Worsening Opioid Epidemic Prompts Action. Am J Nurs 2017; 117(10): 15.
[http://dx.doi.org/10.1097/01.NAJ.0000525858.52569.e6] [PMID: 28957912]

[30] Cheatle MD. Facing the challenge of pain management and opioid misuse, abuse and opioid-related fatalities. Expert Rev Clin Pharmacol 2016; 9(6): 751-4.
[http://dx.doi.org/10.1586/17512433.2016.1160776] [PMID: 26933873]

[31] Hupp JR. The Surgeon's Roles in Stemming the Prescription Opioid Abuse Epidemic. J Oral Maxillofac Surg 2016; 74(7): 1291-3.
[http://dx.doi.org/10.1016/j.joms.2016.05.001] [PMID: 27156949]

[32] Kee JR, Smith RG, Barnes CL. Recognizing and Reducing the Risk of Opioid Misuse in Orthopaedic Practice. J Surg Orthop Adv 2016; 25(4): 238-43.
[PMID: 28244866]

[33] Devin CJ, Chotai S, Parker SL, Tetreault L, Fehlings MG, McGirt MJ. A Cost-Utility Analysis of Lumbar Decompression With and Without Fusion for Degenerative Spine Disease in the Elderly. Neurosurgery 2015; 77 (Suppl. 4): S116-24.
[http://dx.doi.org/10.1227/NEU.0000000000000949] [PMID: 26378349]

[34] Adogwa O, Parker SL, Shau DN, *et al.* Cost per quality-adjusted life year gained of revision neural decompression and instrumented fusion for same-level recurrent lumbar stenosis: defining the value of surgical intervention. J Neurosurg Spine 2012; 16(2): 135-40.
[http://dx.doi.org/10.3171/2011.9.SPINE11308] [PMID: 22054639]

[35] O'Lynnger TM, Zuckerman SL, Morone PJ, Dewan MC, Vasquez-Castellanos RA, Cheng JS. Trends for Spine Surgery for the Elderly: Implications for Access to Healthcare in North America. Neurosurgery 2015; 77 (Suppl. 4): S136-41.
[http://dx.doi.org/10.1227/NEU.0000000000000945] [PMID: 26378351]

[36] Sengupta DK, Herkowitz HN. Lumbar spinal stenosis. Treatment strategies and indications for surgery. Orthop Clin North Am 2003; 34(2): 281-95.
[http://dx.doi.org/10.1016/S0030-5898(02)00069-X] [PMID: 12914268]

[37] Botwin KP, Gruber RD, Bouchlas CG, *et al.* Fluoroscopically guided lumbar transformational epidural steroid injections in degenerative lumbar stenosis: an outcome study. Am J Phys Med Rehabil 2002; 81(12): 898-905.
[http://dx.doi.org/10.1097/00002060-200212000-00003] [PMID: 12447088]

[38]   el-Khoury GY, Ehara S, Weinstein JN, Montgomery WJ, Kathol MH. Epidural steroid injection: a procedure ideally performed with fluoroscopic control. Radiology 1988; 168(2): 554-7.
[http://dx.doi.org/10.1148/radiology.168.2.2969118] [PMID: 2969118]

[39]   Bogduk N, Aprill C, Derby R. Epidural spinal injections.Spinal Care: Diagnosis and Treatment. Mosby 1995; pp. 322-43. https://www.abebooks.com/9780801663284/Spine-Care-Diagnoss-Treatment-Arthur-0801663288/plp

[40]   Huskisson EC, Jones J, Scott PJ. Application of visual-analogue scales to the measurement of functional capacity. Rheumatol Rehabil 1976; 15(3): 185-7.
[http://dx.doi.org/10.1093/rheumatology/15.3.185] [PMID: 968347]

[41]   Pfirrmann CW, Oberholzer PA, Zanetti M, *et al.* Selective nerve root blocks for the treatment of sciatica: evaluation of injection site and effectiveness--a study with patients and cadavers. Radiology 2001; 221(3): 704-11.
[http://dx.doi.org/10.1148/radiol.2213001635] [PMID: 11719666]

[42]   Thomas RJ, McEwen J, Asbury AJ. The Glasgow Pain Questionnaire: a new generic measure of pain; development and testing. Int J Epidemiol 1996; 25(5): 1060-7.
[http://dx.doi.org/10.1093/ije/25.5.1060] [PMID: 8921495]

[43]   Lee IS, Kim SH, Lee JW, *et al.* Comparison of the temporary diagnostic relief of transforaminal epidural steroid injection approaches: conventional *versus* posterolateral technique. AJNR Am J Neuroradiol 2007; 28(2): 204-8.
[PMID: 17296980]

[44]   Macnab I. Negative disc exploration. An analysis of the causes of nerve-root involvement in sixty-eight patients. J Bone Joint Surg Am 1971; 53(5): 891-903.
[http://dx.doi.org/10.2106/00004623-197153050-00004] [PMID: 4326746]

[45]   Lee CK, Rauschning W, Glenn W. Lateral lumbar spinal canal stenosis: classification, pathologic anatomy and surgical decompression. Spine 1988; 13(3): 313-20.
[http://dx.doi.org/10.1097/00007632-198803000-00015] [PMID: 3388117]

[46]   Lee S, Kim SK, Lee SH, *et al.* Percutaneous endoscopic lumbar discectomy for migrated disc herniation: classification of disc migration and surgical approaches. Eur Spine J 2007; 16(3): 431-7.
[http://dx.doi.org/10.1007/s00586-006-0219-4] [PMID: 16972067]

[47]   Hasegawa T, An HS, Haughton VM, Nowicki BH. Lumbar foraminal stenosis: critical heights of the intervertebral discs and foramina. A cryomicrotome study in cadavera. J Bone Joint Surg Am 1995; 77(1): 32-8.
[http://dx.doi.org/10.2106/00004623-199501000-00005] [PMID: 7822353]

[48]   Pfirrmann CW, Metzdorf A, Zanetti M, Hodler J, Boos N. Magnetic resonance classification of lumbar intervertebral disc degeneration. Spine 2001; 26(17): 1873-8.
[http://dx.doi.org/10.1097/00007632-200109010-00011] [PMID: 11568697]

[49]   Lee S, Lee JW, Yeom JS, *et al.* A practical MRI grading system for lumbar foraminal stenosis. AJR Am J Roentgenol 2010; 194(4): 1095-8.
[http://dx.doi.org/10.2214/AJR.09.2772] [PMID: 20308517]

[50]   Hoogland T, Schubert M, Miklitz B, Ramirez A. Transforaminal posterolateral endoscopic discectomy with or without the combination of a low-dose chymopapain: a prospective randomized study in 280 consecutive cases. Spine 2006; 31(24): E890-7.
[http://dx.doi.org/10.1097/01.brs.0000245955.22358.3a] [PMID: 17108817]

[51]   Schubert M, Hoogland T. Endoscopic transforaminal nucleotomy with foraminoplasty for lumbar disk herniation. Oper Orthop Traumatol 2005; 17(6): 641-61.
[http://dx.doi.org/10.1007/s00064-005-1156-9] [PMID: 16369758]

[52]   Kambin P, Casey K, O'Brien E, Zhou L. Transforaminal arthroscopic decompression of lateral recess stenosis. J Neurosurg 1996; 84(3): 462-7.

[http://dx.doi.org/10.3171/jns.1996.84.3.0462] [PMID: 8609559]

[53]   Kambin P, O'Brien E, Zhou L, Schaffer JL. Arthroscopic microdiscectomy and selective fragmentectomy. Clin Orthop Relat Res 1998; (347): 150-67.
[PMID: 9520885]

[54]   Altman DG, Machin D, Bryant TN, Gardner MJ. Statistics with Confidence: Confidence Intervals and Statistical Guidelines. BMJ Books 2nd edition., 2000. https://www.wiley.com/en-us/Statistics+with+Confidence%3A+

[55]   Mercaldo ND, Lau KF, Zhou XH. Confidence intervals for predictive values with an emphasis to case-control studies. Stat Med 2007; 26(10): 2170-83.
[http://dx.doi.org/10.1002/sim.2677] [PMID: 16927452]

[56]   Sigmundsson FG, Kang XP, Jönsson B, Strömqvist B. Correlation between disability and MRI findings in lumbar spinal stenosis: a prospective study of 109 patients operated on by decompression. Acta Orthop 2011; 82(2): 204-10.
[http://dx.doi.org/10.3109/17453674.2011.566150] [PMID: 21434811]

[57]   Vaccaro AR, Rihn JA, Saravanja D, *et al.* Injury of the posterior ligamentous complex of the thoracolumbar spine: a prospective evaluation of the diagnostic accuracy of magnetic resonance imaging. Spine 2009; 34(23): E841-7.
[http://dx.doi.org/10.1097/BRS.0b013e3181bd11be] [PMID: 19927090]

[58]   Lee JC, Cha JG, Yoo JH, Kim HK, Kim HJ, Shin BJ. Radiographic grading of facet degeneration, is it reliable? - a comparison of MR or CT grading with histologic grading in lumbar fusion candidates. Spine J 2012; 12(6): 507-14.
[http://dx.doi.org/10.1016/j.spinee.2012.06.003] [PMID: 22770987]

[59]   Boden SD, Davis DO, Dina TS, Patronas NJ, Wiesel SW. Abnormal magnetic-resonance scans of the lumbar spine in asymptomatic subjects. A prospective investigation. J Bone Joint Surg Am 1990; 72(3): 403-8.
[http://dx.doi.org/10.2106/00004623-199072030-00013] [PMID: 2312537]

[60]   Borenstein DG, O'Mara JW Jr, Boden SD, *et al.* The value of magnetic resonance imaging of the lumbar spine to predict low-back pain in asymptomatic subjects : a seven-year follow-up study. J Bone Joint Surg Am 2001; 83(9): 1306-11.
[http://dx.doi.org/10.2106/00004623-200109000-00002] [PMID: 11568190]

[61]   Lewandrowski KU. Readmissions After Outpatient Transforaminal Decompression for Lumbar Foraminal and Lateral Recess Stenosis. Int J Spine Surg 2018; 12(3): 342-51.
[http://dx.doi.org/10.14444/5040] [PMID: 30276091]

[62]   Lewandrowski KU. Successful outcome after outpatient transforaminal decompression for lumbar foraminal and lateral recess stenosis: The positive predictive value of diagnostic epidural steroid injection. Clin Neurol Neurosurg 2018; 173: 38-45.
[http://dx.doi.org/10.1016/j.clineuro.2018.07.015] [PMID: 30075346]

[63]   Fokter SK, Yerby SA. Patient-based outcomes for the operative treatment of degenerative lumbar spinal stenosis. Eur Spine J 2006; 15(11): 1661-9.
[http://dx.doi.org/10.1007/s00586-005-0033-4] [PMID: 16369827]

[64]   Friedly JL, Comstock BA, Turner JA, *et al.* A randomized trial of epidural glucocorticoid injections for spinal stenosis. N Engl J Med 2014; 371(1): 11-21.
[http://dx.doi.org/10.1056/NEJMoa1313265] [PMID: 24988555]

[65]   Asch HL, Lewis PJ, Moreland DB, *et al.* Prospective multiple outcomes study of outpatient lumbar microdiscectomy: should 75 to 80% success rates be the norm? J Neurosurg 2002; 96(1) (Suppl.): 34-44.
[PMID: 11795712]

[66]   Kim MJ, Lee SH, Jung ES, *et al.* Targeted percutaneous transforaminal endoscopic diskectomy in 295

patients: comparison with results of microscopic diskectomy. Surg Neurol 2007; 68(6): 623-31.
[http://dx.doi.org/10.1016/j.surneu.2006.12.051] [PMID: 18053857]

[67]   Ahn Y, Lee SH, Park WM, Lee HY, Shin SW, Kang HY. Percutaneous endoscopic lumbar discectomy for recurrent disc herniation: surgical technique, outcome, and prognostic factors of 43 consecutive cases. Spine 2004; 29(16): E326-32.
[http://dx.doi.org/10.1097/01.BRS.0000134591.32462.98] [PMID: 15303041]

[68]   Bakeman R, Quera V, McArthur D, Robinson BF. Detecting sequential patterns and determining their reliability with fallible observers. Psychol Methods 1997; 2(4): 357-70.
[http://dx.doi.org/10.1037/1082-989X.2.4.357]

[69]   Sibbald M, Cavalcanti RB. The biasing effect of clinical history on physical examination diagnostic accuracy. Med Educ 2011; 45(8): 827-34.
[http://dx.doi.org/10.1111/j.1365-2923.2011.03997.x] [PMID: 21752079]

[70]   Zwaan L, Monteiro S, Sherbino J, Ilgen J, Howey B, Norman G. Is bias in the eye of the beholder? A vignette study to assess recognition of cognitive biases in clinical case workups. BMJ Qual Saf 2017; 26(2): 104-10.
[http://dx.doi.org/10.1136/bmjqs-2015-005014] [PMID: 26825476]

[71]   Henriksen K, Kaplan H. Hindsight bias, outcome knowledge and adaptive learning 2003.
[http://dx.doi.org/10.1136/qhc.12.suppl_2.ii46]

[72]   Hugh TB, Tracy GD. Hindsight bias in medicolegal expert reports. Med J Aust 2002; 176(6): 277-8.
[http://dx.doi.org/10.5694/j.1326-5377.2002.tb04407.x] [PMID: 11999261]

[73]   Wübken M, Oswald J, Schneider A. Dealing with diagnostic uncertainty in general practice. Z Evid Fortbild Qual Gesundhwes 2013; 107(9-10): 632-7.
[PMID: 24315334]

CHAPTER 9

Cost and Maintenance Management of Endoscopic Spine Systems

Friedrich Tieber[1], **Stefan Hellinger**[2] and **Kai-Uwe Lewandrowski**[3,4,5,*]

[1] *Medical Technologies Consulting, Augsburg, Germany*

[2] *Department of Orthopedic Surgery, Arabellaklinik, Munich, Germany*

[3] *Center for Advanced Spine Care of Southern Arizona and Surgical Institute of Tucson, 4787 E. Camp Lowell Drive, Tucson AZ 85712, USA*

[4] *Associate Professor, Universidad Sanitas, Bogotá, D.C., Colombia, USA*

[5] *Visiting Professor Department Neurosurgery, UNIRIO, Rio de Janeiro, Brazil*

Abstract: Successful implementation of endoscopic spinal surgery programs hinges on reliable performance and case cost similar to traditional decompression surgeries of the lumbar spine. Spinal endoscopes used during routine lumbar decompression surgeries for herniated disc and spinal stenosis should have an estimated life cycle between 150 to 300 surgeries. However, actual numbers may be substantially lower. Abusive use by surgeons, mishandling by staff, and deviation from prescribed cleaning and sterilization protocols may substantially shorten the life cycle. Contingency protocols should be in place to readily replace a broken spinal endoscope during surgery. More comprehensive implementation of endoscopic spine surgery techniques will hinge on technology advancements to make these high-tech surgical instruments more resistant to the stress of daily use and abuse of expanded clinical indications' surgery. The regulatory burden on endoscope makers is likely to increase, calling for increased reimbursement for facilities to cover the added expense for capital equipment purchase, disposables, and the cost of the endoscopic spine surgery program's maintenance. In this chapter, the authors review such maintenance programs' cornerstones in the current regulatory environment that one should implement when attempting to run an endoscopic spinal surgery program at their healthcare facility.

Keywords: Equipment Durability, Cost, Maintenance, Regulatory, Spinal endoscopy.

* **Corresponding author Kai-Uwe Lewandrowski:** Center for Advanced Spine Care of Southern Arizona and Surgical Institute of Tucson, Tucson, AZ, USA, Department of Orthopaedic Surgery, UNIRIO, Rio de Janeiro, Brazil and Department of Orthoapedic Surgery, Fundación Universitaria Sanitas, Bogotá, D.C., Colombia, USA; Tel: +1 520 204-1495; Fax: +1 623 218-1215; E-mail: business@tucsonspine.com

INTRODUCTION

A successfully run endoscopic spinal surgery program depends on reliably performing equipment that can hold up to the abuse of a high-volume clinical program.

Moreover, well-trained and trustworthy staff with dependable knowledge of the cleaning and sterile processing procedures is another crucial element in keeping the cost of maintenance and repairs under control. Everyone partaking in the day-to-day routine of such an endoscopic spine surgery program should understand how this highly sensitive and expensive optical and surgical equipment is custom-built, not easily replaceable, and represents an asset of the healthcare facility whose management requires good stewardship. Team members should employ careful handling of these delicate optical instruments through well-established and uninterrupted custody chains, extending to the end-user surgeons. Practitioners may not always understand the limits of a rigid rod-lens system design of modern spinal endoscopes and their performance limits as they attempt to expand clinical indications of the procedure by trying more complex spinal decompression [1] and increasingly fusion [2 - 7] operations.

High-quality spinal endoscopes are the cornerstone of a well-run spinal endoscopy program. The Instruction For Use (IFU) for modern endoscopes made by various vendors frequently lists a range of 150 to 300 cycles that the end-user should be able to expect before repair or replacement is necessary when employing the recommended intraoperative applications, cleaning- and sterilization procedures. Actual performance cycles may be substantially lower since manufacturers cannot predict actual use patterns by the end-user. Acceptance of surgeons who try to implement endoscopic spinal surgery programs at their respective healthcare facilities may be delayed because of the high implementation cost for capital purchases. It could be further negatively impacted when higher case numbers expose the technology's shortcomings due to added cost for disposables and repairs. Administrators of hospitals and surgery centers are facing lower reimbursement for the standard spinal decompression and fusion codes. Therefore, the higher upfront cost to jumpstart a program that replaces these traditional surgeries with lower or unpredictable payment schedules may pose an insurmountable hurdle that could be hard to overcome.

The affordability of the endoscopic technology for spine surgery is a highly complex problem that not only depends on start-up cost but also on the payer base. The latter is difficult to control, but the cost of maintenance and repair is not. In this chapter, the authors are laying out the highlights of managing the maintenance and the associated cost of endoscopic equipment that is routinely used in spinal endoscopic decompression procedures. The aim was to give the readers insight into what is at stake to be easily replicated in their clinical setting.

COST MANAGEMENT OF MEDICAL DEVICES

Anyone who has used a mechanical or technological device knows that devices tend to break down over time. There are few other industries where managing such resources in the operation is more critical than in healthcare. There are many components associated with medical device management that contribute to high life cycle costs. It is estimated that these costs reach about 100 billion dollars annually. For many healthcare delivery players, this is not just a monetary burden but also requires increasing human resource management dedicated to the maintenance and repair of such high-tech equipment to keep the complex clinical programs going.

Life cycle costs consist of Medical Product Investment (MPI), installation costs, service and repair costs for hard- and software components, and proper ongoing use of the entire equipment. Devices with a high level of complexity typically have high installation and maintenance costs associated with them. The more a hospital or health system spends on these processes, the higher the scrutiny on the clinical and fiduciary performance of such high-tech programs as hospitals and surgery centers are already operating on low margins. Administrators of such organizations may hesitate to implement a novel but costly spinal endoscopy program in their facility if they do not understand the revenue cycle of the new proposed surgical procedure and the ongoing cost for running it either due to maintenance and repairs, or disposables and staff training requirements. Responsible industry partners will help the team leaders at the facility calculate reimbursement of the investment for a complete workstation based on accepted surgical indications. There is an existing time-proven reimbursement coding structure in place.

One way to improve return on investment (ROI) is to set up an endoscopic spinal surgery program with multiple surgeons for the same or for a variety of indications for one and the same workstation to minimize downtime. The other side of the equation is operational cost. The design and build quality of a particular piece of equipment go a long way toward determining its propensity for breakdowns and need for repairs. Some of the products of endoscopic sets and workstations include surgical instruments, endoscopes, video towers and power tools. Surgeons have a significant influence on the product's design. They should work closely with the development team including physicists, electronic engineers, and IT specialists, and the OEM manufacturer and the entity that pro-

provides financing to bring such products to market with appropriate regulatory approval.

EQUIPMENT PROCUREMENT

It is the manufacturers' responsibility to design equipment with a rugged build and as few parts as possible (Fig. **1**). The balance between technology advancement and necessary features should influence the developer, constructor, and company owner's philosophy. One crucial fact is the compatibility of the whole workstation.

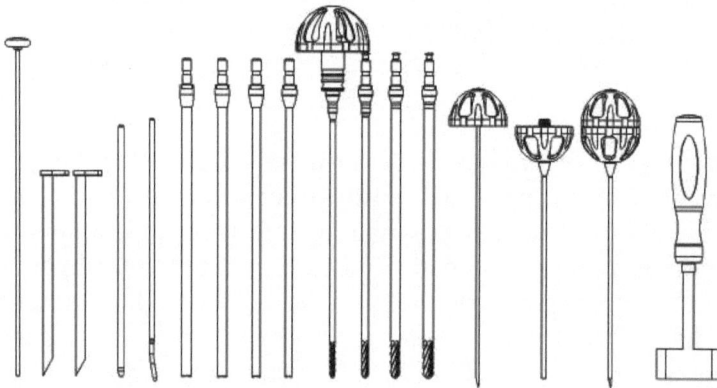

Fig. (1). Schematic of the content of a basic lumbar spinal endoscopy set containing drills, trephines, working sleeves, guide dilators, guide tubes, cannulated bone perforators, and hammer. Additionally, the endoscopic set should be equipped with a minimum of two different sizes of pituitary rongeurs and graspers for the discectomy procedure (not shown).

Many manufacturers point this out and try to force buyers not to have third-party repairs carried out or to procure the entire workstation with them to prevent voiding of the warranty, but even more seriously, the loss of product liability protection. Knowledge of the legal provisions for warranty clauses and early negotiations helps to avoid cost traps later on. In the following Table (**1**), the authors list the basic workstation and instruments for endoscopic spinal surgery interventions:

Table 1. Basic endoscopic spine system without video tower.

Quantity	Description	2018 Pricing by a Legacy Vendor US$
1	Guidance point tip	221,00
1	Guidance drill tip	221,00
1	Guidance blunt tip	221,00

(Table 1) cont.....

Quantity	Description	2018 Pricing by a Legacy Vendor US$
1	Handle for bone drill	770,00
1	Bone drill, 6 mm, manuell	294,00
1	Bone drill, 7 mm, manuell	294,00
1	Bone drill, 8 mm, manuell	294,00
1	Bone drill, 9 mm, manuell	294,00
1	Ball handle	770,00
1	Hammer	237,00
1	Instrument tray	794,00
	Subtotal:	4.410,00
1	Endoscope 3.7 mm standard 6.3 mm 2 including 2 cleaning brushes	9.950,00
1	Endoscope 4.1 mm 7.0 mm incl. including 2 cleaning brushes	11.050,00
	Basic Price for Operation Set	20.128,00
1	Puncture needle set consisting of 1 spinal 18 G needle, 1 22 G needle with guidewires 0.7 mm, 1.0 mm, 1.5 mm with guidewire container	164,00
1	Dilator 6.3 mm	166,00
1	Dilator3.0 mm	158,00
1	Dilator 4.5 mm	158,00
1	Working sleeve 45 degree angle	175,00
1	Working sleeve 0 degree angle	175,00
1	Trephine Set 3,0, 3,5, 4,5 mm	540,00
1	Nerve hook	90,00
1	Spoon forceps 2.7/285	570,00
1	Spoon forceps 3.5/320	785,00
1	Forceps 3.0/320, gezahnt	685,00
1	Kerrison punch 3.5 mm, 90	742,00
1	Instrument tray	1.400,00
-	Subtotal for set of basic instruments:	5.768,00

REPAIR COST OF ENDOSCOPIC INSTRUMENTS

Additional to the investment, repair costs for wear, tear, and damage over the product life cycle will produce additional charges, influencing the case cost. Surgical instruments belong to the category of medium-term capital goods with an expected lifetime of 10 years, related to the service and careful handling.

Endoscopic surgical instruments are divided into the following categories: Scalpel, clamp, scissors, needle holder, punch, rongeur, chisel, hammer, raspatory, drill, cutter, suction tubes, and cannulas. Wear and tear prompting repair takes place on edges, joints, and surfaces. Inadequate treatment leads to rust deposits and damage caused by bending, push, and drop. Ten percent of the investment money for surgical instruments have to be calculated for repair every ten use-cycles, which based on 2018 pricing schedules means approximately 100 US$ per intervention (Table **2**).

Table 2. Estimated repair costs for surgical instruments based on 2018 pricing schedules.

Estimated Repair Costs	Price Per Piece US$
Hook punch, revised, honed and polished	65,00
Spoon forceps, revised, honed and polished	65,00
Grasper, revised and polished	65,00
Needle holder, revised, aligned and polished	75,00
Shaver, revised, honed and polished	70,00
Endoscopic scissor, cutting blades straightened, sharpened and polished	75,00
Bone drill, sharpen and polish	45,00
Trephine, sharpen and polish	45,00
Flushing and suction pipe, revised	20,00

REPAIR COSTS FOR ENDOSCOPES

An increased number of surgical procedures using endoscopic techniques have resulted in the more frequent use of rigid endoscopes. A side effect of this is that more instrument damage has been noticed. Measures must be taken in instrument handling procedures to reduce instrument damage and the cost of instrument repairs. The impacts of such changes are described below. Improved education and training of personnel would help to avoid damage and repair costs. High-temperature damage to lenses could be reduced by adequate use of sterilization apparatus, which will meet the endoscope type's needs. It can be assumed that the reduction of damage to instruments also has a beneficial influence on the quality of the endoscopic surgical procedures because less time is lost, and possibly the image quality can be improved.

DAMAGE RECOGNITION OF DEFECT RIGID ENDOSCOPE

Several tests allow the manufacturer to find out if the damage is caused by misuse of the scope during the operation or bad handling between the operating room and central sterilization or during the sterilization process. At the distal end of the spinal endoscope is the lens which creates the so-called real image. The rod lenses, which are made of glass, transport the image to the eyepiece. They consist of lenses and spacers which are referred to as air lenses. The intermediate image created by each rod lens creates another intermediate image from the air lens and the next rod lens. The endoscope's length dictates the number of rod lenses to the eyepiece from where it is forward to the video camera. The critical parts of a spinal endoscope are illustrated in Fig. (**2**).

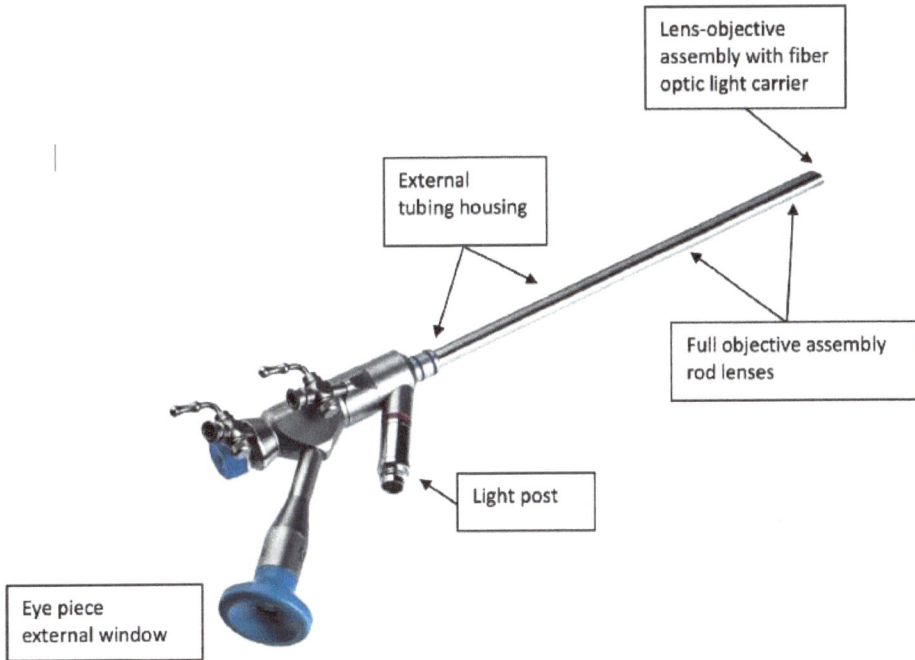

Fig. (2). Shown is the asap foraminoscope with a 20-degree viewing angle. The endoscope's labeled critical portions most susceptible to damage include the external eyepiece or ocular, the light post, the rod-lense assembly, the objective, and the outer tubing.

A common problem prompting repair or replacement of the broken endoscope is the lens's failure by surgical instruments, including power burs, or the repetitive sterilization cycles. Sudden image deterioration during surgery may suggest a leak. Vibration or hammering employing modern motorized endoscopic instruments and tools may cause defects in the inner working channel tube or scratch the lens. Such problems become apparent when assessing the optical image created by the endoscope can for image sharpness error (spherical aberration, astigmatism, field curvature, coma), image scale error (distortion), chromatic aberration, and image illumination error (vignetting, scattered light, and reflections; (Fig. **3**).

Incoming: Outgoing:

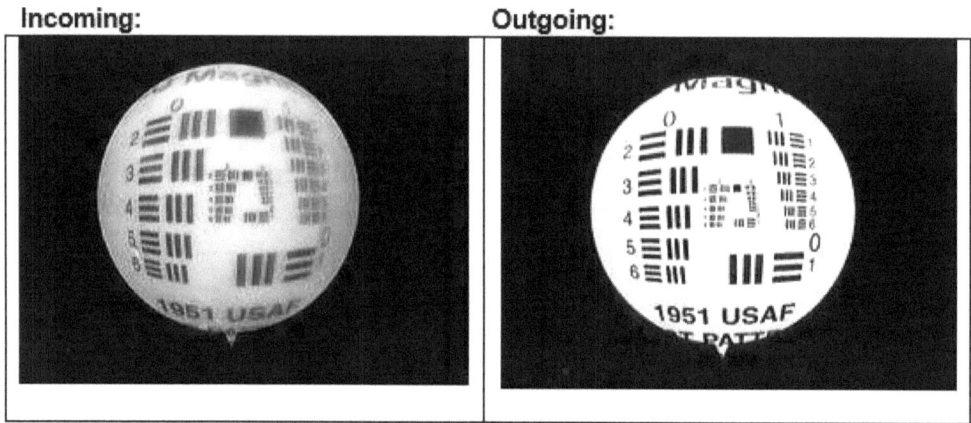

Fig. (3). Damaged endoscopes are examined using "1951 USAF resolution test target". The incoming optical system of the endoscope shows poor contrast and resolution (left side). After repair the outgoing endoscope shows now excellent contrast and resolution (right side).

DAMAGE RECOGNITION OF DEFECT RIGID ENDOSCOPES

Whenever rigid endoscopes are returned to the manufacturer for repair work they are checked for the following problem:

- Front lens: broken or dull, caused by push and drop, or leaking, damaged by instruments, laser, or high-frequency probes (Figs. **4 - 6**),
- Light fibers broken,
- Objective assembly broken or dull,
- Tubing bent or kinked,
- Rod lens system, dull, broken rod lenses, image decentered,
- Light post burned or lens broken,
- Tube passage to the housing kinked,
- Eyepiece dull or broken.

There are many testing procedures at the manufacturer's disposal to determine whether the damage is caused by misuse of the endoscope during the operation, improper staff handing, or the sterile processing department (SPD).

HOW TO REDUCE THE COSTS OF REPAIR AND SERVICE

Certified technicians should recognize the kind of damage and should be able to repair the simple cases corresponding to the manufacturer's repair categories. Small health care organizations may benefit from pooling resources.

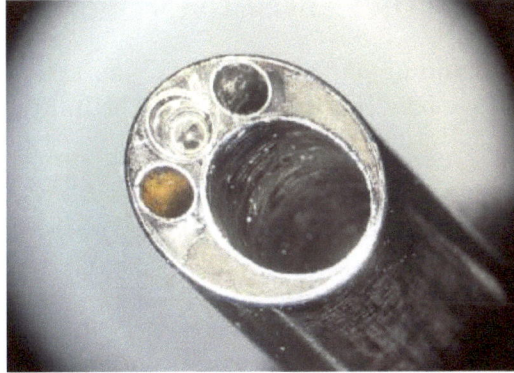

Fig. (4). Microscopic view of a spinal endoscope whose manufacturer advertised superior quality related to the lens's gold-welding. The lens detached from the endoscope had to be retrieved intraoperatively from the patient with a backup endoscope from a different manufacturer.

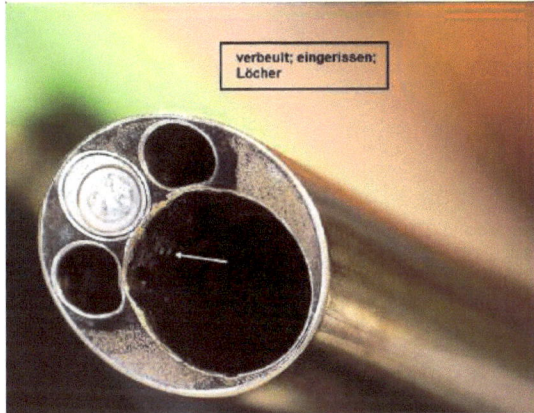

Fig. (5). Common usage-related problems include scratched working channel with tears and leakage of the light fiber.

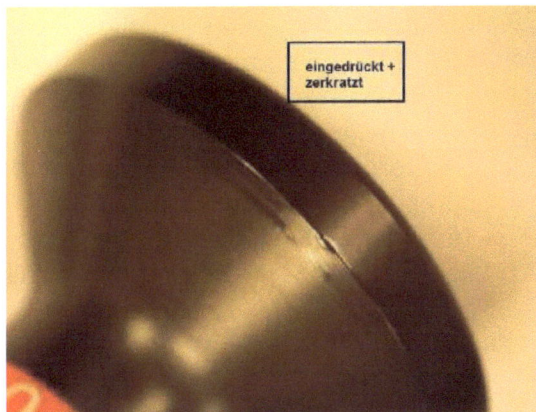

Fig. (6). Common usage-related problems include a scratched ocular.

REPAIR CATEGORIES FOR ENDOSCOPES

The repair technician should give the healthcare organization feedback as to what type of damage to improve handling and service in the following categories:

- Cleaning the outer surfaces,
- Polishing the distal and proximal glass surfaces and of the light post,
- Function control, check of the tightness,
- Opening and exposing the optical system.

The staff of the manufacturer should improve the endoscope by providing service in these following categories:

- Adjustment of the optical system,
- Exchange of the light fibers,
- Exchange of rod lenses,
- Replacement of the objective,
- Close the endoscope vacuum-tight.

The advantage of integrating a hospital certified technician is to check if a repair is more cost-effective or a replacement. Manufacturers often suggest an exchange of the device, even for superficial damages. This will extend the profit of the manufacturer and reduce it for the hospital. Hospitals should consider multiple service partners if possible and negotiate flat fees based on the level of complexity of the repair. Moreover, measuring and negotiating repair turnaround times with partners can minimize excess inventory requirements.

REGULATIONS & LEGAL IMPLICATIONS

In many countries, including the US and Europe, medical devices are regulated by governing administrative bodies regulate medical product affairs to assure their safety and efficacy. Manufacturers must file for approval before marketing and selling their devices. As part of the approval process, the manufacturer's good laboratory and manufacturing procedures (GLMP) must be documented without gaps for quality assurance according to the jurisdictions' law and regulations where the endoscope is to be sold. Therefore, the description of the intended purpose and clinical use in the instructions for use (IFU), the product classification, the risk analysis, and the conformity assessment. This documentation is required to prove that the developed medical product is suitable to achieve the intended purpose by employing validated and verified methods.

In the United States, the necessary legal requirements that manufacturers of medical devices sold must meet are operational registration, a listing of medical devices, premarket notification 510 (k), if not excluded, or premarket approval (PMA), or investigative device exemption (IDE) for clinical studies. In the European Union, medicine products fell under directive 93/42/EEC until 2017 when converted into a regulation, the Medical Device Regulation. The European Medical Device Directive 93/42/EEC requires: Manufacturers must document medical devices' performance and safety in a "clinical evaluation." To this end, the directive requires a "defined and methodically flawless procedure." The MDR 2017 does not differentiate between operators, clinics, hospitals, laboratories, and hospitals. For the EU regulation, these are "health facilities," and this is potentially problematic. The rules set up by the FDA are interpreted by many companies as much easier for companies to understand.

DISCUSSION

Improper handling by surgeons and staff may shorten the predicted life cycle of spinal endoscopes. The added case cost must be taken into account when running an endoscopic spine surgery program at a hospital or an ambulatory surgery center. Under current usage patterns, the reported average life cycle for a spinal endoscope is about 100 cycles. While there is little debate about the benefits of the endoscopic decompression operation, high implementation- and maintenance cost remains of concern since societal cost savings may not be realizable in the same revenue cycle. As a point of fact, endoscopy of the spine is essentially replacing protocols of traditional open and other forms of minimally invasive spinal surgery, which are being performed without the need for additional large upfront capital- and disposable equipment purchases. Most healthcare systems struggle with mandated cost savings. The increasing regulatory burden disproportionally increases the cost of doing business around the world. The CE mark regulation has changed from the Europe Standard EN 60950-1 to EN 62368-1 under which all audio/video (A/V), information and communication technology (ICT) equipment sold in Europe will have to comply with the new EN 62368-1 hazard-based standard by December of 2020. This also applies to all existing equipment currently CE marked under EN 60950-1. In 2017, the European Parliament passed legislation to transition the EU's medical device directive (MDD) to the more rigorous medical device regulation (MDR). The net effect is a significant expansion of accountability for future legal damages to any operators, including authorized representatives, importers, and distributors. The reporting requirements and accountability criteria have increased the scrutiny of risk assessment documentation on the manufacturer's part, who now have to create and maintain technical files more meticulously. Quality control processes raise production costs. This cost increase may push the makers of spinal endoscopes who operate in a small niche market out of business since they operate in a small market with inconsistent demand. Technological innovation may be stifled as the cost of change is too high. Moreover, repair and maintenance costs may go up since the margins on new sales are dwindling. Therefore, developing well-run maintenance and repair protocols is essential to operators in hospitals and surgery centers to keep the case cost under control by maximizing the existing endoscopic equipment's life cycle.

CONCLUSION

To understand the FDA's control process, the responsible legislator, a "Guidance Document" has been published. The critical part of product service and repair is the requirement of risk analyses and "Post Market Surveillance." A certified Regulatory Affairs Manager must be employed to fulfill these requirements. This manager is expected to work closely with surgeons who carry out studies to prove the safety of the products offered.

CONSENT FOR PUBLICATION

Not applicable.

CONFLICT OF INTEREST

The authors declare no conflict of interest, financial or otherwise.

ACKNOWLEDGEMENT

Declared none.

REFERENCES

[1]   Wang B, Lü G, Patel AA, Ren P, Cheng I. An evaluation of the learning curve for a complex surgical technique: the full endoscopic interlaminar approach for lumbar disc herniations. Spine J 2011; 11(2): 122-30.
[http://dx.doi.org/10.1016/j.spinee.2010.12.006] [PMID: 21296295]

[2]   Xu B, Xu H, Ma X, *et al.* Bilateral decompression and intervertebral fusion via unilateral fenestration for complex lumbar spinal stenosis with a mobile microendoscopic technique. Medicine (Baltimore) 2018; 97(4): e9715.
[http://dx.doi.org/10.1097/MD.0000000000009715] [PMID: 29369203]

[3]   Heo DH, Park CK. Clinical results of percutaneous biportal endoscopic lumbar interbody fusion with application of enhanced recovery after surgery. Neurosurg Focus 2019; 46(4): E18.
[http://dx.doi.org/10.3171/2019.1.FOCUS18695] [PMID: 30933919]

[4]   Heo DH, Son SK, Eum JH, Park CK. Fully endoscopic lumbar interbody fusion using a percutaneous unilateral biportal endoscopic technique: technical note and preliminary clinical results. Neurosurg Focus 2017; 43(2): E8.
[http://dx.doi.org/10.3171/2017.5.FOCUS17146] [PMID: 28760038]

[5]   Lewandrowski K-U, Ransom NA, Yeung A. Subsidence induced recurrent radiculopathy after staged

two-level standalone endoscopic lumbar interbody fusion with a threaded cylindrical cage: a case report. J Spine Surg 2020; 6 (Suppl. 1): S286-93.
[http://dx.doi.org/10.21037/jss.2019.09.25] [PMID: 32195435]

[6]   Lewandrowski KU, Ransom NA, Yeung A. Subsidence induced recurrent radiculopathy after staged two-level standalone endoscopic lumbar interbody fusion with a threaded cylindrical cage: a case report. J Spine Surg 2020; 6 (Suppl. 1): S286-93.
[http://dx.doi.org/10.21037/jss.2019.09.25] [PMID: 32195435]

[7]   Wang MY, Grossman J. Endoscopic minimally invasive transforaminal interbody fusion without general anesthesia: initial clinical experience with 1-year follow-up. Neurosurg Focus 2016; 40(2): E13.
[http://dx.doi.org/10.3171/2015.11.FOCUS15435] [PMID: 26828882]

CHAPTER 10

Regenerative Medicine and Interventional Endoscopic Pain Surgery for Degenerative Conditions of the Spine

Álvaro Dowling[1], Juan Carlos Vera[2] and **Kai-Uwe Lewandrowski**[3,4,5,*]

[1] *Orthopaedic Spine Surgeon, Director of Endoscopic Spine Clinic, Santiago, Chile. Visiting Professor, Department of Orthopaedic Surgery, USP, Ribeirão Preto, Brazil*

[2] *Molecular Biotechnology Engineer, Universidad de Chile Business Development Manager-VidaCel, Chile*

[3] *Center for Advanced Spine Care of Southern Arizona and Surgical Institute of Tucson, Tucson AZ, USA*

[4] *Associate Professor of Orthopaedic Surgery, Universidad Colsanitas, Bogota, Colombia, USA*

[5] *Visiting Professor, Department Orthopaedic Surgery, UNIRIO, Rio de Janeiro, Brazil*

Abstract: Regenerative medicine is a subspecialty of medicine that seeks to recruit and enhance the body's own inherent healing armamentarium in the treatment of patient pathology. In regenerative spine care, the intention is to assist in the repair and potentially replace or restore damaged tissue through autologous or allogenic biologics. In the authors' opinion, future spine care will likely evolve into a blend of prevailing strategies from interventional pain management and minimally invasive spine surgery. This form of spine care nowadays is commonly called interventional pain surgery. The interest in regenerative medicine in general and in interventional pain surgery of the spine is growing given the high patient awareness of problems with traditional spine surgery, whose focus is on decompression of pinched nerves and correction of spinal instability and deformity. However, reoperation- and complication rates are high with those open corrective spine surgeries as many of the spine's degenerative conditions are being only treated surgically when the disease has progressed to its end-stage. The sole application of image-based medical necessity criteria for surgical intervention in the spine seems slightly out of step with the growing demand for less aggressive and burdensome procedures that could perhaps be instituted earlier in the disease process where the goal is to heal the spinal injury or repair damage from the degenerative process more naturally. In this chapter, the authors review and discuss the current state of the art in regenerative biologic therapies and interventional pain care of the

* **Corresponding author Kai-Uwe Lewandrowski:** Center for Advanced Spine Care of Southern Arizona and Surgical Institute of Tucson, Tucson, AZ, USA, Department of Orthopaedic Surgery, UNIRIO, Rio de Janeiro, Brazil and Department of Orthoapedic Surgery, Fundación Universitaria Sanitas, Bogotá, D.C., Colombia, USA; Tel: +1 520 204-1495; Fax: +1 623 218-1215; E-mail: business@tucsonspine.com

spine from their perspective as endoscopic spine surgeons. Simplifying therapeutic measures and strategies are at the heart of what patients request of us as surgeons. This field's applications in modern spine care are clearly in their infancy, except for fusion. The authors will discuss potential applications of select advanced biologics technologies and their attempts at integrating them into their endoscopic spinal stenosis surgery program to treat degenerative spinal disease and instability-related symptomatic end-stage degenerative vacuum disc disease in the elderly.

Keywords: Biologics, Endoscopic spine care, Regenerative technologies.

INTRODUCTION

Numerous treatments and therapeutics have been applied to manage chronic spinal pain ranging from over the counter medications and devices, a variety of image-guided interventional pain management techniques, to complex spinal fusion. The emerging field of regenerative medicine is likely to become the next frontier in musculoskeletal and spinal care models [1 - 3]. According to the recent statistics, Americans already spent some 87.6 billion on self-directed management of low back and neck pain and another 95.9 billion on musculoskeletal pain. These numbers account for the third and fourth highest health care expenditure among all disease categories.

Despite numerous alternative therapy techniques to spinal fusion, this aggressive and disruptive way of treating common degenerative conditions of the lumbar spine remains the mainstay of modern spine care. Although clinical outcomes with spinal fusion are well studied and its indications well understood, it remains riddled with blood loss, persistent postoperative pain, a relatively high complication- and reoperation rate due to adjacent segment disease, and junctional instability and deformity. The stigma of overall high cost and continued medical service utilization even after extensive surgery, persistent disability, and low return-to-work rates remain. Evidence-based clinical treatment guidelines published by several professional organizations have attempted to outline appropriate medical necessity guidelines for surgical spine care to achieve more consistent clinical improvements in a more cost-effective manner. However, such medical societies' clinical treatment- or insurance companies' coverage guidelines may also hamper innovation. Nowadays, regenerative medicine is still a stepchild of spine care and is often declared experimental. It is typically only made available to those who can afford it. Success stories of such regenerative therapies in professional athletes will likely facilitate bringing it to the forefront of accepted medical care by incorporating biomechanical, biochemical, biomedical technology advancements to improve cellular replication migration, restitution, and modelling [4 - 11].

While there is no doubt that regenerative medicine will play an increasing role in modern spine care, the burden of proof will always rest on the innovators. Desperate patients, sometimes driven by media hype, will always seek out promising treatments even if the clinical evidence in their support is weak. Therefore, adherence to the highest ethical standards in any other medical research area is the foundation for conducting clinical outcome research with commonly pursued regenerative therapeutic strategies, including medicinal signaling, mesenchymal- and stem cells [12] and platelet-enriched plasma [13 - 16] injections. Injections of these remedies in facet joints and discs [3, 12, 14, 17] of the lumbar spine and the sacroiliac joints [18, 19] and paraspinal muscles [20], ligaments [16, 21, 22], and tendons [23 - 25] have been tried. This chapter will review the current state-of-the-art regenerative therapies of the intervertebral disc and enhancement of interbody fusion as they apply to endoscopic spine surgery. Regarding the latter, the authors present their clinical experience with platelet enriched application allograft corticocancellous chips in un-instrumented spinal fusions intended for the elderly as one example of simplified spine care.

REGENERATIVE MEDICINE STRATEGIES

Biological therapies help heal tissues damaged acutely or chronically, including ligaments, menisci, articular cartilage, tendons, discs, and joints. While various biologicals are utilized in regenerative therapy of the spine and other musculoskeletal disorders, platelet rich plasma (PRP) and mesenchymal stem cells (MSCs) are the current mainstays of regenerative medicine treatments.

Platelet Rich Plasma

PRP's regenerative benefits occur *via* the increased concentration of growth factors secreted by platelets in an inflammatory environment [26]. It may be derived from autologous or allogeneic derivatives of whole blood and contains very high concentrations of platelets. These growth factors are essential to the healing process, as they increase fibroblast and osteoblast metabolic activity while reducing cell apoptosis. They are promoting angiogenesis, thereby increasing blood flow and circulation to the newly formed tissues and increasing the expression of the pro-collagen gene and collagen-derived growth factors, which increase the tensile strength of the new tissue (Fig. **1**) [27 - 29].

The α-granules have been recognized to provide the growth factors and cytokines essential to normal wound healing [30]. PRP derived factors play a role in local angiogenesis, proliferation, differentiation, and homing of local and stem cells. They also are responsible for local production of matrix proteins, including collagen, which are the building blocks of normal tissue restoration. The net effect on the local tissue environment is regeneration. Exciting its regenerative effects on bone, cartilage, skin, tendon, and muscle has motivated several orthopedic and spinal surgery applications. Stimulation of angiogenesis with the reconstitution of the vascular supply to an injured or degenerated area seems to be impacting clinical outcomes reported by patients (PROMs) the most [31 - 35].

PLATELET ACTION

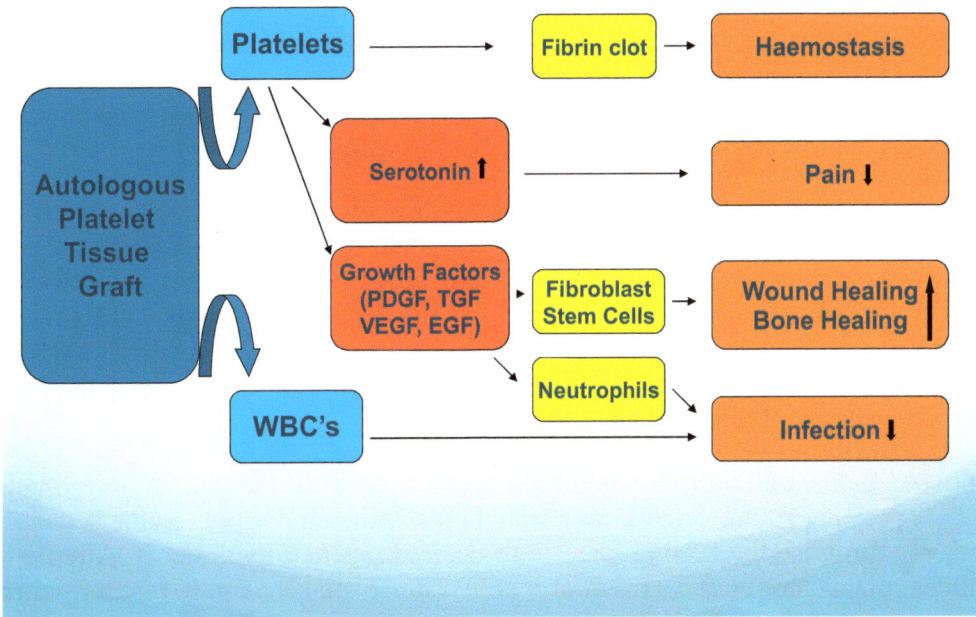

Fig. (1). Schematic of some of the platelet derived actions on the healing process of musculoskeletal tissues [26].

While the benefit has been demonstrated in many orthopaedic applications, quantifying it with disease-specific outcome tools commonly used in clinical spine research is problematic. Determining the PRP-related additional effect size increase of a beneficial therapy or reconstructive procedure depends on designing well-controlled and matched study cohorts to avoid overestimating its benefit [36]. Additional errors in the clinical outcome analysis may come from a lack of standardization and variability in the PRP generation. Moreover, the inconsistent use of terminology and inconsistent purity standards may affect the PRP. These variations in standards reflect themselves in the use of various terminologies, including "… platelet-enriched plasma, platelet-rich concentrate, platelet concentrate, leukocyte-rich PRP, platelet-rich fibrin, PRP rich in growth factors, platelet-rich fibrin matrix, autologous concentrated plasma, platelet gel, pure PRP, platelet release..." and others [24, 37 - 40]. A classification system for PRP has therefore been suggested by Harrison *et al.* in an attempt to provide a "... clear definition or quantification of the PRP biological properties..." [24] which incorporated elements of previous classification systems [37 - 39, 41]. The Harrison classification includes elements of PRP activation, concentration, and the preparation method [24]. By activation method, Harrison identified PRP application with and without and frozen-thawed preparations. By concentration, the suggested subcategories were group A with a platelet count of $< 900 \times 103$ μL^{-1}, group B - $900–1700 \times 103$ μL^{-1}, and group C with a platelet count of > 1700 $\times 103$ μL^{-1}. Classification by method of preparation Harrison suggested sub classifying preparations using gravitational centrifugation techniques, standard cell separators, and autologous selective filtration technology (plateletpheresis) [24].

The commercially available PRP preparation devices also lack standardization [42]. PRP regenerative properties are determined by growth- and differentiation factors being released when the platelets are activated. Leukocytes and red blood cells may also play a role in modulating the local antibacterial and immune response [43]. The PRP induced creation of a fibrin scaffold in the wound or at the application site location provides the primary structure to facilitate the repair and regeneration of the local tissues.

Anticoagulants are required when PRP is prepared from the patient (autologous) in the operating room. Trisodium citrate is the anticoagulant of choice because it does not diminish the PRP preparation's desired regenerative effects. Alternative anticoagulants commonly used are acid citrate dextrose (ACD) and citrate phosphate dextrose (CPD) with and without adenine. The commonly used chelator EDTA provokes platelet swelling and activation and is therefore unsuitable for PRP preparation. In the operating room, high purity PRP preparations can be produced by single-step gravitational centrifugation at $170–200 \times g$ for 10 min, which is one of three methods to produce PRP [24]. Alternative methods are cell separators and plateletpheresis – a form of autologous selective filtration. The cell separation is typically performed using a full unit of blood. Adjusting the g-force and centrifugation time will affect platelet concentration, purity, viability, and activation status. Ultimately, these parameters determine its efficacy in the desired clinical setting. Once the surgeon is ready to apply the PRP during his procedure, the PRP preparation must be activated. During this activation, platelets release the content of their α-granules. The generated clot provides a scaffold to capture and retain the secreted proteins wherever they are applied during the surgical procedure. Platelets can be activated by thrombin or recalcification. The duration and time of the activation are controversial. The entire PRP preparation process and activation process lacks standardization, which makes assessing the benefits of PRP in patient outcomes difficult [44, 45]. Attempts at formulating consensus recommendations for standardizing the use of platelets in regenerative medicine have been made and subsequently published since 2016 [24]. Standard protocols for PRP preparations for orthopaedic application in the treatment of hip and knee osteoarthritis have been described by others [46].

ACTIVE FACTORS IN PRP

Only a few studies have analyzed the active components released by platelets from their alpha granules upon activation of the PRP preparations [47 - 49]. With the commonly employed intraoperative preparation methods PRP preparations can also be divided into leukocyte poor (LP)-PRP and leukocyte rich (LR)-PRP preparations [50]. The most commonly employed commercial systems are ACP (LP-PRP) made by Arthrex (Naples, FL, USA) and GPS III (LR-PRP) made by Biomet Biologics Co., (Warsaw, IN, USA [51].

Lee *et al.* identified proteins in PRP preparations through two-dimensional gel electrophoresis, followed by gene ontology (GO) analysis using the ACP and the GPS systems [52]. The complete blood cell count (CBC) test done immediately on prepared PRP samples to investigate the cell composition, including leukocytes and platelets. The authors then extracted proteins by size-fractionating by one-dimensional-sodium dodecyl sulfate-polyacrylamide gel electrophoresis (SDS-PAGE) from isolated and lysed platelets. Proteins were then identified using liquid chromatography-tandem mass spectrometry. The gene ontology analysis was performed to classify proteins according to their functions employing the AmioGo2 GO database (https://www.AmiGO.geneontology.org) [53]. The extracted PRP proteins' tasks were assigned by utilizing keywords describing tissue healing, angiogenesis, fibroblasts proliferation, and upregulation of collagen and glycosaminoglycan production [54]. Of the 1555 isolated proteins, 778 proteins were implied in wound healing. A total of 285 proteins were isolated exclusively from leukocyte-rich PRP preparations. Namely, the ANXA2, CAPZA1, anxa6, SERPING1, TF, Naca, krt5, MYL12A, WDR1, F9, KNG1, FGG, HSPA5, Gp1bb, Rac2, VCL, C4BPB, FLNA, Arpc4, TUBA4A, Pdia6, CPB2, Aqp1, CFL1, CFD, GNAI2, ITGB3, COL1A2, LAMP2, Gp9, CSRP1, MYL9, RAP1B, CALM1, DMTN, PRTN3 proteins were involved in wound healing. Angiogenesis proteins including GPX1, H3BM21, and ITGB3 were isolated from both LP-PRP and LR-PRP preparations. The THBS1 and DMTN proteins responsible for fibroblast migration were identified in both LP-PRP and LR-PRP [52]. Many more proteins involved in the biosynthesis of collagen and glycosaminoglycan binding were determined by Lee *et al.* The authors recommend that the readers of this chapter read the source reference article by

Lee *et al.* for a more detailed review of the complex protein analysis results from LR- and LP-PRP preparations. In this chapter, the focus is on the PRP technology's clinical application with endoscopic spinal fusion.

PRP SPINAL FUSION APPLICATION

PRP's healing effect has been the subject of a recent meta-analysis of five retrospective studies enrolling 253 patients and nine prospective cohort studies, which enrolled a total of 460 patients.. [55] The spinal fusion was rated as excellent in those studies that used a high concentration of PRP compared to controls with an odds ratio (OR) = 4.35, 95% confidence interval (CI) (2.13, 8.83), and $P < 0.05$). PRP's fusion promoting effect was further corroborated by finding poor bony fusion in those studies in whom low dose PRP was used compared to control groups. The rate of new bone formation was high in the PRP group compared to the control group based on computed tomography evaluation of bone formation. The mean difference in the Hounsfield unit (HU) was 144.91 (95% CI (80.63, 209.18), $P < 0.05$). PRP also accelerated the fusion, which occurred in the PRP group within six months after surgery compared to the control group with a mean difference of -2.03 (95% CI (-2.35, -1.7); $P < 0.05$). However, no difference was found in patient self-reported reduction in the visual analog pain scores (VAS) between the PRP group and control.

MESENCHYMAL STEM CELLS & DEGENERATIVE DISC DISEASE

Zeckser *et al.* (169) have stated that all interventional therapies should optimally strive to fulfill a trilogy of treatment objectives [56]:

1. Decline and resolution of primary nociceptive disc pain with functional improvement
2. Reversal or slowing catabolism
3. Partial or complete restoration of the disc tissue.

Currently, stem cell-based therapy is in full development [57 - 59]. Its use aims to replace degenerated human cells, tissues, and organs, restoring their physiological functions [60 - 64]. This therapeutic option is on the rise, becoming an alternative for various clinical and research applications. Since the inception of this strategy to date, numerous pre-clinical and clinical studies have shown that mesenchymal stem cells are safe for both autologous and allogeneic use, in addition to being easy to isolate and expand *in vitro* in sufficient quantities for the doses that are required [65 - 69]. Recent studies show that, above the differentiation capacity as the primary mechanism to promote tissue regeneration, the therapeutic effects of mesenchymal cells are a consequence of the paracrine and autocrine mechanisms resulting from the set of bioactive factors secreted in soluble form to the extracellular space that they include soluble proteins, nucleic acids, lipids, cytokines, neurotrophins, growth factors, and active extracellular vesicles secreted or through extracellular vesicles (EV) [63, 67, 69 - 72]. Through stem cell-based regenerative therapy, the treatment of degenerative intervertebral disc disease is being investigated, modulating the inflammatory response and restoring cellular homeostasis within the disc. Currently, it focuses on the use of cells extracted from intervertebral discs or stem cells from bone marrow, fat, or umbilical cord, whether they are autologous or allogeneic. The effects of MSCs to delay and even reverse the degenerative cascade in intervertebral discs have been well documented in many experimental studies that include different animal models before being translated for clinical use [73 - 81].

Mesenchymal stem cells are believed to promote proteoglycan synthesis [82 - 84], and type II collagen [76, 85 - 87] decreased with degenerative disc disease, thus reversing or stopping the process of disc degeneration [88 - 93]. Mesenchymal stem cells could be influencing the pro-inflammatory state of the intervertebral disc through negative feedback provided by the production of anti-inflammatory cytokines [94, 95], growth factors [96 - 99], and anti-catabolic factors [100, 101]. There are signaling and interaction patterns between stem cells and their environment (Fig. **2**) [102 - 106]. In this sense, if the microenvironment is mildly inflammatory, these cells can have a pro-inflammatory behavior. However, in a highly inflammatory setting, they play an essential immunoregulatory effect [107 - 110]. Two-way communication is established between stem cells in contact with nucleus pulposus cells [76, 111], which is diminished in advanced stages of intervertebral disc degeneration [112]. The communication signals could be a stimulus to mesenchymal stem cells to differentiate into cells similar to nucleus pulposus cells [76, 92, 113]. Another action that could be occurring is a reprogramming of the cells of the nucleus pulposus as a result of the paracrine effects of mesenchymal stem cells [114]. In short, a wide variety of stem cell-based approaches for treating disc degeneration and fusion already exist and are commercially available.

The International Society for Cell Therapy (ISCT) states that mesenchymal stem cells possess a morphology similar to fibroblasts and adherence to plastic when cultured in standard terms, expressing the surface markers CD73, CD90, and CD105, as well as adhesion molecules CD106, CD166), intercellular adhesion molecule one and CD29. MSCs lack hematopoietic markers CD45, CD34, CD14, CD11b, CD79a, and CD19 and the major histocompatibility complex (MHC) II, nor co-stimulatory molecules, and express MHC I low [115]. Mesenchymal stem cells generate immunomodulatory effects through cell-to-cell contact and the secretion of various paracrine factors [65, 116, 117]. There is also evidence that they generate a therapeutic effect through direct cell fusion [118], mitochondrial transfer [119, 120], and microvesicle production [65, 121, 122].

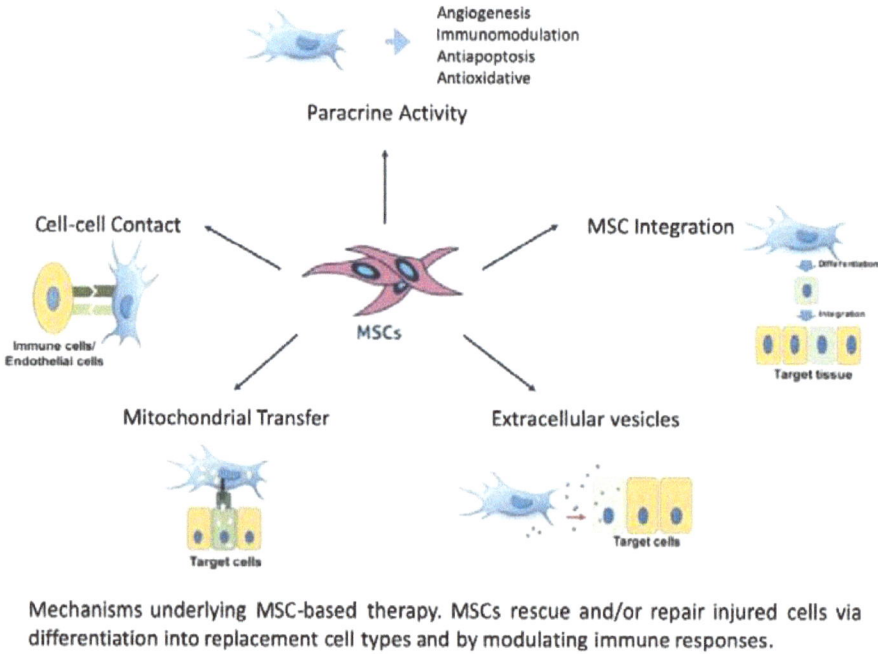

Mechanisms underlying MSC-based therapy. MSCs rescue and/or repair injured cells via differentiation into replacement cell types and by modulating immune responses.

Fig. (2). Schematic of some of the mesenchymal stem cells signaling and interaction patterns with their environment.

Umbilical cord MSCs were studied in the treatment of degenerative disc disease (Fig. **1**) with favorable results concerning pain and disability according to the Visual Analogue Score (VAS) survey and the Oswestry functional score [123 - 128]. These MSCs can be easily obtained by treating the umbilical cord or cord blood of newborns and stored in nitrogen until use. These cells show a low power of immunogenicity and a lower risk of rejection after transplantation compared to other stem cells [129]. Recent work conducted a systemic review of autologous MSC injections for intervertebral disc regeneration in a total of 98 patients and 122 levels treated in seven studies [130]. Patients with low back pain due to initial intervertebral disc degeneration and low-stage radiological degeneration were eligible for stem cell infiltration. Average Oswestry disability index and visual analog scale scores improved at one-year follow-up. Quantitative improvements such as T2-weighted magnetic resonance imaging scans, bulge sizes, and disc bulges also improved. MSC injection is a safe and feasible option for intervertebral disc regeneration in patients with early degeneration. Regardless of the origin of the MSCs, a general clinical and radiological improvement in the patients has been demonstrated combined with a low complication rate during follow-up observation.

According to the author's experience and the clinical evidence of published experimental works, it seems safe in treating low back pain, the local administration (intradiscal) of a certain amount of mesenchymal stem cells, in the order of 5 to 10 million cells by intervened disc (Fig. **3**). During the same procedure, it is also recommended to complement this infiltration with PRP's application, as suggested by various guidelines for the management of low back pain, such as the guidelines of the American Society of Interventional Pain Physicians (ASIPP) published in 2019 [131]. A formal review of the author's clinical results with the MSCs is currently underway and will be reported in due time.

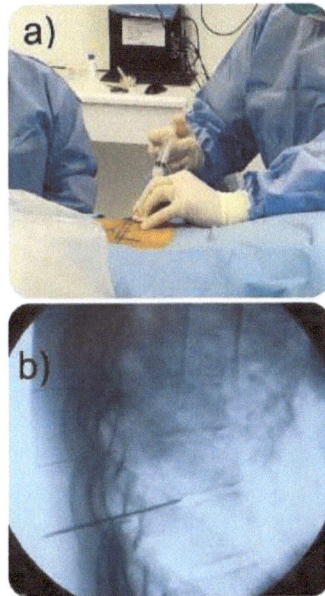

Fig. (3). Stem cells injection Posterolateral approach (**a**) with the spinal needle positioned in the symptomatic degenerative intervertebral disc.

GENE THERAPY FOR INTERVERTEBRAL DISC DEGENERATION

Gene therapy is defined as the transfer of either RNA or DNA to treat or prevent disease. Once a therapeutic gene is successfully transferred into the target cells, genetically modified cells produce the gene products (RNA or Proteins). Chronic conditions such as disc degeneration are good candidates for gene therapy. In 1998, the first report of successful *in vivo* sustained B-galactosidase expression after gene transfer with adenovirus in rabbits. Viral or nonviral vectors must transfer the gene into the target cells expressing their genes as a part of the life cycle. Gene therapy is an ideal method to treat disc degeneration because of his avascular environment. While clinical applications of gene therapy to date are limited, a limited review of some of the emerging techniques seems worthwhile for discussion purposes.

Retroviral therapies have been applied in the study of the degenerative disc disease process. A study by Wehling *et al. via* retrovirus transfer two exogenous genes to chondrocyte cells from bovine. This study concluded that local gene therapy is effective for disc degeneration [132]. Adenovirus has been used by Nishida *et al. in vivo* and *in vitro* and it was observed that Ad-lacZ injected into the nucleus pulposus of the lumbar intervertebral disc. Rabbit were successfully transferred to the disc *via* adenovirus [133]. A study by Liu *et al.* reported the utility of the green fluorescence protein transfer with baculovirus. It concluded baculovirus might be useful as a gene therapy vector for degenerative disc disease [134]. Liu *et al.* demonstrated the feasibility of multiple gene expression using the lentivirus. They determined it can transfer a substantial amount of exogenous genes and has an advantage in multiple gene expression capabilities in intervertebral disc cells [135].

Non-virus therapies are alternatives to viral gene transfer. There is increasing attention due to its safety and simplicity, which comes with lower efficacy. Examples include RNA interference, which aims at upregulating genes to stimulate matrix synthesis. RNA interference is also an essential biological approach for specific gene silencing. Several studies demonstrated that siRNA-mediated gene silencing in rat and human disc cells *in vitro* is feasible and effective in downregulating specific gene expression [136 - 138]. Sudo and Yamada *et al.* similarly demonstrated the effects of caspase-3 siRNA *in vitro* and *in vivo* [139]. After confirming the antiapoptotic effect of caspase-3 siRNA *in vitro*, they performed an *in vivo* study using an annular puncture model and external compression model, respectively. They demonstrated suppression of degenerative change and inhibition of apoptosis.

Microbubble-enhanced ultrasound technique has been applied to increase permeability of the cell membrane of the nucleus cells by sonoporation or cavitation. Nishida *et al.* demonstrated this microbubble-enhanced ultrasound gene therapy in the intervertebral disc [140]. The ultrasound group demonstrated approximately an 11-fold increase in luciferase activity compared to the plasmid DNA-only group. Another promising technique is the application of polyplex micelle demonstrated by *in vitro* experiments with rabbit disc NP cells and *in vivo* analysis with Sprague Dawley rats demonstrated that miR-29a effectively silenced MMP-2 expression, inhibited the fibrosis process, and reversed disc degeneration in animal models by blocking the β-catenin translocation pathway from the cytoplasm to the nucleus.

SPINAL FUSION BIOLOGY & REGENERATIVE STRATEGIES

Biologics in lumbar fusion have always been an essential element. In the past, there were few options. Autograft was the primary choice of many surgeons. The removal of bone from the iliac crest may still be the preferred method of harvesting autograft but has fallen out of favor due to donor site problems, including persistent pain, infections, palpable defect, fracture at the donor site, and its limited availability. Besides, there are many commercially available alternative products. The problems are Cortical allografts have considerable structural strength and are suitable for vertebral interbody fusion. Strong evidence only for osteoinductive proteins including rhBMP-2 [141] and OP-1 [142 - 149] shows that they can be used as bone enhancers and spinal fusion substitutes. The available clinical evidence in adults for rh-BMP-2 has been graded 1A and 2B for platelet gel as an enhancer of the effect of autografts applied in posterior and anterior lumbar fusion.

Autologous Bone Marrow Aspiration (BMA) is an autogenic source of osteogenic precursors cells that can differentiate into osteoblasts and other mesenchymal cells. The disadvantage is obtaining sufficient progenitor cells. To achieve lumbar fusion needs scaffolds including autograft, allografts, or ceramics. Many studies show the use of BMA as an adjunct to fusion with local bone graft in MISS TLIF [125, 150], and OLLIF [151], ceramics in XLIF [152, 153], and allograft in OLIF [154, 155]. These studies reported fusion rates in the range of 86% to 97% of Fusion in MISS [156].

In comparison to autografts, allografts are a type of bone graft obtained from either a cadaverous donor tissue. It has osteoconductive action by providing a scaffold. However, it is associated with weak osteoinductive properties that depend on preserving growth factors within the graft [154]. Allografts are used as alternatives to autografts because of their availability in larger quantities and the absence of donor site problems. The potential risks of viral infection and disease transmission have been discussed in the literature, but these are extremely rare. Allograft bone graft materials are frequently used combined with BMA or in combination with rh-BMP-2 in MISS spinal fusion surgeries. Only one apparent study reported the exclusive use of allograft alone with a 90% of fusion rate.

Demineralized bone matrix (DBM) was introduced in 1991 as a commercially available bone graft as a substitute or additive to the autologous bone [157, 158]. The donor's bone is treated with hydrochloric acid to remove the mineralized portion maintaining the collagen type 1 structure. This demineralized scaffold also contains some types of IV and X collagen. Non-collagenous proteins and some growth factors are also present. The organic matrix provides osteoconductive properties while growth factors including transforming growth factors beta, fibroblast growth factors, and other GFs. One of the main problems is the variability inefficiency [157, 158]. Therefore, DBM is rarely used alone. Cammisa *et al.* compared ICBG to DBM (Grafton)/autograft composite in 102 patients where the two types of grafts were implanted on either side of the patient's lumbar spine [159]. Two-year follow-up radiographic studies revealed almost equal fusion rates of 54% for ICBG and 52% for DBM, suggesting the efficacy of DBM as a bone graft extender is equally successful as autograft. Analysis of another 203 patients who received DBM combined with other biologics revealed fusion rates of 98% (97-98%). These rates were significantly higher than any other bone graft extender material (p < 0.05) except for BMA and rhBMP-2 alone when used in anterior and lateral interbody fusion applications.

Ceramics are synthetic bone grafts that have only osteoconductive properties [160, 161]. The significant advantage of ceramics is its immediate strength. Additional upsides include the lack of risk of disease transmission, long shelf life, an unlimited supply. The disadvantage is the lack of cortical stability [160 - 164]. Commercially available forms include hydroxyapatite (HA), tricalcium phosphate (TCP), calcium phosphate, and calcium sulfate. In the three studies that used ceramics as extenders combined with osteoinductive local autograft, a fusion rate of 86% (83–88%) was observed (98). In a study using ceramics in combination with rh-BMP-2, the fusion rate was 76% [64].

BMP-2 is a member of the transforming growth factor B (TFG-B) family. They are involved in the proliferation, differentiation, maturation of mesenchymal stem cells. In 1965, Marshall Urist extracted BMP from a partially purified extract of DBM [165 - 169]. Since then, over 20 BMPs have been identified to play an active role in fracture healing and new bone formation [170]. When applied in contained applications, clinical outcomes are favorable. Off-label applications may lead to problems including postoperative breathing problems following uncontained use in anterior cervical spine surgery. The FDA subsequently issued a warning of using rh-BMP-2 in the cervical spine because of airway edema and dysphagia [171 - 174].

CLINICAL SERIES

The authors applied the PRP technologies in patients with painful end-stage lumbar degenerative disc disease who often have vacuum disc disease and complain of a combination of mechanical- and sciatica-type low back and leg pain [175]. These painful collapsed and rigid lumbar motion segments were treated with endoscopic decompression and interbody fusion by placing bone allograft enriched with PRP prepared from the same patients to evoke an interbody fusion to achieve a more reliable resolution of symptoms. These patients were worked up to validate the painful level with diagnostic injections before treating the end-stage degenerative disc endoscopically with the PRP-enhanced allograft (Fig. **4**). The endoscopic transforaminal intradiscal decompression and fusion surgery were performed under local anesthesia in the sedated yet awake patient [176].

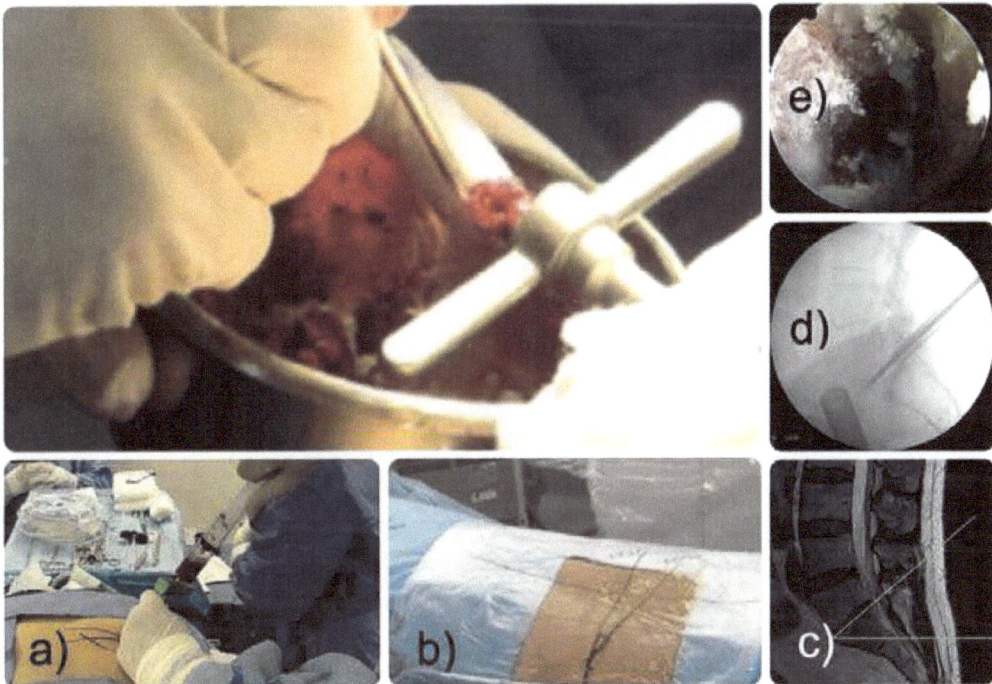

Fig. (4). Autologous bone marrow was extracted from the patient's iliac crest using two syringes (15 to 30 cc) to extract the same amount of bone marrow tissue from the patient's iliac crest, typically containing an average of ~200,000/μL (**a**). The surgical interspace was accessed with the transforaminal endoscopic approach (**b, d**). The preoperative MRI scan confirmed endstage degenerative disc disease (**c**). This PRP enriched allograft was placed and compacted into the intervertebral disc space (**e**) starting on the far-side opposite of the annulotomy (**d**) by impacting the cancellous bone allograft chips with a mallet through a funnel system consisting of a tubular retractor with a conical attachment and an impactor (large top left panel).

A total of 29 patients, 16 of which were male, and another 13 were female were included [175]. All patients were determined to have a vacuum end-stage degenerative intervertebral disc either on preoperative imaging studies, or during a previous endoscopic transforaminal discectomy procedure. The PRP enhanced allograft interbody fusion was performed with the inside-out technique. Cancellous allograft chips enriched with bone marrow concentrate and activated platelet-derived growth factor (PRP) served as an interbody fusion graft. Fifteen to 30 cc of autologous bone marrow was extracted from the patient's iliac crest using two syringes to extract the same amount of bone marrow tissue from the patient's iliac crest typically containing an average of ~200,000/μL.

This PRP enriched allograft was placed and compacted into the intervertebral disc space starting on the far-side opposite of the annulotomy by impacting the cancellous bone allograft chips with a mallet through a funnel system consisting of a tubular retractor with a conical attachment and an impactor. Care was taken to avoid any voids in the bone graft deposit to minimize postoperative graft resorption or dislodgement from the disc space. Before removal of the working cannula from the triangular safe zone, the impacted bone graft was inspected to ascertain that no graft was protruding beyond the annulotomy site or was dislodged between the exiting or traversing nerve root.

The average age was 53.48 years ranging from 31 to 78 years of age. The average follow-up was 33.41 months ranging from 24 to 43 months. The interbody fusion was evaluated using the Brantigan, Steffee, Fraser – BSF – classification [177]. A BSF-1:grade was assigned if there was a collapse of the graft, loss of disc height, vertebral slip, significant resorption of the bone graft, or lucency suggesting pseudarthrosis. A BSF-2 grade was given if radiographic imaging showed lucency within the compacted allograft spacer but solid bone growing connecting the vertebral endplate. A BSF-3 grade was assigned if bony bridges were noted in at least half of the fusion area with a similar density achieved initially during the endoscopic interbody fusion surgery. Radiographical fusion through half of the fusion area is considered to be mechanically solid fusion, even if there is lucency on the opposite side.

Outcomes were favorable with a mean VAS score reduction of 5.72 and ODI reductions of 43.34. The Macnab ranking was also reduced by 1.69 grades at the final follow up [175]. These reductions were statistically significant ($p < 0.0001$). Preoperatively 69% of patients ranked themselves as *"Fair,"* and 31% as *"Poor"* according to Macnab criteria. Postoperatively, 34.5% of patients had *"Excellent,"* and 62.1% of patients had *"Good"* clinical outcomes, respectively. All improved patients experienced improvement of their claudication symptoms and mechanical back pain. The fusion was rated as BSF 2 in six and as BSF 3 in another 23 patients. Each of the 5 patients with BSF 2 had *"Excellent"* or *"Good"* outcomes according to the Macnab criteria. The authors concluded that the procedure may be a valuable adjunct to the endoscopic decompression procedure. Their fusion method appears attractive because of its simplicity, and the use of biologically active grafting material consisting of a combination of PRP and allograft cancellous chips. A large percentage of patients experienced a significant resolution of their symptoms even though the interbody fusion may be incomplete in most patients. This PRP augmented simplified endoscopically assisted interbody fusion provides patients with good pain relief after a short convalescence period without serious short, or unmanageable long-term complications [175].

DISCUSSION

Pain caused by degenerative disc disease generates the highest health costs for society, estimated only in the US between $19.6 and $118.8 billion [178]. Various studies have characterized the biochemical pathways and the biomechanical forces involved in the intervertebral disc, raising theories about the relationship between structure, functionality, and damage [179 - 181]. Regenerative medicine applications in the spine are already here. The PRP-based technologies and cell-based therapies have successfully demonstrated the efficacy of disc regeneration treatments or enhanced fusion in humans. These treatments have employed various cell types, including those obtained from both homologous (disc) and non-homologous sources (*e.g.*, knee cartilage, adipose tissue). They have used both autologous and allogeneic approaches. Some examples of these results are those provided by an Australian company that has shown promising results using immunoselected adipose tissue-derived mesenchymal stem cells (MSC) injected into patients' discs, generating pain relief and improving the water content in the treated discs compared to controls [182 - 184]. It has currently reached an agreement with a legacy healthcare company to commercialize this product in Europe and the Americas. It is in phase III clinical trials comparing it to spinal fusion.

Another example is the use of modified cells from adult disc tissue from a US company. It also is carrying out clinical trials of the candidate product IDCT (injectable discogenic cell therapy). This injectable contains a mixture of specialized therapeutic progenitor cells engineered from donated adult disc tissue, or "discogenic" cells, and a carrier material. Promising data in animals suggests a potential therapeutic benefit of IDCT, including improved disc height and normalization of disc architecture. Hydrogel based therapies already in clinical use in treating knee articular cartilage defects in combination with autologous disc chondrocytes are also under investigation.

The majority of regenerative therapies still produce suboptimal outcomes because they do not fulfill the three criteria of Zeckser *et al.* discussed earlier in this chapter [56]. A systematic review of 53 manuscripts of MSC use in the treatment of spinal cord injury, intervertebral disc repair, and spinal fusion demonstrated regeneration in both mice and rats following the injections of MSCs [74]. Another study demonstrated regeneration following bone marrow MSCs implanted into the tail discs of rodents, which resulted in the proliferation of nucleus pulposus cells, an increase in disc height, and a decreased concentration of MSCs for four weeks post-injection [185]. However, none of these studies have met the clinical application threshold, except for MSCs derived from umbilical cords. These were safely transplanted into patients, resulting in decreased pain and improved lumbar function [186]. Wang *et al.* demonstrated that MSCs derived from 4 origins (nucleus pulposus, annulus fibrosus, cartilage endplate, and bone marrow) showed similar capabilities to differentiate into the appropriate cell required for intervertebral disc regeneration [187]. Long-term studies of MSC intradiscal therapy are being conducted, but at this time, the most significant duration of study length is 24 months. Noriega *et al.* found that injection of 25 x 1010 allogeneic cells per disc segment achieved faster and more significant improvement than controls [188]. Allogeneic MSCs should be considered for patient comfort, procedural convenience, and stem cell deficiency cases. Pettine *et al.* showed that of 26 surgical candidates for spinal fusion or disc replacement surgery, 24 (92%) were able to avoid surgery for 12 months, and 21 patients (81%) were able to avoid surgery by two years following intradiscal bone marrow mesenchymal cell implantation [128, 189]. While no patient worsened, some improved on the MRI-based Pfirrmann grading system.

CONCLUSION

Currently, the PRP technology is closest to routine clinical use. It is used combined with other bone grafts or extenders in spinal fusion and other regenerative applications of the spine. The authors present their clinical experience with the PRP technology in enhanced clinical outcomes with the endoscopic stand-alone interbody fusion procedure in the elderly. The simplification of spinal decompression and fusion is the stepping stone to future regenerative spine care, which will likely change clinical practice standards widely accepted today.

CONSENT FOR PUBLICATION

Not applicable.

CONFLICT OF INTEREST

The authors declare no conflict of interest, financial or otherwise.

ACKNOWLEDGEMENT

Declared none.

REFERENCES

[1]   Everts PA, van Erp A, DeSimone A, Cohen DS, Gardner RD. Platelet rich plasma in orthopedic surgical medicine. Platelets 2021; 32(2): 163-74.
       [http://dx.doi.org/10.1080/09537104.2020.1869717] [PMID: 33400591]

[2]   Bowers RL, Troyer WD, Mason RA, Mautner KR. Biologics. Tech Vasc Interv Radiol 2020; 23(4): 100704.
       [http://dx.doi.org/10.1016/j.tvir.2020.100704] [PMID: 33308583]

[3]   Bąkowski P, Kaszyński J, Wałecka J, Ciemniewska-Gorzela K, Bąkowska-Żywicka K, Piontek T. Autologous adipose tissue injection *versus* platelet-rich plasma (PRP) injection in the treatment of knee osteoarthritis: a randomized, controlled study - study protocol. BMC Musculoskelet Disord 2020; 21(1): 314.
       [http://dx.doi.org/10.1186/s12891-020-03345-8] [PMID: 32434498]

[4]   Noback PC, Donnelley CA, Yeatts NC, Parisien RL, Fleischli JE, Ahmad CS, *et al.* Utilization of orthobiologics by sports medicine physicians: a survey-based study. J Am Acad Orthop Surg Glob Res Rev 2021; 5(1): e20.00185.

[5]   Seow D, Shimozono Y, Tengku Yusof TNB, Yasui Y, Massey A, Kennedy JG. Platelet-rich plasma injection for the treatment of hamstring injuries: a systematic review and meta-analysis with best-worst case analysis. Am J Sports Med 2020; 363546520916729.
       [PMID: 32427520]

[6]   A Hamid MS, Hussein KH, Helmi Salim AM, *et al.* Study protocol for a double-blind, randomised placebo-controlled trial evaluating clinical effects of platelet-rich plasma injection for acute grade-2 hamstring tear among high performance athletes. BMJ Open 2020; 10(8): e039105.
       [http://dx.doi.org/10.1136/bmjopen-2020-039105] [PMID: 32820000]

[7]   Makaram NS, Murray IR, Rodeo SA, *et al.* The use of biologics in professional and Olympic sport: a scoping review protocol. Bone Jt Open 2020; 1(11): 715-9.
       [http://dx.doi.org/10.1302/2633-1462.111.BJO-2020-0159] [PMID: 33241221]

[8]   Lee KY, Baker HP, Hanaoka CM, Tjong VK, Terry MA. Treatment of patellar and hamstring tendinopathy with platelet-rich plasma in varsity collegiate athletes: A case series. J Orthop 2019; 18: 91-4.
       [http://dx.doi.org/10.1016/j.jor.2019.10.007] [PMID: 32189891]

[9]   Bradley JP, Lawyer TJ, Ruef S, Towers JD, Arner JW. Platelet-rich plasma shortens return to play in national football league players with acute hamstring injuries. Orthop J Sports Med 2020; 8(4): 2325967120911731.
       [http://dx.doi.org/10.1177/2325967120911731] [PMID: 32341927]

[10]   Conant BJ, German NA, David SL. The use of platelet-rich plasma for conservative treatment of partial ulnar collateral ligament tears in overhead athletes: a critically appraised topic. J Sport Rehabil 2019; 29(4): 509-14.
       [http://dx.doi.org/10.1123/jsr.2018-0174] [PMID: 31653802]

[11]   Chauhan A, McQueen P, Chalmers PN, *et al.* Nonoperative treatment of elbow ulnar collateral ligament injuries with and without platelet-rich plasma in professional baseball players: a comparative and matched cohort analysis. Am J Sports Med 2019; 47(13): 3107-19.
       [http://dx.doi.org/10.1177/0363546519876305] [PMID: 31589470]

[12]   Dregala RC, Uribe Y, Bodor M. Human mesenchymal stem cells respond differentially to platelet preparations and synthesize hyaluronic acid in nucleus pulposus extracellular matrix. Spine J 2020; 20(11): 1850-60.
       [http://dx.doi.org/10.1016/j.spinee.2020.06.011] [PMID: 32565315]

[13]   Shehadi JA, Elzein SM, Beery P, Spalding MC, Pershing M. Combined administration of platelet rich plasma and autologous bone marrow aspirate concentrate for spinal cord injury: a descriptive case series. Neural Regen Res 2021; 16(2): 362-6.

[http://dx.doi.org/10.4103/1673-5374.290903] [PMID: 32859799]

[14] Wu TJ, Hung CY, Lee CW, Lam S, Clark TB, Chang KV. Ultrasound-guided lumbar intradiscal injection for discogenic pain: technical innovation and presentation of two cases. J Pain Res 2020; 13: 1103-7.
[http://dx.doi.org/10.2147/JPR.S253047] [PMID: 32547174]

[15] Ruiz-Lopez R, Tsai YC. A randomized double-blind controlled pilot study comparing leucocyte-rich platelet-rich plasma and corticosteroid in caudal epidural injection for complex chronic degenerative spinal pain. Pain Pract 2020; 20(6): 639-46.
[http://dx.doi.org/10.1111/papr.12893] [PMID: 32255266]

[16] Liu W, Xie X, Wu J. Platelet-rich plasma promotes spinal ligament healing after injury. Clin Lab 2020; 66(7).
[http://dx.doi.org/10.7754/Clin.Lab.2019.191154] [PMID: 32658438]

[17] Wolff M, Shillington JM, Rathbone C, Piasecki SK, Barnes B. Injections of concentrated bone marrow aspirate as treatment for Discogenic pain: a retrospective analysis. BMC Musculoskelet Disord 2020; 21(1): 135.
[http://dx.doi.org/10.1186/s12891-020-3126-7] [PMID: 32111220]

[18] Wallace P, Bezjian Wallace L, Tamura S, Prochnio K, Morgan K, Hemler D. Effectiveness of ultrasound-guided platelet-rich plasma injections in relieving sacroiliac joint dysfunction. Am J Phys Med Rehabil 2020; 99(8): 689-93.
[http://dx.doi.org/10.1097/PHM.0000000000001389] [PMID: 31972616]

[19] Sussman WI, Jerome MA, Foster L. Platelet-rich plasma for the treatment of coccydynia: a case report and review of regenerative medicine for coccydynia. Regen Med 2019; 14(12): 1151-4.
[http://dx.doi.org/10.2217/rme-2019-0102] [PMID: 31960759]

[20] Borrione P, Gianfrancesco AD, Pereira MT, Pigozzi F. Platelet-rich plasma in muscle healing. Am J Phys Med Rehabil 2010; 89(10): 854-61.
[http://dx.doi.org/10.1097/PHM.0b013e3181f1c1c7] [PMID: 20855985]

[21] Zhang J, Liu Z, Tang J, *et al.* Fibroblast growth factor 2-induced human amniotic mesenchymal stem cells combined with autologous platelet rich plasma augmented tendon-to-bone healing. J Orthop Translat 2020; 24: 155-65.
[http://dx.doi.org/10.1016/j.jot.2020.01.003] [PMID: 33101966]

[22] Hexter AT, Sanghani-Kerai A, Heidari N, *et al.* Mesenchymal stromal cells and platelet-rich plasma promote tendon allograft healing in ovine anterior cruciate ligament reconstruction. Knee Surg Sports Traumatol Arthrosc 2020; 29(11): 3678-88.
[PMID: 33331973]

[23] Hurley ET, Colasanti CA, Anil U, Luthringer TA, Alaia MJ, Campbell KA, *et al.* The effect of platelet-rich plasma leukocyte concentration on arthroscopic rotator cuff repair: a network meta-analysis of randomized controlled trials. Am J Sports Med 2020; 363546520975435.
[PMID: 33332160]

[24] Harrison P, Didembourg M, Wood A, Devi A, Dinsdale R, Hazeldine J, *et al.* Characteristics of L-PRP preparations for treating Achilles tendon rupture within the PATH-2 study. Platelets 2020; 1-7.
[PMID: 33242293]

[25] Gleich J, Milz S, Ockert B. Principles of tendon healing at the shoulder and consequences for their treatment: Importance of platelet-rich plasma and regenerative medicine. Unfallchirurg 2020; 124(2): 89-95.

[26] Alves R, Grimalt R. A review of platelet-rich plasma: history, biology, mechanism of action, and classification. Skin Appendage Disord 2018; 4(1): 18-24.
[http://dx.doi.org/10.1159/000477353] [PMID: 29457008]

[27] Akbas F, Ozdemir B, Bahtiyar N, Arkan H, Onaran I. Platelet-rich plasma and platelet-derived lipid

factors induce different and similar gene expression responses for selected genes related to wound healing in rat dermal wound environment. Mol Biol Res Commun 2020; 9(4): 145-53.
[PMID: 33344661]

[28]   Arora G, Arora S. Platelet-rich plasma-Where do we stand today? A critical narrative review and analysis. Dermatol Ther 2021; 34(1): e14343.
[http://dx.doi.org/10.1111/dth.14343] [PMID: 32979292]

[29]   Qian Z, Wang H, Bai Y, *et al.* Improving chronic diabetic wound healing through an injectable and self-healing hydrogel with platelet-rich plasma release. ACS Appl Mater Interfaces 2020; 12(50): 55659-74.
[http://dx.doi.org/10.1021/acsami.0c17142] [PMID: 33327053]

[30]   Nurden AT. Platelets, inflammation and tissue regeneration. Thromb Haemost 2011; 105 (Suppl. 1): S13-33.
[http://dx.doi.org/10.1160/THS10-11-0720] [PMID: 21479340]

[31]   Andia I, Abate M. Platelet-rich plasma: combinational treatment modalities for musculoskeletal conditions. Front Med 2018; 12(2): 139-52.
[http://dx.doi.org/10.1007/s11684-017-0551-6] [PMID: 29058255]

[32]   Dai WL, Zhou AG, Zhang H, Zhang J. Efficacy of platelet-rich plasma in the treatment of knee osteoarthritis: a meta-analysis of randomized controlled trials. Arthroscopy 2017; 33(3): 659-670.e1.
[http://dx.doi.org/10.1016/j.arthro.2016.09.024] [PMID: 28012636]

[33]   Fitzpatrick J, Bulsara M, Zheng MH. The effectiveness of platelet-rich plasma in the treatment of tendinopathy: a meta-analysis of randomized controlled clinical trials. Am J Sports Med 2017; 45(1): 226-33.
[http://dx.doi.org/10.1177/0363546516643716] [PMID: 27268111]

[34]   Sheth U, Dwyer T, Smith I, *et al.* Does platelet-rich plasma lead to earlier return to sport when compared with conservative treatment in acute muscle injuries? a systematic review and meta-analysis. Arthroscopy 2018; 34(1): 281-288.e1.
[http://dx.doi.org/10.1016/j.arthro.2017.06.039] [PMID: 28800920]

[35]   Martinez-Zapata MJ, Martí-Carvajal AJ, Solà I, *et al.* Autologous platelet-rich plasma for treating chronic wounds. Cochrane Database Syst Rev 2016; (5): CD006899.
[http://dx.doi.org/10.1002/14651858.CD006899.pub3] [PMID: 27223580]

[36]   Rachul C, Rasko JEJ, Caulfield T. Implicit hype? Representations of platelet rich plasma in the news media. PLoS One 2017; 12(8): e0182496.
[http://dx.doi.org/10.1371/journal.pone.0182496] [PMID: 28792974]

[37]   Dohan Ehrenfest DM, Bielecki T, Mishra A, *et al.* In search of a consensus terminology in the field of platelet concentrates for surgical use: platelet-rich plasma (PRP), platelet-rich fibrin (PRF), fibrin gel polymerization and leukocytes. Curr Pharm Biotechnol 2012; 13(7): 1131-7.
[http://dx.doi.org/10.2174/138920112800624328] [PMID: 21740379]

[38]   Dohan Ehrenfest DM, Andia I, Zumstein MA, Zhang CQ, Pinto NR, Bielecki T. Classification of platelet concentrates (Platelet-Rich Plasma-PRP, Platelet-Rich Fibrin-PRF) for topical and infiltrative use in orthopedic and sports medicine: current consensus, clinical implications and perspectives. Muscles Ligaments Tendons J 2014; 4(1): 3-9.
[http://dx.doi.org/10.32098/mltj.01.2014.02] [PMID: 24932440]

[39]   Mishra A, Harmon K, Woodall J, Vieira A. Sports medicine applications of platelet rich plasma. Curr Pharm Biotechnol 2012; 13(7): 1185-95.
[http://dx.doi.org/10.2174/138920112800624283] [PMID: 21740373]

[40]   De Pascale MR, Sommese L, Casamassimi A, Napoli C. Platelet derivatives in regenerative medicine: an update. Transfus Med Rev 2015; 29(1): 52-61.
[http://dx.doi.org/10.1016/j.tmrv.2014.11.001] [PMID: 25544600]

[41] Dohan Ehrenfest DM, Rasmusson L, Albrektsson T. Classification of platelet concentrates: from pure platelet-rich plasma (P-PRP) to leucocyte- and platelet-rich fibrin (L-PRF). Trends Biotechnol 2009; 27(3): 158-67.
[http://dx.doi.org/10.1016/j.tibtech.2008.11.009] [PMID: 19187989]

[42] Magalon J, Chateau AL, Bertrand B, *et al.* DEPA classification: a proposal for standardising PRP use and a retrospective application of available devices. BMJ Open Sport Exerc Med 2016; 2(1): e000060.
[http://dx.doi.org/10.1136/bmjsem-2015-000060] [PMID: 27900152]

[43] D'asta F, Halstead F, Harrison P, Zecchi Orlandini S, Moiemen N, Lord J. The contribution of leucocytes to the antimicrobial activity of platelet-rich plasma preparations: A systematic review. Platelets 2018; 29(1): 9-20.
[http://dx.doi.org/10.1080/09537104.2017.1317731] [PMID: 28681651]

[44] Chahla J, Cinque ME, Piuzzi NS, *et al.* A call for standardization in platelet-rich plasma preparation protocols and composition reporting: a systematic review of the clinical orthopaedic literature. J Bone Joint Surg Am 2017; 99(20): 1769-79.
[http://dx.doi.org/10.2106/JBJS.16.01374] [PMID: 29040132]

[45] Murray IR, Geeslin AG, Goudie EB, Petrigliano FA, LaPrade RF. Minimum information for studies evaluating biologics in orthopaedics (MIBO): Platelet-rich plasma and mesenchymal stem cells. J Bone Joint Surg Am 2017; 99(10): 809-19.
[http://dx.doi.org/10.2106/JBJS.16.00793] [PMID: 28509821]

[46] Caiado A, Ferreira-Dos-Santos G, Gonçalves S, Horta L, Soares Branco P. Proposal of a new standardized freeze-thawing technical protocol for leucocyte-poor platelet-rich plasma preparation and cryopreservation. Cureus 2020; 12(7): e8997-e.
[http://dx.doi.org/10.7759/cureus.8997]

[47] Maynard DM, Heijnen HF, Horne MK, White JG, Gahl WA. Proteomic analysis of platelet *alpha*-granules using mass spectrometry. J Thromb Haemost 2007; 5(9): 1945-55.
[http://dx.doi.org/10.1111/j.1538-7836.2007.02690.x] [PMID: 17723134]

[48] Maguire PB, Wynne KJ, Harney DF, O'Donoghue NM, Stephens G, Fitzgerald DJ. Identification of the phosphotyrosine proteome from thrombin activated platelets. Proteomics 2002; 2(6): 642-8.
[http://dx.doi.org/10.1002/1615-9861(200206)2:6<642::AID-PROT642>3.0.CO;2-I] [PMID: 12112843]

[49] García A, Prabhakar S, Hughan S, *et al.* Differential proteome analysis of TRAP-activated platelets: involvement of DOK-2 and phosphorylation of RGS proteins. Blood 2004; 103(6): 2088-95.
[http://dx.doi.org/10.1182/blood-2003-07-2392] [PMID: 14645010]

[50] Harmon KG, Rao AL. The use of platelet-rich plasma in the nonsurgical management of sports injuries: hype or hope? Hematology (Am Soc Hematol Educ Program) 2013; 2013: 620-6.
[http://dx.doi.org/10.1182/asheducation-2013.1.620] [PMID: 24319241]

[51] Fitzpatrick J, Bulsara MK, McCrory PR, Richardson MD, Zheng MH. Analysis of platelet-rich plasma extraction: variations in platelet and blood components between 4 common commercial kits. Orthop J Sports Med 2017; 5(1): 2325967116675272.
[http://dx.doi.org/10.1177/2325967116675272] [PMID: 28210651]

[52] Lee HW, Choi K-H, Kim J-Y, *et al.* Proteomic classification and identification of proteins related to tissue healing of platelet-rich plasma . Clin Orthop Surg 2020; 12(1): 120-9.
[http://dx.doi.org/10.4055/cios.2020.12.1.120] [PMID: 32117548]

[53] Carbon S, Ireland A, Mungall CJ, Shu S, Marshall B, Lewis S. AmiGO: online access to ontology and annotation data. Bioinformatics 2009; 25(2): 288-9.
[http://dx.doi.org/10.1093/bioinformatics/btn615] [PMID: 19033274]

[54] Graziani F, Ivanovski S, Cei S, Ducci F, Tonetti M, Gabriele M. The *in vitro* effect of different PRP concentrations on osteoblasts and fibroblasts. Clin Oral Implants Res 2006; 17(2): 212-9.

[http://dx.doi.org/10.1111/j.1600-0501.2005.01203.x] [PMID: 16584418]

[55]   Manini DR, Shega FD, Guo C, Wang Y. Role of platelet-rich plasma in spinal fusion surgery: systematic review and meta-analysis. Adv Orthop 2020; 2020: 8361798.
[http://dx.doi.org/10.1155/2020/8361798] [PMID: 32455028]

[56]   Zeckser J, Wolff M, Tucker J, Goodwin J. Multipotent mesenchymal stem cell treatment for discogenic low back pain and disc degeneration. Stem Cells Int 2016; 2016: 3908389.
[http://dx.doi.org/10.1155/2016/3908389] [PMID: 26880958]

[57]   Berebichez-Fridman R, Montero-Olvera PR. Sources and clinical applications of mesenchymal stem cells: state-of-the-art review. Sultan Qaboos Univ Med J 2018; 18(3): e264-77.
[http://dx.doi.org/10.18295/squmj.2018.18.03.002] [PMID: 30607265]

[58]   Ding DC, Shyu WC, Lin SZ. Mesenchymal stem cells. Cell Transplant 2011; 20(1): 5-14.
[http://dx.doi.org/10.3727/096368910X] [PMID: 21396235]

[59]   Samsonraj RM, Raghunath M, Nurcombe V, Hui JH, van Wijnen AJ, Cool SM. Concise review: multifaceted characterization of human mesenchymal stem cells for use in regenerative medicine. Stem Cells Transl Med 2017; 6(12): 2173-85.
[http://dx.doi.org/10.1002/sctm.17-0129] [PMID: 29076267]

[60]   Fu X, Liu G, Halim A, Ju Y, Luo Q, Song AG. Mesenchymal stem cell migration and tissue repair. Cells 2019; 8(8): E784.
[http://dx.doi.org/10.3390/cells8080784] [PMID: 31357692]

[61]   Li N, Hua J. Interactions between mesenchymal stem cells and the immune system. Cell Mol Life Sci 2017; 74(13): 2345-60.
[http://dx.doi.org/10.1007/s00018-017-2473-5] [PMID: 28214990]

[62]   Lv FJ, Tuan RS, Cheung KM, Leung VY. Concise review: the surface markers and identity of human mesenchymal stem cells. Stem Cells 2014; 32(6): 1408-19.
[http://dx.doi.org/10.1002/stem.1681] [PMID: 24578244]

[63]   Mushahary D, Spittler A, Kasper C, Weber V, Charwat V. Isolation, cultivation, and characterization of human mesenchymal stem cells. Cytometry A 2018; 93(1): 19-31.
[http://dx.doi.org/10.1002/cyto.a.23242] [PMID: 29072818]

[64]   Uccelli A, Moretta L, Pistoia V. Mesenchymal stem cells in health and disease. Nat Rev Immunol 2008; 8(9): 726-36.
[http://dx.doi.org/10.1038/nri2395] [PMID: 19172693]

[65]   Gomzikova MO, James V, Rizvanov AA. Therapeutic application of mesenchymal stem cells derived extracellular vesicles for immunomodulation. Front Immunol 2019; 10: 2663.
[http://dx.doi.org/10.3389/fimmu.2019.02663] [PMID: 31849929]

[66]   Mazini L, Rochette L, Amine M, Malka G. Regenerative capacity of Adipose Derived Stem Cells (ADSCs), comparison with Mesenchymal Stem Cells (MSCs). Int J Mol Sci 2019; 20(10): E2523.
[http://dx.doi.org/10.3390/ijms20102523] [PMID: 31121953]

[67]   Murphy MB, Moncivais K, Caplan AI. Mesenchymal stem cells: environmentally responsive therapeutics for regenerative medicine. Exp Mol Med 2013; 45(11): e54.
[http://dx.doi.org/10.1038/emm.2013.94] [PMID: 24232253]

[68]   Song Y, Du H, Dai C, *et al.* Human adipose-derived mesenchymal stem cells for osteoarthritis: a pilot study with long-term follow-up and repeated injections. Regen Med 2018; 13(3): 295-307.
[http://dx.doi.org/10.2217/rme-2017-0152] [PMID: 29417902]

[69]   Vizoso FJ, Eiro N, Cid S, Schneider J, Perez-Fernandez R. Mesenchymal stem cell secretome: toward cell-free therapeutic strategies in regenerative medicine. Int J Mol Sci 2017; 18(9): E1852.
[http://dx.doi.org/10.3390/ijms18091852] [PMID: 28841158]

[70]   Caseiro AR, Santos Pedrosa S, Ivanova G, *et al.* Mesenchymal stem/ stromal cells metabolomic and

bioactive factors profiles: a comparative analysis on the umbilical cord and dental pulp derived stem/stromal cells secretome. PLoS One 2019; 14(11): e0221378.
[http://dx.doi.org/10.1371/journal.pone.0221378] [PMID: 31774816]

[71] Harrell CR, Jovicic N, Djonov V, Arsenijevic N, Volarevic V. Mesenchymal stem cell-derived exosomes and other extracellular vesicles as new remedies in the therapy of inflammatory diseases. Cells 2019; 8(12): E1605.
[http://dx.doi.org/10.3390/cells8121605] [PMID: 31835680]

[72] Meyerrose T, Olson S, Pontow S, *et al.* Mesenchymal stem cells for the sustained *in vivo* delivery of bioactive factors. Adv Drug Deliv Rev 2010; 62(12): 1167-74.
[http://dx.doi.org/10.1016/j.addr.2010.09.013] [PMID: 20920540]

[73] Cheng X, Zhang G, Zhang L, *et al.* Mesenchymal stem cells deliver exogenous miR-21 *via* exosomes to inhibit nucleus pulposus cell apoptosis and reduce intervertebral disc degeneration. J Cell Mol Med 2018; 22(1): 261-76.
[http://dx.doi.org/10.1111/jcmm.13316] [PMID: 28805297]

[74] Khan S, Mafi P, Mafi R, Khan W. A systematic review of mesenchymal stem cells in spinal cord injury, intervertebral disc repair and spinal fusion. Curr Stem Cell Res Ther 2018; 13(4): 316-23.
[http://dx.doi.org/10.2174/1574888X11666170907120030] [PMID: 28891440]

[75] Liao Z, Luo R, Li G, *et al.* Exosomes from mesenchymal stem cells modulate endoplasmic reticulum stress to protect against nucleus pulposus cell death and ameliorate intervertebral disc degeneration *in vivo.* Theranostics 2019; 9(14): 4084-100.
[http://dx.doi.org/10.7150/thno.33638] [PMID: 31281533]

[76] Lu K, Li HY, Yang K, *et al.* Exosomes as potential alternatives to stem cell therapy for intervertebral disc degeneration: in-vitro study on exosomes in interaction of nucleus pulposus cells and bone marrow mesenchymal stem cells. Stem Cell Res Ther 2017; 8(1): 108.
[http://dx.doi.org/10.1186/s13287-017-0563-9] [PMID: 28486958]

[77] Richardson SM, Kalamegam G, Pushparaj PN, *et al.* Mesenchymal stem cells in regenerative medicine: Focus on articular cartilage and intervertebral disc regeneration. Methods 2016; 99: 69-80.
[http://dx.doi.org/10.1016/j.ymeth.2015.09.015] [PMID: 26384579]

[78] Tam WK, Cheung KM, Leung VY. Intervertebral disc engineering through exploiting mesenchymal stem cells: progress and perspective. Curr Stem Cell Res Ther 2016; 11(6): 505-12.
[http://dx.doi.org/10.2174/1574888X10666141126112755] [PMID: 25429703]

[79] Vadalà G, Ambrosio L, Russo F, Papalia R, Denaro V. Interaction between mesenchymal stem cells and intervertebral disc microenvironment: from cell therapy to tissue engineering. Stem Cells Int 2019; 2019: 2376172.
[http://dx.doi.org/10.1155/2019/2376172] [PMID: 32587618]

[80] Vadalà G, Russo F, Ambrosio L, Papalia R, Denaro V. Mesenchymal stem cells for intervertebral disc regeneration. J Biol Regul Homeost Agents 2016; 30(4) (Suppl. 1): 173-9.
[PMID: 28002916]

[81] Xia C, Zeng Z, Fang B, *et al.* Mesenchymal stem cell-derived exosomes ameliorate intervertebral disc degeneration *via* anti-oxidant and anti-inflammatory effects. Free Radic Biol Med 2019; 143: 1-15.
[http://dx.doi.org/10.1016/j.freeradbiomed.2019.07.026] [PMID: 31351174]

[82] Arasu UT, Kärnä R, Härkönen K, *et al.* Human mesenchymal stem cells secrete hyaluronan-coated extracellular vesicles. Matrix Biol 2017; 64: 54-68.
[http://dx.doi.org/10.1016/j.matbio.2017.05.001] [PMID: 28483644]

[83] Götting C, Prante C, Kuhn J, Kleesiek K. Proteoglycan biosynthesis during chondrogenic differentiation of mesenchymal stem cells. ScientificWorldJournal 2007; 7: 1207-10.
[http://dx.doi.org/10.1100/tsw.2007.231] [PMID: 17704854]

[84] Narakornsak S, Poovachiranon N, Peerapapong L, Pothacharoen P, Aungsuchawan S. Mesenchymal

stem cells differentiated into chondrocyte-Like cells. Acta Histochem 2016; 118(4): 418-29.
[http://dx.doi.org/10.1016/j.acthis.2016.04.004] [PMID: 27087049]

[85] Heck BE, Park JJ, Makani V, Kim EC, Kim DH. PPAR-δ agonist with mesenchymal stem cells induces type II collagen-producing chondrocytes in human arthritic synovial fluid. Cell Transplant 2017; 26(8): 1405-17.
[http://dx.doi.org/10.1177/0963689717720278] [PMID: 28901183]

[86] Hsueh CM, Lin HM, Tseng TY, Huang YD, Lee HS, Dong CY. Dynamic observation and quantification of type I/II collagen in chondrogenesis of mesenchymal stem cells by second-order susceptibility microscopy. J Biophotonics 2019; 12(2): e201800097.
[http://dx.doi.org/10.1002/jbio.201800097] [PMID: 29920965]

[87] Qi L, Wang R, Shi Q, Yuan M, Jin M, Li D. Umbilical cord mesenchymal stem cell conditioned medium restored the expression of collagen II and aggrecan in nucleus pulposus mesenchymal stem cells exposed to high glucose. J Bone Miner Metab 2019; 37(3): 455-66.
[http://dx.doi.org/10.1007/s00774-018-0953-9] [PMID: 30187277]

[88] Cao C, Zou J, Liu X, et al. Bone marrow mesenchymal stem cells slow intervertebral disc degeneration through the NF-κB pathway. Spine J 2015; 15(3): 530-8.
[http://dx.doi.org/10.1016/j.spinee.2014.11.021] [PMID: 25457469]

[89] Perez-Cruet M, Beeravolu N, McKee C, et al. Potential of human nucleus pulposus-like cells derived from umbilical cord to treat degenerative disc disease. Neurosurgery 2019; 84(1): 272-83.
[http://dx.doi.org/10.1093/neuros/nyy012] [PMID: 29490072]

[90] Urits I, Capuco A, Sharma M, et al. Stem cell therapies for treatment of discogenic low back pain: a comprehensive review. Curr Pain Headache Rep 2019; 23(9): 65.
[http://dx.doi.org/10.1007/s11916-019-0804-y] [PMID: 31359164]

[91] Wei A, Shen B, Williams L, Diwan A. Mesenchymal stem cells: potential application in intervertebral disc regeneration. Transl Pediatr 2014; 3(2): 71-90.
[PMID: 26835326]

[92] Xia K, Gong Z, Zhu J, et al. Differentiation of pluripotent stem cells into nucleus pulposus progenitor cells for intervertebral disc regeneration. Curr Stem Cell Res Ther 2019; 14(1): 57-64.
[http://dx.doi.org/10.2174/1574888X13666180918095121] [PMID: 30227822]

[93] Zhao Y, Qin Y, Wu S, et al. Mesenchymal stem cells regulate inflammatory milieu within degenerative nucleus pulposus cells via p38 MAPK pathway. Exp Ther Med 2020; 20(5): 22.
[http://dx.doi.org/10.3892/etm.2020.9150] [PMID: 32934687]

[94] Chen S, Cui G, Peng C, et al. Transplantation of adipose-derived mesenchymal stem cells attenuates pulmonary fibrosis of silicosis via anti-inflammatory and anti-apoptosis effects in rats. Stem Cell Res Ther 2018; 9(1): 110.
[http://dx.doi.org/10.1186/s13287-018-0846-9] [PMID: 29673394]

[95] Liu H, Li D, Zhang Y, Li M. Inflammation, mesenchymal stem cells and bone regeneration. Histochem Cell Biol 2018; 149(4): 393-404.
[http://dx.doi.org/10.1007/s00418-018-1643-3] [PMID: 29435765]

[96] Danišovič L, Varga I, Polák S. Growth factors and chondrogenic differentiation of mesenchymal stem cells. Tissue Cell 2012; 44(2): 69-73.
[http://dx.doi.org/10.1016/j.tice.2011.11.005] [PMID: 22185680]

[97] Endo K, Fujita N, Nakagawa T, Nishimura R. Comparison of the effect of growth factors on chondrogenesis of canine mesenchymal stem cells. J Vet Med Sci 2019; 81(8): 1211-8.
[http://dx.doi.org/10.1292/jvms.18-0551] [PMID: 31167981]

[98] Gilevich IV, Fedorenko TV, Pashkova IA, Porkhanov VA, Chekhonin VP. Effects of growth factors on mobilization of mesenchymal stem cells. Bull Exp Biol Med 2017; 162(5): 684-6.
[http://dx.doi.org/10.1007/s10517-017-3687-0] [PMID: 28361423]

[99]   Sinclair KL, Mafi P, Mafi R, Khan WS. The use of growth factors and mesenchymal stem cells in orthopaedics: in particular, their use in fractures and non-unions: a systematic review. Curr Stem Cell Res Ther 2017; 12(4): 312-25.
[http://dx.doi.org/10.2174/1574888X11666160614104500] [PMID: 27306399]

[100]   Mang T, Kleinschmidt-Dörr K, Ploeger F, Lindemann S, Gigout A. The GDF-5 mutant M1673 exerts robust anabolic and anti-catabolic effects in chondrocytes. J Cell Mol Med 2020; 24(13): 7141-50.
[http://dx.doi.org/10.1111/jcmm.15149] [PMID: 32497388]

[101]   Niada S, Giannasi C, Gomarasca M, Stanco D, Casati S, Brini AT. Adipose-derived stromal cell secretome reduces TNFα-induced hypertrophy and catabolic markers in primary human articular chondrocytes. Stem Cell Res (Amst) 2019; 38: 101463.
[http://dx.doi.org/10.1016/j.scr.2019.101463] [PMID: 31108390]

[102]   Bessa-Gonçalves M, Silva AM, Brás JP, *et al.* Fibrinogen and magnesium combination biomaterials modulate macrophage phenotype, NF-kB signaling and crosstalk with mesenchymal stem/stromal cells. Acta Biomater 2020; 114: 471-84.
[http://dx.doi.org/10.1016/j.actbio.2020.07.028] [PMID: 32688091]

[103]   Chaudhuri O, Cooper-White J, Janmey PA, Mooney DJ, Shenoy VB. Effects of extracellular matrix viscoelasticity on cellular behaviour. Nature 2020; 584(7822): 535-46.
[http://dx.doi.org/10.1038/s41586-020-2612-2] [PMID: 32848221]

[104]   Pinho S, Frenette PS. Haematopoietic stem cell activity and interactions with the niche. Nat Rev Mol Cell Biol 2019; 20(5): 303-20.
[http://dx.doi.org/10.1038/s41580-019-0103-9] [PMID: 30745579]

[105]   Wang X, Shah FA, Vazirisani F, *et al.* Exosomes influence the behavior of human mesenchymal stem cells on titanium surfaces. Biomaterials 2020; 230: 119571.
[http://dx.doi.org/10.1016/j.biomaterials.2019.119571] [PMID: 31753474]

[106]   Xin S, Gregory CA, Alge DL. Interplay between degradability and integrin signaling on mesenchymal stem cell function within poly(ethylene glycol) based microporous annealed particle hydrogels. Acta Biomater 2020; 101: 227-36.
[http://dx.doi.org/10.1016/j.actbio.2019.11.009] [PMID: 31711899]

[107]   Dabrowska S, Andrzejewska A, Lukomska B, Janowski M. Neuroinflammation as a target for treatment of stroke using mesenchymal stem cells and extracellular vesicles. J Neuroinflammation 2019; 16(1): 178.
[http://dx.doi.org/10.1186/s12974-019-1571-8] [PMID: 31514749]

[108]   Duan Y, Li X, Zuo X, *et al.* Migration of endothelial cells and mesenchymal stem cells into hyaluronic acid hydrogels with different moduli under induction of pro-inflammatory macrophages. J Mater Chem B Mater Biol Med 2019; 7(36): 5478-89.
[http://dx.doi.org/10.1039/C9TB01126A] [PMID: 31415053]

[109]   Ye F, Jiang J, Zong C, *et al.* Sirt1-overexpressing mesenchymal stem cells drive the anti-tumor effect through their pro-inflammatory capacity. Mol Ther 2020; 28(3): 874-88.
[http://dx.doi.org/10.1016/j.ymthe.2020.01.018] [PMID: 32027844]

[110]   Zheng J, Zhu L, Iok In I, Chen Y, Jia N, Zhu W. Bone marrow-derived mesenchymal stem cells-secreted exosomal microRNA-192-5p delays inflammatory response in rheumatoid arthritis. Int Immunopharmacol 2020; 78: 105985.
[http://dx.doi.org/10.1016/j.intimp.2019.105985] [PMID: 31776092]

[111]   Lehmann TP, Jakub G, Harasymczuk J, Jagodziński PP. Transforming growth factor β mediates communication of co-cultured human nucleus pulposus cells and mesenchymal stem cells. J Orthop Res 2018; 36(11): 3023-32.
[http://dx.doi.org/10.1002/jor.24106] [PMID: 29999195]

[112]   Smith LJ, Gorth DJ, Showalter BL, *et al. in vitro* characterization of a stem-cell-seeded triple-

interpenetrating-network hydrogel for functional regeneration of the nucleus pulposus. Tissue Eng Part A 2014; 20(13-14): 1841-9.
[http://dx.doi.org/10.1089/ten.tea.2013.0516] [PMID: 24410394]

[113] Hua J, Shen N, Wang J, *et al.* Small molecule-based strategy promotes nucleus pulposus specific differentiation of adipose-derived mesenchymal stem cells. Mol Cells 2019; 42(9): 661-71.
[PMID: 31564076]

[114] Gnecchi M, Danieli P, Malpasso G, Ciuffreda MC. Paracrine mechanisms of mesenchymal stem cells in tissue repair. Methods Mol Biol 2016; 1416: 123-46.
[http://dx.doi.org/10.1007/978-1-4939-3584-0_7] [PMID: 27236669]

[115] Viswanathan S, Shi Y, Galipeau J, *et al.* Mesenchymal stem *versus* stromal cells: International Society for Cell & Gene Therapy (ISCT®) Mesenchymal Stromal Cell committee position statement on nomenclature. Cytotherapy 2019; 21(10): 1019-24.
[http://dx.doi.org/10.1016/j.jcyt.2019.08.002] [PMID: 31526643]

[116] Jayaramayya K, Mahalaxmi I, Subramaniam MD, *et al.* Immunomodulatory effect of mesenchymal stem cells and mesenchymal stem-cell-derived exosomes for COVID-19 treatment. BMB Rep 2020; 53(8): 400-12.
[http://dx.doi.org/10.5483/BMBRep.2020.53.8.121] [PMID: 32731913]

[117] Nojehdehi S, Soudi S, Hesampour A, Rasouli S, Soleimani M, Hashemi SM. Immunomodulatory effects of mesenchymal stem cell-derived exosomes on experimental type-1 autoimmune diabetes. J Cell Biochem 2018; 119(11): 9433-43.
[http://dx.doi.org/10.1002/jcb.27260] [PMID: 30074271]

[118] Zhang LN, Kong CF, Zhao D, *et al.* Fusion with mesenchymal stem cells differentially affects tumorigenic and metastatic abilities of lung cancer cells. J Cell Physiol 2019; 234(4): 3570-82.
[http://dx.doi.org/10.1002/jcp.27011] [PMID: 30417342]

[119] Li C, Cheung MKH, Han S, *et al.* Mesenchymal stem cells and their mitochondrial transfer: a double-edged sword. Biosci Rep 2019; 39(5): BSR20182417.
[http://dx.doi.org/10.1042/BSR20182417] [PMID: 30979829]

[120] Paliwal S, Chaudhuri R, Agrawal A, Mohanty S. Regenerative abilities of mesenchymal stem cells through mitochondrial transfer. J Biomed Sci 2018; 25(1): 31.
[http://dx.doi.org/10.1186/s12929-018-0429-1] [PMID: 29602309]

[121] Keshtkar S, Azarpira N, Ghahremani MH. Mesenchymal stem cell-derived extracellular vesicles: novel frontiers in regenerative medicine. Stem Cell Res Ther 2018; 9(1): 63.
[http://dx.doi.org/10.1186/s13287-018-0791-7] [PMID: 29523213]

[122] Rani S, Ryan AE, Griffin MD, Ritter T. Mesenchymal stem cell-derived extracellular vesicles: toward cell-free therapeutic applications. Mol Ther 2015; 23(5): 812-23.
[http://dx.doi.org/10.1038/mt.2015.44] [PMID: 25868399]

[123] Amirdelfan K, Bae H, McJunkin T, *et al.* Allogeneic mesenchymal precursor cells treatment for chronic low back pain associated with degenerative disc disease: a prospective randomized, placebo-controlled 36-month study of safety and efficacy. Spine J 2020; 21(2): 212-30.
[PMID: 33045417]

[124] Blanco JF, Villarón EM, Pescador D, *et al.* Autologous mesenchymal stromal cells embedded in tricalcium phosphate for posterolateral spinal fusion: results of a prospective phase I/II clinical trial with long-term follow-up. Stem Cell Res Ther 2019; 10(1): 63.
[http://dx.doi.org/10.1186/s13287-019-1166-4] [PMID: 30795797]

[125] García de Frutos A, González-Tartière P, Coll Bonet R, *et al.* Randomized clinical trial: expanded autologous bone marrow mesenchymal cells combined with allogeneic bone tissue, compared with autologous iliac crest graft in lumbar fusion surgery. Spine J 2020; 20(12): 1899-910.
[http://dx.doi.org/10.1016/j.spinee.2020.07.014] [PMID: 32730985]

[126] Kumar H, Ha DH, Lee EJ, *et al.* Safety and tolerability of intradiscal implantation of combined autologous adipose-derived mesenchymal stem cells and hyaluronic acid in patients with chronic discogenic low back pain: 1-year follow-up of a phase I study. Stem Cell Res Ther 2017; 8(1): 262.
[http://dx.doi.org/10.1186/s13287-017-0710-3] [PMID: 29141662]

[127] Migliorini F, Rath B, Tingart M, Baroncini A, Quack V, Eschweiler J. Autogenic mesenchymal stem cells for intervertebral disc regeneration. Int Orthop 2019; 43(4): 1027-36.
[http://dx.doi.org/10.1007/s00264-018-4218-y] [PMID: 30415465]

[128] Pettine KA, Murphy MB, Suzuki RK, Sand TT. Percutaneous injection of autologous bone marrow concentrate cells significantly reduces lumbar discogenic pain through 12 months. Stem Cells 2015; 33(1): 146-56.
[http://dx.doi.org/10.1002/stem.1845] [PMID: 25187512]

[129] Yaghoubi Y, Movassaghpour A, Zamani M, Talebi M, Mehdizadeh A, Yousefi M. Human umbilical cord mesenchymal stem cells derived-exosomes in diseases treatment. Life Sci 2019; 233: 116733.
[http://dx.doi.org/10.1016/j.lfs.2019.116733] [PMID: 31394127]

[130] Rozier P, Maria A, Goulabchand R, Jorgensen C, Guilpain P, Noël D. Mesenchymal stem cells in systemic sclerosis: allogenic or autologous approaches for therapeutic use? Front Immunol 2018; 9: 2938.
[http://dx.doi.org/10.3389/fimmu.2018.02938] [PMID: 30619298]

[131] Navani A, Manchikanti L, Albers SL, *et al.* Responsible, safe, and effective use of biologics in the management of low back pain: American Society of Interventional Pain Physicians (ASIPP) guidelines. Pain Physician 2019; 22(1S): S1-S74.
[PMID: 30717500]

[132] Wehling P, Schulitz KP, Robbins PD, Evans CH, Reinecke JA. Transfer of genes to chondrocytic cells of the lumbar spine. Proposal for a treatment strategy of spinal disorders by local gene therapy. Spine 1997; 22(10): 1092-7.
[http://dx.doi.org/10.1097/00007632-199705150-00008] [PMID: 9160467]

[133] Nishida K, Kang JD, Suh JK, Robbins PD, Evans CH, Gilbertson LG. Adenovirus-mediated gene transfer to nucleus pulposus cells. Implications for the treatment of intervertebral disc degeneration. Spine 1998; 23(22): 2437-42.
[http://dx.doi.org/10.1097/00007632-199811150-00016] [PMID: 9836359]

[134] Liu X, Li K, Song J, Liang C, Wang X, Chen X. Efficient and stable gene expression in rabbit intervertebral disc cells transduced with a recombinant baculovirus vector. Spine 2006; 31(7): 732-5.
[http://dx.doi.org/10.1097/01.brs.0000206977.61305.43] [PMID: 16582845]

[135] Liu Y, Yu T, Ma XX, Xiang HF, Hu YG, Chen BH. Lentivirus-mediated TGF-β3, CTGF and TIMP1 gene transduction as a gene therapy for intervertebral disc degeneration in an *in vivo* rabbit model. Exp Ther Med 2016; 11(4): 1399-404.
[http://dx.doi.org/10.3892/etm.2016.3063] [PMID: 27073456]

[136] Kakutani K, Nishida K, Uno K, *et al.* Prolonged down regulation of specific gene expression in nucleus pulposus cell mediated by RNA interference *in vitro*. J Orthop Res 2006; 24(6): 1271-8.
[http://dx.doi.org/10.1002/jor.20171] [PMID: 16705690]

[137] Nishida K, Suzuki T, Kakutani K, Yurube T, Maeno K, Kurosaka M, *et al.* Gene therapy approach for disc degeneration and associated spinal disorders. Eur Spine J 2008; 17 Suppl 4(Suppl 4): 459-66.
[http://dx.doi.org/10.1007/s00586-008-0751-5]

[138] Yurube T, Ito M, Kakiuchi Y, Kuroda R, Kakutani K. Autophagy and mTOR signaling during intervertebral disc aging and degeneration. JOR Spine 2020; 3(1): e1082.
[http://dx.doi.org/10.1002/jsp2.1082] [PMID: 32211593]

[139] Yamada K, Sudo H, Iwasaki K, *et al.* Caspase 3 silencing inhibits biomechanical overload-induced intervertebral disk degeneration. Am J Pathol 2014; 184(3): 753-64.

[http://dx.doi.org/10.1016/j.ajpath.2013.11.010] [PMID: 24389166]

[140] Nishida K, Doita M, Takada T, *et al.* Sustained transgene expression in intervertebral disc cells *in vivo* mediated by microbubble-enhanced ultrasound gene therapy. Spine 2006; 31(13): 1415-9.
[http://dx.doi.org/10.1097/01.brs.0000219945.70675.dd] [PMID: 16741448]

[141] Hurlbert RJ, Alexander D, Bailey S, *et al.* rhBMP-2 for posterolateral instrumented lumbar fusion: a multicenter prospective randomized controlled trial. Spine 2013; 38(25): 2139-48.
[http://dx.doi.org/10.1097/BRS.0000000000000007] [PMID: 24296479]

[142] Bomback DA, Grauer JN, Lugo R, Troiano N, Patel TCh, Friedlaender GE. Comparison of posterolateral lumbar fusion rates of Grafton Putty and OP-1 Putty in an athymic rat model. Spine 2004; 29(15): 1612-7.
[http://dx.doi.org/10.1097/01.BRS.0000132512.53305.A1] [PMID: 15284503]

[143] Bright C, Park YS, Sieber AN, Kostuik JP, Leong KW. *In vivo* evaluation of plasmid DNA encoding OP-1 protein for spine fusion. Spine 2006; 31(19): 2163-72.
[http://dx.doi.org/10.1097/01.brs.0000232721.59901.45] [PMID: 16946649]

[144] Delawi D, Jacobs W, van Susante JL, *et al.* OP-1 Compared with Iliac Crest Autograft in Instrumented Posterolateral Fusion: A Randomized, Multicenter Non-Inferiority Trial. J Bone Joint Surg Am 2016; 98(6): 441-8.
[http://dx.doi.org/10.2106/JBJS.O.00209] [PMID: 26984911]

[145] Furlan JC, Perrin RG, Govender PV, *et al.* Use of osteogenic protein-1 in patients at high risk for spinal pseudarthrosis: a prospective cohort study assessing safety, health-related quality of life, and radiographic fusion. Invited submission from the Joint Section on Disorders of the Spine and Peripheral Nerves, March 2007. J Neurosurg Spine 2007; 7(5): 486-95.
[http://dx.doi.org/10.3171/SPI-07/09/486] [PMID: 17977189]

[146] Guerado E, Cervan AM, Bertrand ML, Benitez-Parejo N. Allograft plus OP-1 enhances ossification in posterolateral lumbar fusion: A seven year follow-up. Injury 2016; 47 (Suppl. 3): S78-82.
[http://dx.doi.org/10.1016/S0020-1383(16)30611-8] [PMID: 27692113]

[147] Leach J, Bittar RG. BMP-7 (OP-1) safety in anterior cervical fusion surgery. J Clin Neurosci 2009; 16(11): 1417-20.
[http://dx.doi.org/10.1016/j.jocn.2009.02.012] [PMID: 19665382]

[148] Paramore CG, Lauryssen C, Rauzzino MJ, *et al.* The safety of OP-1 for lumbar fusion with decompression-- a canine study. Neurosurgery 1999; 44(5): 1151-5.
[http://dx.doi.org/10.1097/00006123-199905000-00134] [PMID: 10232555]

[149] White AP, Vaccaro AR, Hall JA, Whang PG, Friel BC, McKee MD. Clinical applications of BMP-7/OP-1 in fractures, nonunions and spinal fusion. Int Orthop 2007; 31(6): 735-41.
[http://dx.doi.org/10.1007/s00264-007-0422-x] [PMID: 17962946]

[150] Ichiyanagi T, Anabuki K, Nishijima Y, Ono H. Isolation of mesenchymal stem cells from bone marrow wastes of spinal fusion procedure (TLIF) for low back pain patients and preparation of bone dusts for transplantable autologous bone graft with a serum glue. Biosci Trends 2010; 4(3): 110-8.
[PMID: 20592461]

[151] Abbasi H, Abbasi A. Oblique Lateral Lumbar Interbody Fusion (OLLIF): Technical notes and early results of a single surgeon comparative study. Cureus 2015; 7(10): e351.
[http://dx.doi.org/10.7759/cureus.351] [PMID: 26623206]

[152] Becker S, Maissen O, Ponomarev I, Stoll T, Rahn B, Wilke I. Osteopromotion by a beta-tricalcium phosphate/bone marrow hybrid implant for use in spine surgery. Spine 2006; 31(1): 11-7.
[http://dx.doi.org/10.1097/01.brs.0000192762.40274.57] [PMID: 16395170]

[153] Nickoli MS, Hsu WK. Ceramic-based bone grafts as a bone grafts extender for lumbar spine arthrodesis: a systematic review. Global Spine J 2014; 4(3): 211-6.
[http://dx.doi.org/10.1055/s-0034-1378141] [PMID: 25083364]

[154] Ajiboye RM, Hamamoto JT, Eckardt MA, Wang JC. Clinical and radiographic outcomes of concentrated bone marrow aspirate with allograft and demineralized bone matrix for posterolateral and interbody lumbar fusion in elderly patients. Eur Spine J 2015; 24(11): 2567-72.
[http://dx.doi.org/10.1007/s00586-015-4117-5] [PMID: 26169879]

[155] Ploumis A, Albert TJ, Brown Z, Mehbod AA, Transfeldt EE. Healos graft carrier with bone marrow aspirate instead of allograft as adjunct to local autograft for posterolateral fusion in degenerative lumbar scoliosis: a minimum 2-year follow-up study. J Neurosurg Spine 2010; 13(2): 211-5.
[http://dx.doi.org/10.3171/2010.3.SPINE09603] [PMID: 20672956]

[156] Chang KY, Hsu WK. Spinal biologics in minimally invasive lumbar surgery. Minim Invasive Surg 2018; 2018: 5230350.
[http://dx.doi.org/10.1155/2018/5230350] [PMID: 29850240]

[157] Gruskin E, Doll BA, Futrell FW, Schmitz JP, Hollinger JO. Demineralized bone matrix in bone repair: history and use. Adv Drug Deliv Rev 2012; 64(12): 1063-77.
[http://dx.doi.org/10.1016/j.addr.2012.06.008] [PMID: 22728914]

[158] Zhang H, Yang L, Yang XG, *et al.* Demineralized bone matrix carriers and their clinical applications: an overview. Orthop Surg 2019; 11(5): 725-37.
[http://dx.doi.org/10.1111/os.12509] [PMID: 31496049]

[159] Cammisa FP Jr, Lowery G, Garfin SR, *et al.* Two-year fusion rate equivalency between Grafton DBM gel and autograft in posterolateral spine fusion: a prospective controlled trial employing a side-by-side comparison in the same patient. Spine 2004; 29(6): 660-6.
[http://dx.doi.org/10.1097/01.BRS.0000116588.17129.B9] [PMID: 15014276]

[160] D'Souza M, Macdonald NA, Gendreau JL, Duddleston PJ, Feng AY, Ho AL. Graft materials and biologics for spinal interbody fusion. Biomedicines 2019; 7(4): E75.
[http://dx.doi.org/10.3390/biomedicines7040075] [PMID: 31561556]

[161] Duarte RM, Varanda P, Reis RL, Duarte ARC, Correia-Pinto J. Biomaterials and bioactive agents in spinal fusion. Tissue Eng Part B Rev 2017; 23(6): 540-51.
[http://dx.doi.org/10.1089/ten.teb.2017.0072] [PMID: 28514897]

[162] Cottrill E, Pennington Z, Lankipalle N, *et al.* The effect of bioactive glasses on spinal fusion: A cross-disciplinary systematic review and meta-analysis of the preclinical and clinical data. J Clin Neurosci 2020; 78: 34-46.
[http://dx.doi.org/10.1016/j.jocn.2020.04.035] [PMID: 32331941]

[163] Khan SN, Fraser JF, Sandhu HS, Cammisa FP Jr, Girardi FP, Lane JM. Use of osteopromotive growth factors, demineralized bone matrix, and ceramics to enhance spinal fusion. J Am Acad Orthop Surg 2005; 13(2): 129-37.
[http://dx.doi.org/10.5435/00124635-200503000-00006] [PMID: 15850370]

[164] Xue QY, Ji Q, Li HS, *et al.* Alendronate treatment does not inhibit bone formation within biphasic calcium phosphate ceramics in posterolateral spinal fusion: an experimental study in porcine model. Chin Med J (Engl) 2009; 122(22): 2770-4.
[PMID: 19951612]

[165] Urist MR. Bone histogenesis and morphogenesis in implants of demineralized enamel and dentin. J Oral Surg 1971; 29(2): 88-102.
[PMID: 4927173]

[166] Urist MR, Mikulski A, Lietze A. Solubilized and insolubilized bone morphogenetic protein. Proc Natl Acad Sci USA 1979; 76(4): 1828-32.
[http://dx.doi.org/10.1073/pnas.76.4.1828] [PMID: 221908]

[167] Urist MR, Mikulski AJ, Nakagawa M, Yen K. A bone matrix calcification-initiator noncollagenous protein. Am J Physiol 1977; 232(3): C115-27.
[http://dx.doi.org/10.1152/ajpcell.1977.232.3.C115] [PMID: 190900]

[168] Urist MR, Sato K, Brownell AG, *et al.* Human bone morphogenetic protein (hBMP). Proc Soc Exp Biol Med 1983; 173(2): 194-9.
[http://dx.doi.org/10.3181/00379727-173-41630] [PMID: 6866999]

[169] Urist MR, Strates BS. Bone formation in implants of partially and wholly demineralized bone matrix. Including observations on acetone-fixed intra and extracellular proteins. Clin Orthop Relat Res 1970; 71(71): 271-8.
[PMID: 5433388]

[170] Chen D, Zhao M, Mundy GR. Bone morphogenetic proteins. Growth Factors 2004; 22(4): 233-41.
[http://dx.doi.org/10.1080/08977190412331279890] [PMID: 15621726]

[171] Epstein NE. Complications due to the use of BMP/INFUSE in spine surgery: The evidence continues to mount. Surg Neurol Int 2013; 4 (Suppl. 5): S343-52.
[http://dx.doi.org/10.4103/2152-7806.114813] [PMID: 23878769]

[172] Guzman JZ, Merrill RK, Kim JS, *et al.* Bone morphogenetic protein use in spine surgery in the United States: how have we responded to the warnings? Spine J 2017; 17(9): 1247-54.
[http://dx.doi.org/10.1016/j.spinee.2017.04.030] [PMID: 28456674]

[173] James AW, LaChaud G, Shen J, *et al.* A review of the clinical side effects of bone morphogenetic protein-2. Tissue Eng Part B Rev 2016; 22(4): 284-97.
[http://dx.doi.org/10.1089/ten.teb.2015.0357] [PMID: 26857241]

[174] Poeran J, Opperer M, Rasul R, *et al.* Change in off-label use of bone morphogenetic protein in spine surgery and associations with adverse outcome. Global Spine J 2016; 6(7): 650-9.
[http://dx.doi.org/10.1055/s-0036-1571284] [PMID: 27781184]

[175] Dowling Á, Bárcenas JGH, Lewandrowski KU. Transforaminal endoscopic decompression and uninstrumented allograft lumbar interbody fusion: A feasibility study in patients with end-stage vacuum degenerative disc disease. Clin Neurol Neurosurg 2020; 196: 106002.
[http://dx.doi.org/10.1016/j.clineuro.2020.106002] [PMID: 32562950]

[176] Abrão Jo. Dowling Al, León JFRr, Lewandrowski K-U. Anesthesia for endoscopic spine surgery of the spine in an ambulatory surgery center. Global Journal of Anesthesia & Pain Medicine 2020; 3(5): 326-36. [GJAPM].

[177] Brantigan JW, Steffee AD, Lewis ML, Quinn LM, Persenaire JM. Lumbar interbody fusion using the Brantigan I/F cage for posterior lumbar interbody fusion and the variable pedicle screw placement system: two-year results from a Food and Drug Administration investigational device exemption clinical trial. Spine 2000; 25(11): 1437-46.
[http://dx.doi.org/10.1097/00007632-200006010-00017] [PMID: 10828927]

[178] Dagenais S, Caro J, Haldeman S. A systematic review of low back pain cost of illness studies in the United States and internationally. Spine J 2008; 8(1): 8-20.
[http://dx.doi.org/10.1016/j.spinee.2007.10.005] [PMID: 18164449]

[179] Dowdell J, Erwin M, Choma T, Vaccaro A, Iatridis J, Cho SK. Intervertebral disk degeneration and repair. Neurosurgery 2017; 80(3S): S46-54.
[http://dx.doi.org/10.1093/neuros/nyw078] [PMID: 28350945]

[180] Hemanta D, Jiang XX, Feng ZZ, Chen ZX, Cao YW. Etiology for degenerative disc disease. Chin Med Sci J 2016; 31(3): 185-91.
[http://dx.doi.org/10.1016/S1001-9294(16)30049-9] [PMID: 27733227]

[181] Kos N, Gradisnik L, Velnar T. A brief review of the degenerative intervertebral disc disease. Med Arh 2019; 73(6): 421-4.
[http://dx.doi.org/10.5455/medarh.2019.73.421-424] [PMID: 32082013]

[182] Freeman BJC, Kuliwaba JS, Jones CF, *et al.* Allogeneic mesenchymal precursor cells promote healing in postero-lateral annular lesions and improve indices of lumbar intervertebral disc degeneration in an ovine model. Spine 2016; 41(17): 1331-9.

[http://dx.doi.org/10.1097/BRS.0000000000001528] [PMID: 26913464]

[183] Shu CC, Dart A, Bell R, *et al.* Efficacy of administered mesenchymal stem cells in the initiation and co-ordination of repair processes by resident disc cells in an ovine (Ovis aries) large destabilizing lesion model of experimental disc degeneration. JOR Spine 2018; 1(4): e1037.
[http://dx.doi.org/10.1002/jsp2.1037] [PMID: 31463452]

[184] Shu CC, Smith MM, Smith SM, Dart AJ, Little CB, Melrose J. A histopathological scheme for the quantitative scoring of intervertebral disc degeneration and the therapeutic utility of adult mesenchymal stem cells for intervertebral disc regeneration. Int J Mol Sci 2017; 18(5): E1049.
[http://dx.doi.org/10.3390/ijms18051049] [PMID: 28498326]

[185] Ishiguro H, Kaito T, Yarimitsu S, *et al.* Intervertebral disc regeneration with an adipose mesenchymal stem cell-derived tissue-engineered construct in a rat nucleotomy model. Acta Biomater 2019; 87: 118-29.
[http://dx.doi.org/10.1016/j.actbio.2019.01.050] [PMID: 30690206]

[186] Anderson DG, Markova D, An HS, *et al.* Human umbilical cord blood-derived mesenchymal stem cells in the cultured rabbit intervertebral disc: a novel cell source for disc repair. Am J Phys Med Rehabil 2013; 92(5): 420-9.
[http://dx.doi.org/10.1097/PHM.0b013e31825f148a] [PMID: 23598901]

[187] Wang F, Nan LP, Zhou SF, *et al.* Injectable hydrogel combined with nucleus pulposus-derived mesenchymal stem cells for the treatment of degenerative intervertebral disc in rats. Stem Cells Int 2019; 2019: 8496025.
[http://dx.doi.org/10.1155/2019/8496025] [PMID: 31737077]

[188] Noriega DC, Ardura F, Hernández-Ramajo R, *et al.* Intervertebral disc repair by allogeneic mesenchymal bone marrow cells: a randomized controlled trial. Transplantation 2017; 101(8): 1945-51.
[http://dx.doi.org/10.1097/TP.0000000000001484] [PMID: 27661661]

[189] Pettine K, Suzuki R, Sand T, Murphy M. Treatment of discogenic back pain with autologous bone marrow concentrate injection with minimum two year follow-up. Int Orthop 2016; 40(1): 135-40.
[http://dx.doi.org/10.1007/s00264-015-2886-4] [PMID: 26156727]

CHAPTER 11

Transforaminal Epiduroscopic Basivertebral Nerve Laser Ablation for Chronic Low Back Pain Associated with Modic Changes

Byapak Paudel[1, 2], **Nitin Maruti Adsul**[1,3], **Hyeun Sung Kim**[1,*] and **Il-Tae Jang**[1]

[1] *Department of Neurosurgery, Nanoori Gangnam Hospital, Seoul, Republic of Korea*

[2] *Department of Orthopaedics & Traumatology, Grande International Hospital, Kathmandu, Nepal*

[3] *Sir Ganga Ram Hospital, Ortho-Spine Surgery, New Delhi, India*

Abstract: Among different causes of chronic low back pain, Modic changes of the endplates have been identified as an MRI-image representation of end stage degenerative disc disease. Painful innervation of these degenerative endplates from within the vertebral body by arborization of the basivertebral nerve towards these endplates has been demonstrated. Ablation of the basivertebral nerve has been identified as one possible way to treat chronic low back pain. This chapter describes the transforaminal epiduroscopic laser ablation of the basivertebral nerve and its associated clinical outcomes.

Keywords: Basivertebral nerve, Chronic low back pain, Epiduroscopy, Laser ablation, Modic changes, Transforaminal approach.

INTRODUCTION

Chronic back pain is a disabling condition affecting large portions of the aging population the world over. It is associated with decreased quality of life and loss of economic status. Pain in the spine may arise from any of the three columns. Pain in the anterior column may be from discal pressure changes and is commonly referred to as discogenic low back pain. Stimulation of neural structures around the disc and vertebral endplate and symptomatic disc degeneration in the middle column in conjunction with chemical changes and mechanical pressure on the neural structures are leading pain generators in the middle column. Similarly, pain in the posterior column may arise in facet joints, muscles, and ligaments.

* **Corresponding author Hyeun Sung Kim:** Department of Neurosurgery, Nanoori Gangnam Hospital, Seoul, Republic of Korea; Tel: +82-10-2440-2631; E-mail: neurospinekim@gmail.com

Kai-Uwe Lewandrowski, Jorge Felipe Ramírez León, Anthony Yeung, Gun Choi, Stefan Hellinger and Álvaro Dowling (Eds.)

These conditions may cause axial back pain with or without radiation along recognized dermatomes. It can also cause referred pain – the so-called sclerotomal pain, which patients may describe as local or referred deep-seated bone pain referred from degenerated vertebral segments.

Modic changes of the degenerated vertebral endplates have been associated with an MRI-image correlated with such sclerotomal pain [1]. There are three types of Modic changes [2]. In type one, the T1-weighted image series shows a hypointensity signal, and T2 weighted images show a hyperintensity signal in the endplates. These findings are believed to be structurally related to acute disruption and fissuring of endplates. This condition leads to vascularized fibrous tissue's ingrowth into the marrow of the corresponding adjacent vertebral body. Type two Modic changes represent chronic degeneration, and the MRI image correlates hyperintensity in T1- and isointensity in T2-weighted series. Histologically there is the fatty degeneration of the vertebral bone marrow. Type three Modic changes represent bony sclerosis. Its MRI image correlate shows hypointense T1- and T2-weighted image series. Modic changes are associated with chronic low back pain [3]. Especially, type 1 and 2 Modic changes have been identified as most painful [4, 5].

A painful symptomatic lumbar motion segment may be the sensitized ingrowth of nerve fibers from the sinuvertebral- and the basivertebral nerve. The sinuvertebral nerve is densely located at the posterior annulus and posterior longitudinal ligament, whereas the basivertebral nerve preferentially innervates the endplates. (6) Therefore, the authors stipulated that the transforaminal epiduroscopic laser ablation of the basivertebral nerve may be a viable alternative to more aggressive spinal surgeries, including fusion to treat chronic back pain associated.

THE RATIONALE OF TRANSFORAMINAL LASER ABLATION OF THE BASIVERTEBRAL NERVE

The vertebral endplate is richly innervated by free nerve endings that arborize the basivertebral nerve. This neoinnervation may be sensitized and stimulated by inflammatory mediators. When the basivertebral nerve is sensitized, it may produce disabling chronic low back pain. Pain may be associated with or without Modic changes. Conceptionally, the ablation of the basivertebral nerve disrupts nociceptors' signal path, thereby producing pain relief (Fig. **1**).

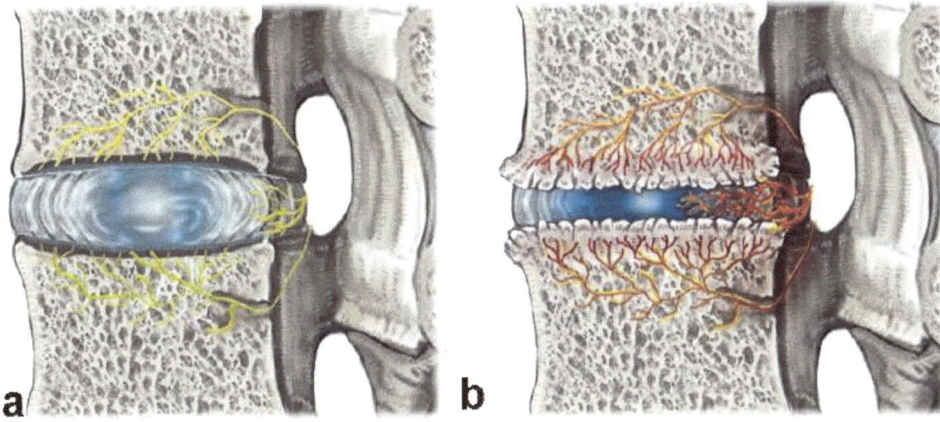

Fig. (1). Illustration of pathologic innervation of degenerative endplates by the basivertebral nerve: **a)** normal innervation, **b)** pathologic innervation.

SURGICAL SETUP

The transforaminal laser ablation of the basivertebral nerve is indicated in patients with severe low back pain associated with positive discography. Other etiologies should be ruled out with clinical investigations, including advanced CT or MRI imaging and diagnostic spinal injections. After diagnostic confirmation of discogenic low back pain associated with end-stage degenerative disc disease with Modic changes of the endplates on MRI scanning, patients may consent for the interventional surgical basivertebral nerve ablation. The authors developed a clinical protocol consisting of directly visualized transforaminal endoscopic laser ablation of the basivertebral nerve. The transforaminal endoscopy platform lends itself well for the epiduroscopic laser ablation as it provides easy access to the epidural space surrounding the disc space. The epiduroscopic laser ablation technology uses a small flexible epiduroscopic catheter system through which the laser fiber can be introduced and directed under continued direct visualization onto the basivertebral nerve. Therefore, this hybrid procedure requires that the surgeon understand both the transforaminal endoscopic anatomy and the technical and procedural aspects of spinal endoscopic and epiduroscopic procedures. Characteristics of patient positioning OR setup, incision access planning by identifying surgical landmarks. The docking points at the spine for the endoscopic working cannula have been described in other chapters of this Bentham text series on spinal endoscopy. The authors also emphasize the need for high-quality endoscopes, endoscopic instruments, and videoendoscopic tower systems to support this delicate detail-driven operation.

EQUIPMENT AND INSTRUMENTS

Many devices for ablation of the basivertebral nerve are commercially available. Most of them are designed for the transpedicular intraosseous route. In comparison, the authors employ a system - NeedleView CH (Lutronic®, Ilsan, South Korea) - designed for the transforaminal epidural and extraosseous route. This system operates at a wavelength of 1414nm with 0.75–12 watt and allows to advance the side-firing Nd: YAG laser fiber to the target area. The laser system has the ability for both thermos-vibration and ablation. The laser-tissue interactions, including the Moses effect, have been described in another chapter of volume three of the Bentham text series on contemporary spinal endoscopy. The Nd: YAG laser employed in the authors' clinical series can ablate a spherical area of approximately 10mm in diameter. The procedure is done under continuous irrigation with a constant flow of normal saline at about a pressure of 40 mm of Hg. This hydrostatic pressure can typically be achieved by gravity. However, more exact pressures may be generated by an irrigation pump. Irrigation also helps with improved visualization of the surgical field.

PATIENT POSITIONING

The patient is placed in a prone position on a lordotic spinal frame on top of a radiolucent operating table making abdominal content free from compression. Alternatively, chest rolls and pelvic support cushions may be used. This will ensure less bleeding during surgery by reducing venous pressure.

ANESTHESIA

The epiduroscopic basivertebral nerve ablation can typically be done under local anesthesia using 7 to 10 cc of 1% lidocaine. Initially, the surgeon should inject the skin and infiltrate the surgical corridor muscles from the skin to the surgical neuroforamen. Another injection of local anesthetic is done after the first one has taken effect some 3 to 5 minutes later. Approximately 2 to 3 cc of 1.6% lidocaine are mixed with epinephrine and injected directly into the foraminal area. Additional use of sedation may be used at the discretion of the anesthesiologist. Some patients with medical comorbidities may be better off with a secured airway and other forms of anesthesia. The reader may find additional information on anesthesia's appropriate choice in a chapter in volume 1 of this Bentham text.

LANDMARKS

The surgical level is identified under fluoroscopic C-arm control. The transforaminal approach's skin entry point is marked by employing access strategies described in other chapters in this text. The most appropriate attack angles are measured on the patient using the iliac crest in relationship to the surgical level by drawing intersecting lines in the anteroposterior (AP) and lateral (LAT) views.

DOCKING POINTS

A Quincke tip BD Spinal needle 18 G measuring 15 cm in length is docked at suprapedicular notch to access the rostral vertebral endplate at the surgical level. Both AP and LAT fluoroscopy images are used to ensure proper docking (Fig. **2**).

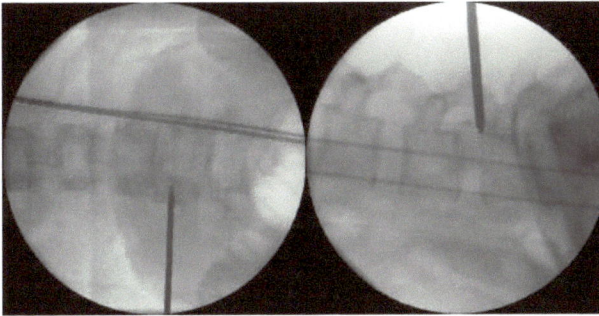

Fig. (2). Intraoperative AP and LAT fluoroscopy images to verify targeting of the suprapedicular notch with the spinal needle and dilator which should be docked at the rostral vertebral endplate at the surgical level.

A guidewire is inserted through the spinal needle. Serial dilators are passed over the guidewire allowing to place the working channel facing the target area. The endoscope is then inserted through the working channel enabling direct visualization of the target area (Fig. **3**).

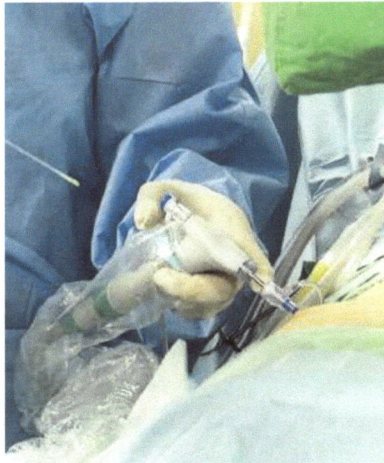

Fig. (3). Intraoperative view of a transforaminal endoscopy with the NeedleView CH system (Lutronic®, Ilsan, South Korea). The surgeon is holding the laser fiber in his right hand.

BASIVERTEBRAL NERVE ABLATION

The ablation of the basivertebral nerve is then carried out by directing the laser fiber under direct epiduroscopic visualization, illustrated in Figs. (**4** and **5**).

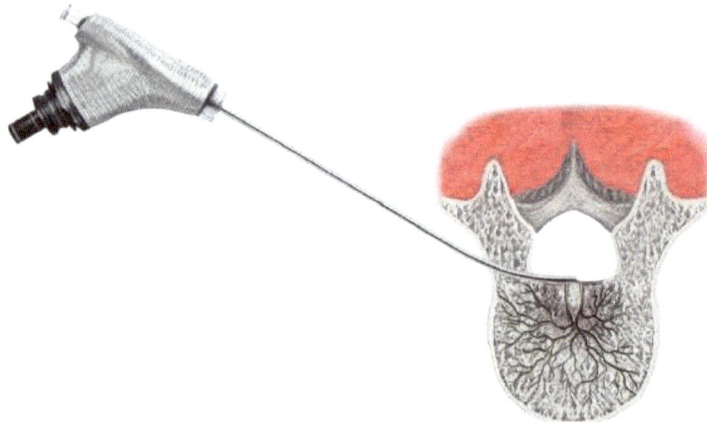

Fig. (4). Schematic axial view through a lumbar vertebral body where the flexible epiduroscopic laser ablation system targets the entry point of the basivertebral nerve in the midline and just below the ring apophysis of the rostral endplate of the distal vertebral body.

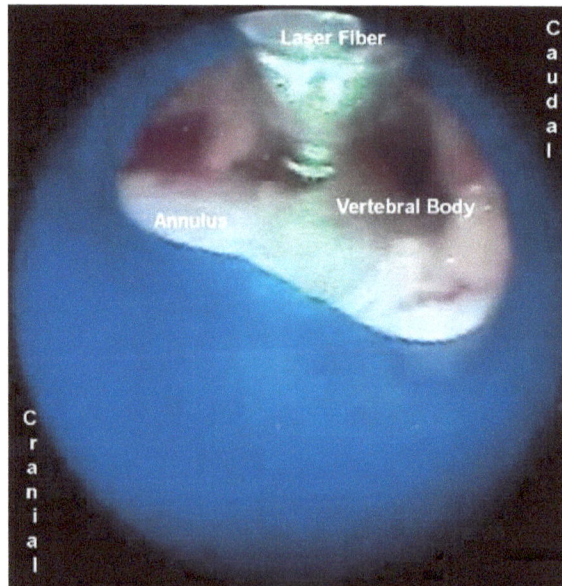

Fig. (5). Intraoperative epiduroscopic view showing the laser fiber in the center aiming at the basivertebral nerve entering the vertebral body at the basivertebral foramen in the midline and just below the ring apophysis of the rostral endplate of the distal vertebral body which can be found at the junction between the annulus and the endplate.

We operate the Nd: YAG laser with energy settings of 4.5-6 W. Intraoperatively, the preoperative workup of the painful endplate with Modic changes on the corresponding MRI scans once more verified by attempting to replicate the patient's response observed during provocative preoperative discography by provoking the same endplate with the laser. For this protocol to work, the slightly sedated patient should communicate with the surgeon during these provocative maneuvers. Moreover, local anesthesia should only be injected into the neuroforamen but not into the central epidural space underneath the dural sac. The patient should be reassessed intraoperatively for pain relief to determine the completion of the procedure.

CLINICAL SERIES

We studied this technique in 14 consecutive patients (6 men and eight women) whose MRI findings correlated with clinical findings. Our patients had chronic LBP with mean symptoms duration of 21.21 ± 21.87 (range: 4–84) months. The mean age and follow-up period were 46 ± 9.95 (range: 31 -63) years and 15.3 ± 2.67 months (range: 12–20 months). According to Pfirmann's grade, disc degeneration grade was grade IV in 8 (57.14%) patients and grade V in 6 (42.85%) patients. Eight had type 1 Modic changes, and the remaining six patients had type 2 Modic changes.

The preoperative VAS score changed from 7.79 ± 0.98 (range: 6–10) to the immediate postoperative score of 1.93 ± 1.39 (range: 1–6). Which was significant statistically (P < 0.0001)). This improvement was maintained at third month with score of 2.21 ± 0.89 (range: 1–5; P < 0.0001) and at final follow up with score of 2.36 ± 1.01 (range: 1–5; P < 0.0001). We had good to excellent results in 92.85% according to Macnab's criteria (7 patients (50%) had excellent, six patients (42.85%) had good), and one patient (7.14%) had a fair outcome. We had no device- or procedure-related serious adverse events. We did not have infections, discitis, paresis, dural tears, vascular injuries, or systemic complications until the latest follow-up.

ILLUSTRATIVE CASE

Our illustrative case is a 31 years old female patient who had chronic low back pain for the last two years and demonstrated Modic change in MRI and concordant pain on provocative discography. She had undergone Transforaminal epiduroscopic laser ablation of the basivertebral nerve after the procedure patient has remained pain-free for the last four years (Fig. **6**). Please click on this link to view this illustrative case.

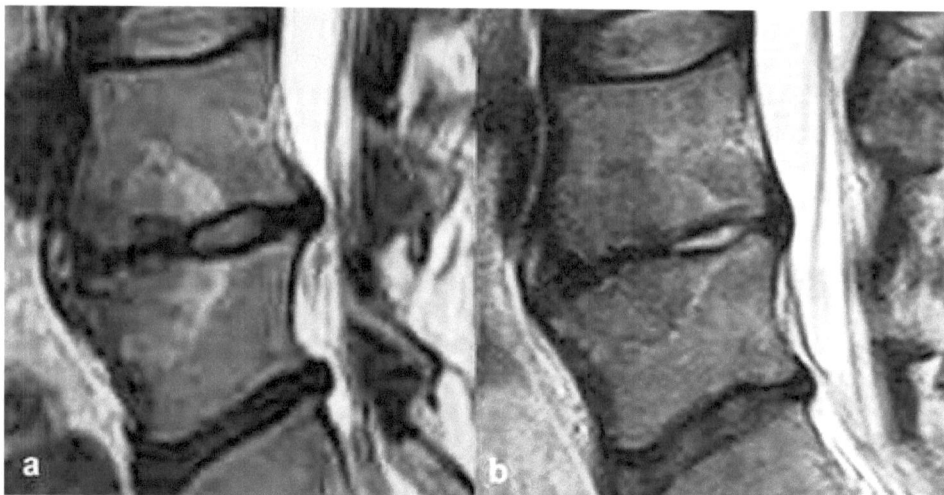

Fig. (6). Pre **(a)**- and postoperative 1yr follow up **(b)** MRI scan of our illustrative case-patient. This 35-year old female underwent basivertebral nerve laser ablation. The one-year follow-up MRI scan shows the ablation denervation effect of the transforaminal epiduroscopic basivertebral laser ablation (TEBLA).

DISCUSSION

Modic change in MRI signal intensity changes in the vertebral bone marrow is not related to marrow malignancy, pyogenesis, or seropositive rheumatic disorders. It is an independent risk factor for severe and disabling episodes of LBP [3, 6]. It is associated with both disc degeneration and the presence and severity of LBP [7]. LBP associated with Modic changes is characterized by pain at all times of the day, night pain, and morning pain/stiffness [8, 9]. Chronic LBP associated with Modic changes has poor outcome with conservative treatment [10, 11]. The pathogenesis of Modic change is not clear yet. But mechano-immunological, infectious, genetic etiologies are postulated [12, 13]. The least requirement for Modic change is disc/endplate damage with persistent stimulus [3]. Different treatment modalities, from conservative with physiotherapy, pain medications, intradiscal steroid injections, Bisphosphonates, and Anti-TNF-α antibodies, are done, but these modalities have a very short-term effect [3].

Recently ablation of the basivertebral nerve has emerged as a new modality of treatment for chronic low back pain [14 - 18]. There are two different types of ablation approaches. The first one is intraosseous ablation done through transpedicular route by radiofrequency [15, 18 - 21], and the second one is extraosseous ablation done through transforaminal route by laser [17, 22, 23]. We perform extraosseous ablation done through transforaminal epiduroscopic route using the laser [17, 22, 23]. Our technique differs from the existing intraosseous technique in the literature:

1. First, our approach is extraosseous through the transforaminal epiduroscopic route with proper visualization of anatomy

2. Second, we use a laser instead of radiofrequency.

3. Third, our approach is very close to the basivertebral nerve endings compared to other intraosseous approaches. Ablation ours distant from the nerve endings at the center of the vertebral body.

4. Fourth, we have added the thermo-vibration effect to provoke pain by stimulating the basivertebral nerve.

5. Fifth, we can ablate a small spherical region of approximately 10 mm in diameter.

6. Sixth, we can control ablation in one direction because of the laser cable end's side-firing property.

7. Seventh, with this technique, most importantly, we can do three steps of provocation tests to check the Modic changes as the source of pain. The three steps are as follows: (a) provocative preoperative discography, (b) intraoperative laser provocation into the basivertebral nerve of the vertebral body with Modic changes, and (c) intraoperative relief of pain assessment by laser provocation of the same painful area after completion of the laser ablation procedure.

CONCLUSION

Transforaminal epiduroscopic laser ablation of the basivertebral nerve is a promising technique to treat patients with chronic low back pain associated with Modic changes that may consider as an alternative to fusion. This minimally invasive epiduroscopic procedure falls into interventional pain surgeries, which may ultimately replace traditional open spine surgery protocols. Comparative analysis of radiofrequency *versus* laser use may shed light on the merits of these two widely available technologies.

CONSENT FOR PUBLICATION

Not applicable.

CONFLICT OF INTEREST

The authors declare no conflict of interest, financial or otherwise.

ACKNOWLEDGEMENT

Declared none.

REFERENCES

[1]   de Roos A, Kressel H, Spritzer C, Dalinka M. MR imaging of marrow changes adjacent to end plates in degenerative lumbar disk disease. AJR Am J Roentgenol 1987; 149(3): 531-4.
[http://dx.doi.org/10.2214/ajr.149.3.531] [PMID: 3497539]

[2]   Modic MT, Steinberg PM, Ross JS, Masaryk TJ, Carter JR. Degenerative disk disease: assessment of changes in vertebral body marrow with MR imaging. Radiology 1988; 166(1 Pt 1): 193-9.
[http://dx.doi.org/10.1148/radiology.166.1.3336678] [PMID: 3336678]

[3]   Dudli S, Fields AJ, Samartzis D, Karppinen J, Lotz JC. Pathobiology of Modic changes. Eur Spine J 2016; 25(11): 3723-34.
[http://dx.doi.org/10.1007/s00586-016-4459-7] [PMID: 26914098]

[4]   Määttä JH, Wadge S, MacGregor A, Karppinen J, Williams FM. ISSLS Prize Winner: Vertebral Endplate (Modic) Change is an Independent Risk Factor for Episodes of Severe and Disabling Low Back Pain. Spine 2015; 40(15): 1187-93.
[http://dx.doi.org/10.1097/BRS.0000000000000937] [PMID: 25893353]

[5]   Ohtori S, Inoue G, Ito T, *et al.* Tumor necrosis factor-immunoreactive cells and PGP 9.5-immunoreactive nerve fibers in vertebral endplates of patients with discogenic low back Pain and Modic Type 1 or Type 2 changes on MRI. Spine 2006; 31(9): 1026-31.
[http://dx.doi.org/10.1097/01.brs.0000215027.87102.7c] [PMID: 16641780]

[6]   Manniche C, O'Neill S. New insights link low-virulent disc infections to the etiology of severe disc degeneration and Modic changes. Future Sci OA 2019; 5(5): FSO389.
[http://dx.doi.org/10.2144/fsoa-2019-0022] [PMID: 31245043]

[7]   Mok FP, Samartzis D, Karppinen J, Fong DY, Luk KD, Cheung KM. Modic changes of the lumbar spine: prevalence, risk factors, and association with disc degeneration and low back pain in a large-scale population-based cohort. Spine J 2016; 16(1): 32-41.
[http://dx.doi.org/10.1016/j.spinee.2015.09.060] [PMID: 26456851]

[8]   Bailly F, Maigne JY, Genevay S, *et al.* Inflammatory pain pattern and pain with lumbar extension associated with Modic 1 changes on MRI: a prospective case-control study of 120 patients. Eur Spine J 2014; 23(3): 493-7.
[http://dx.doi.org/10.1007/s00586-013-3036-6] [PMID: 24221918]

[9]   Arnbak B, Jurik AG, Jensen TS, Manniche C. Association Between Inflammatory Back Pain Characteristics and Magnetic Resonance Imaging Findings in the Spine and Sacroiliac Joints. Arthritis Care Res (Hoboken) 2018; 70(2): 244-51.
[http://dx.doi.org/10.1002/acr.23259] [PMID: 28426912]

[10]   Jensen RK, Leboeuf-Yde C. Is the presence of modic changes associated with the outcomes of different treatments? A systematic critical review. BMC Musculoskelet Disord 2011; 12(1): 183.
[http://dx.doi.org/10.1186/1471-2474-12-183] [PMID: 21831312]

[11]   Jensen OK, Nielsen CV, Sørensen JS, Stengaard-Pedersen K. Type 1 Modic changes was a significant risk factor for 1-year outcome in sick-listed low back pain patients: a nested cohort study using magnetic resonance imaging of the lumbar spine. Spine J 2014; 14(11): 2568-81.
[http://dx.doi.org/10.1016/j.spinee.2014.02.018] [PMID: 24534386]

[12]   Rajasekaran S, Tangavel C, Aiyer SN, *et al.* ISSLS PRIZE IN CLINICAL SCIENCE 2017: Is infection the possible initiator of disc disease? An insight from proteomic analysis. Eur Spine J 2017; 26(5): 1384-400.
[http://dx.doi.org/10.1007/s00586-017-4972-3] [PMID: 28168343]

[13]   Nguyen C, Poiraudeau S, Rannou F. From Modic 1 vertebral-endplate subchondral bone signal changes detected by MRI to the concept of 'active discopathy'. Ann Rheum Dis 2015; 74(8): 1488-94.
[http://dx.doi.org/10.1136/annrheumdis-2015-207317] [PMID: 25977562]

[14]   Wong DA. Basivertebral nerve ablation: does the path followed suggest this technology is ready for adoption into clinical practice?: COMMENTARY ON: Khalil J et al. A prospective, randomized, multicenter study of intraosseous basivertebral nerve ablation for the treatment of chronic low back pain. SpineJ. 2019;10:1620-1632. 2019. Spine J. 2020;20(2):154-5.
[http://dx.doi.org/10.1016/j.spinee.2019.05.598]

[15]   Truumees E, Macadaeg K, Pena E, *et al.* A prospective, open-label, single-arm, multi-center study of intraosseous basivertebral nerve ablation for the treatment of chronic low back pain. Eur Spine J 2019; 28(7): 1594-602.
[http://dx.doi.org/10.1007/s00586-019-05995-2] [PMID: 31115683]

[16]   Khalil JG, Smuck M, Koreckij T, *et al.* A prospective, randomized, multicenter study of intraosseous basivertebral nerve ablation for the treatment of chronic low back pain. Spine J 2019; 19(10): 1620-32.
[http://dx.doi.org/10.1016/j.spinee.2019.05.598] [PMID: 31229663]

[17]   Kim HS, Adsul N, Yudoyono F, *et al.* Transforaminal Epiduroscopic Basivertebral Nerve Laser Ablation for Chronic Low Back Pain Associated with Modic Changes: A Preliminary Open-Label Study. Pain Res Manag 2018; 2018: 6857983.
[http://dx.doi.org/10.1155/2018/6857983] [PMID: 30186540]

[18]   Becker S, Hadjipavlou A, Heggeness MH. Ablation of the basivertebral nerve for treatment of back pain: a clinical study. Spine J 2017; 17(2): 218-23.
[http://dx.doi.org/10.1016/j.spinee.2016.08.032] [PMID: 27592808]

[19]   Fischgrund JS, Rhyne A, Franke J, *et al.* Intraosseous Basivertebral Nerve Ablation for the Treatment of Chronic Low Back Pain: 2-Year Results From a Prospective Randomized Double-Blind Sham-Controlled Multicenter Study. Int J Spine Surg 2019; 13(2): 110-9.
[http://dx.doi.org/10.14444/6015] [PMID: 31131209]

[20]   Lorio M, Clerk-Lamalice O, Beall DP, Julien T. International Society for the Advancement of Spine Surgery Guideline-Intraosseous Ablation of the Basivertebral Nerve for the Relief of Chronic Low Back Pain. Int J Spine Surg 2020; 14(1): 18-25.
[http://dx.doi.org/10.14444/7002] [PMID: 32128298]

[21]   Fischgrund JS, Rhyne A, Franke J, *et al.* Intraosseous basivertebral nerve ablation for the treatment of chronic low back pain: a prospective randomized double-blind sham-controlled multi-center study. Eur Spine J 2018; 27(5): 1146-56.
[http://dx.doi.org/10.1007/s00586-018-5496-1] [PMID: 29423885]

[22]   Kim HS, Wu PH, Jang IT. Lumbar Degenerative Disease Part 1: Anatomy and Pathophysiology of Intervertebral Discogenic Pain and Radiofrequency Ablation of Basivertebral and Sinuvertebral Nerve Treatment for Chronic Discogenic Back Pain: A Prospective Case Series and Review of Literature. Int J Mol Sci 2020; 21(4): E1483.
[http://dx.doi.org/10.3390/ijms21041483] [PMID: 32098249]

[23]   Wu PH, Kim HS, Jang IT. Intervertebral Disc Diseases PART 2: A Review of the Current Diagnostic and Treatment Strategies for Intervertebral Disc Disease. Int J Mol Sci 2020; 21(6): E2135.
[http://dx.doi.org/10.3390/ijms21062135] [PMID: 32244936]

CHAPTER 12

Uniportal Endoscopic Transforaminal Decompression Associated with Cylindrical Percutaneous Interspinous Spacer

R. Cantú-Leal[1,*] and **R. Cantu-Longoria[2]**

[1] *Department of Spine Surgery, Hospital Christus Muguerza Alta Especialidad in Monterrey, Mexico*

[2] *Orthopaedic Spine Surgeon, Hospital Christus Muguerza Alta Especialidad, Villa Alegre C.P. 64130 Monterrey. N.L., Mexico*

Abstract: Combining the percutaneous transforaminal endoscopic decompression (PTED) with interspinous process distraction systems (ISP) may offer additional benefits in treating spinal stenosis in patients who have failed conservative treatment. We retrospectively investigated the medical records of 152 patients who underwent transforaminal endoscopic decompression with simultaneous ISP placement through the same incision. Patients were operated on from January 2008 to June 2016 and included 80 males, and 72 patients were females. Clinical data analysis was done on 142 patients two years postoperatively since ten patients were lost in follow-up. Primary outcome measures were pre-and postoperative visual analog scale (VAS) criteria and the Oswestry Disability Index. Only patients with a minimum follow-up of 2 years were included. The analysis included 224 patients who underwent interspinous spacers during the transforaminal endoscopic decompression. Of the 152 patients, 84 complained of axial facet-related pain syndromes *versus* the remaining 68 patients who chiefly complained of radicular symptoms. The postoperative VAS reduction at two-year follow-up for the low back was 6.4. The patient-reported ODI reductions were of a similar magnitude at 40.4%. According to Macnab criteria, the percentage of patients who graded their surgical results as excellent or good was 90%. At two-year follow-up, 5 percent of patients required another operation to deal with failure to cure or recurrent symptoms due to implant subsidence. The authors concluded that adding an interspinous process spacer to the endoscopic decompression in patients treated for lateral lumbar stenosis and foraminal stenosis with low-grade spondylolisthesis might improve clinical outcomes by stabilizing the posterior column.

Keywords: Endoscopic spine surgery, Interspinous process distraction, Lumbar lateral recess and foraminal stenosis.

* **Corresponding author R. Cantú-Leal:** Department of Spine Surgery, Hospital Christus Muguerza Alta Especialidad, Monterrey, Mexico; Tel: +52 81 8333 1216; E-mail: dr_robertocantu@yahoo.com

Kai-Uwe Lewandrowski, Jorge Felipe Ramírez León, Anthony Yeung, Gun Choi, Stefan Hellinger and Álvaro Dowling (Eds.)

INTRODUCTION

The authors of this chapter explored the feasibility and clinical benefits of a transforaminal decompression procedure combined with a percutaneous threaded cylindrical interspinous process spacer placed through the same lateral portal for better relief of both radicular leg and axial back pain symptoms stemming from the resulting decrease in the remaining nucleus pulposus and decreased pressure on arthritic facet joints. The authors are well-recognized key opinion leaders (KOLs) known for having pioneered endoscopic spinal surgery in Mexico, starting in an academic hospital-based setting with an orthopaedic residency program over 20 years ago. The endoscopic spine surgery program began with simple transforaminal decompression surgeries employing the "inside-out" technique popularized by Yeung *et al.* in the late 1990ies [1 - 5]. The authors soon realized that the transforaminal discectomy effectively relieves sciatica-type leg- and back pain but had limitations. That definition of appropriate patient selection criteria was directly related to the surgeons' skill level and the availability of advanced endoscopic equipment. With the evolution of more advanced video-endoscopic equipment and more effective decompression tools, indications for endoscopic spinal surgery have expanded from simple herniated disc to include sciatica stemming from boney or ligamentous stenosis. The latter condition is often associated with more advanced degeneration of the lumbar motion segment involving the facet joint complex and the intervertebral disc itself. Advanced disc degeneration may be associated with increased intradiscal pressures and progressive vertical collapse. In the end-stage of the degenerative process, the intervertebral disc may even be void of any functional tissue and has been reported to be hollow at times. The concept of vertical instability has been introduced by Luk *et al.* to characterize this process [6]. It essentially implies dynamic lateral recess and foraminal stenosis due to a mechanically incompetent disc that others have associated with the vacuum phenomenon [7 - 9]. In the opinion of this team of authors, this process may contribute to less favorable clinical outcomes. It stimulated the interest in combining the endoscopic three transforaminal decompression procedure with other ancillary procedures that could aid in the stabilization of the lumbar motion segment, perhaps earlier in the disease process, without exposing the patient to the burden of a traditional instrumented fusion. Therefore, the idea of combining the endoscopic transforaminal decompression with an interspinous process spacer was entertained.

INTERSPINOUS PROCESS SPACERS

Knowles introduced the first lumbar interspinous process spacer (IPS) in the '50s [10]. In the last decade, many ISPs have been marketed. However, only the following implants have been approved by the FDA: X-STOP® Interspinous Process Decompression (IPD®) System, Coflex® Interlaminar Technology implant (formerly known as Interspinous U), and the Superion® Interspinous Spacer (ISS, VertiFlex [11]. The approved surgical indication is for treating symptoms related to central canal-, foraminal stenosis, or Grade I degenerative spondylolisthesis in patients over 50 years [12].

Numerous other devices have been approved for clinical use in Latin America and Europe, some for additional indications. In general, osteoporosis, spondylolisthesis grade 2 and above, pars defects, ankylosis of the spinous processes, infection, severe neural element compression causing cauda equina, and excessive spinal deformity are contraindications to the procedure [12 - 15]. Some unpublished clinical trials have been started in the United States. Two Coflex® trials have been completed [16, 17], and another two Coflex® trials are scheduled for completion in June of 2022 and 2023, respectively (Table **1**) [18, 19]. The intradiscal and annular pressure have been shown to vary inversely between the extension and neutral position of the lumbar spine. Paolo *et al.* reported a 63% increase in posterior annular pressure in extension and 38% in the standing position with a simultaneous decrease of intranuclear pressure of 41% and 20%, respectively [20]. The authors demonstrated that most ISP increases spinal stability in extension, while a few also stabilize in flexion. However, none protected against instability in axial rotation or lateral stability [20].

Table 1. National Clinical Trial (NCT) on interspinous spacers.

NCT No.	Trial Name	Planned Enrollment	Completion Date
*NCT03041896	Retrospective Evaluation of the Clinical and Radiographic Performance of Coflex® Interlaminer Technology *versus* Decompression With or Without Fusion	5000	Oct 2017
*NCT01316211	Comparative Evaluation of Clinical Outcome in the Treatment of Degenerative Spinal Stenosis With Concomitant Low Back Pain by Decompression With and Without Additional Stabilization Using the CoflexTM Interlaminar Technology	245	Dec 2017
*NCT02555280	A 2 and 5 Year Comparative Evaluation of Clinical Outcomes in the Treatment of Degenerative Spinal Stenosis With Concomitant Low Back Pain by Decompression With and Without Additional Stabilization Using the Coflex® Interlaminar Technology for FDA Real Conditions of Use Study (Post-Approval 'Real Conditions of Use' Study)	345	Jun 2022

(Table 1) cont.....

NCT No.	Trial Name	Planned Enrollment	Completion Date
NCT02457468	The Coflex®COMMUNITY Study: An Observational Study of Coflex® Interlaminar Technology	500	Jun 2023

*Denotes industry-sponsored or cosponsored trial. Reproduced from Medical Policy – 7.01.107 Interspinous and Interlaminar Stabilization/Distraction Devices (Spacers) BCBSA Ref. Policy: 7.01.107 Effective Date: Last Revised: Replaces: July 1, 2021 June 1, 2021 N/A. https://www.premera.com/medicalpolicies/7.01.107.pdf

Presumably, ISP functions have been introduced to stabilize the spine with less aggressive means by restricting extension and thereby reducing axial back and neurogenic claudication pain by increasing neuroforaminal volume, and diminishing intradiscal pressure, and compression forces across arthritic facet joints *via* distraction of the adjacent lamina or spinous processes. During implantation between the spinous processes or the adjacent laminae, devices are typically expanded to increase the neuroforaminal volume by distraction while maintaining the supraspinous ligament assisting in holding the implant in place. Devices have been used as a simplified treatment for stenosis-related claudication symtoms when compared to traditional decompression procedures. ISP implantation without concomittant decompression has the advantage of the operation not causing epidural scarring or being associated with a cerebrospinal fluid leakage risk. Outcomes with ISP have been variable, particularly in patients in whom ISP was used as a stand- alone solution to treat their spinal stenosis with up to grade 1 spondylolisthesis. Randomized controlled trials (RCTs) on the Superion® Interspinous Spacer (ISS) and the coflex® interlaminar implant using primary 5 outcome measures assessing symptoms resolution, functional outcomes, quality of adjusted life years, show a high failure and complication rate whenever ISP are used as an alternative to spinal decompression. One pivotal FDA trial studied clinical outcomes with the Superion® ISP compared to the X-STOP without any control groups of non-operative care or traditional open surgery [21]. Results suggested a higher (80%) success rate with the Superion® ISS in some primary outcome measures than with the X- STOP, which is no longer on the market [22]. In comparison, the multicenter, double-blind FELIX trial evaluated clinical outcomes with the coflex® interlaminar implant (also called the interspinous U) [23 - 25]. Standardized functional clinical outcomes measures were compared in patients who were treated with decompression alone *versus* placement the coflex® interlaminar implant. While outcomes were reportedly similar between patients treated with decompression and patients in the Coflex® group at 2-year follow-up, 1-year reoperation rates were significantly higher in patients who were solely treated with interlaminar placement of the coflex® (29%) than in patients who underwent a primary decompression (8%) without an IPS [26]. The reliability of the coflex® was slightly worse in patients who underwent a two-level procedure with a 1-year reoperation rate of 38%, compared to decompression alone remaining at 6%, respectively. Similarly, two-year reoperation rates were also higher if patients had ISP placed at two levels - 33% for patients who had coflex® alone *versus* 8% for patients who had the coflex® with a concomitant decompression [27]. Other studies have looked at the 3 to 5-year clinical outcomes with the coflex® device [28 - 30]. One study even reported heterotopic ossification as an unintended consequence of the implantation of an IPS [31]. As a result, many health care plans have equivocal coverage determinations. Most of them in the United States advised that the clinical evidence is insufficient for definitive treatment recommendation.

ISP REGULATORY APPROVAL STATUS

The FDA granted premarket approval for the Superion® Interspinous Spacer (ISS, VertiFlex) in 2015. Its instructions for use (IFU) indicated that ISS was meant treat adults who have achieved skeletal maturity and are suffering from lumbar neurogenic claudication symptoms relieved by flexion, including pain, numbness, and cramping legs. The approval allows for a maximum of two level surgery from L1 to L5. The ISS was limited to patients without back pain who failed six months of non-operative care and whose preoperative cross-sectional imaging studies demonstrated moderate central or lateral canal spinal stenosis due to thickening of the ligamentum flavum without instability in excess of grade 1 spondylolisthesis or foraminal stenosis [32]. The post-approval evaluation of ISS for continued FDA approval is ongoing with two separate trails currently underway: 1) the Superion® Post-Approval Clinical Evaluation and Review (SPACER), and 2) the Superion® New Enrollment Study [23]. The first study comparing the Superion® device with the X-STOP is scheduled for 60-month [29]. The second study has a minimum requirement of 358 patients undergoing decompression alone having to be enrolled. The FDA has approved the coflex® for clinical use in single- or two-level surgeries for similar spinal stenosis indications in skeletally mature patients levels L1 to L5 [33, 34]. The coflex® is not an actual ISP but is intended as an interlaminar stabilization device following a lumbar decompression. The coflex® has a long list of contraindications mandated by the FDA and listed in the IFU, including prior fusion or decompressive laminectomy at any lumbar index level, trauma or tumor at any lumbar level(s), severe facet hypertrophy requiring substantial bony resection, which could prompt postoperative instability, spondylolisthesis (greater than grade II), spondylolysis, scoliosis (> 25 degrees), osteoporosis, axial back without radicular pain, obesity, (body mass index > 40), active or chronic systemic or local, infection, cauda equina, titanium alloys allergy, gandolinium precluding magnetic resonance imaging. The FDA labeling also warns against the risk of spinous process fracture. Post-marketing contingency studies required for continued FDA approval of the coflex® hinges on annual reporting two long-term follow-up studies [28, 29]. Five-year follow-up has been reported by one of the original investigational device exemption (IDE) studies with up to [30].

The Wallis® System was first marketed in Europe in 1986. It is currently undergoing FDA-regulated clinical trials in the United States - was initially sold by Abbott Spine and is now commercially distributed through Zimmer Spine. The device consists of a body (first generation titanium; second generation polyetheretherketone - PEEK), which is held between two adjacent spinous processes by a flat dacron band.

The DIAM™ Spinal Stabilization System (Medtronic Sofamor Danek) is another ISP with a soft silicone core. It is also undergoing clinical trials regulated by the FDA. The DIAM™ ISP system differs from most devices since it requires resection of the interspinous ligament. Fixation to the spinous processes is achieved with laces. The In-Space (Synthes) and FLEXUS™ (Globus Medical) devices is another FDA trial underway in the US at this time. Its focus is the implant's comparison to historical X-STOP data. In Europe, clinical trials employing the NL-Prow™ (Non-Linear Technologies), Aperius® (Medtronic Spine), and Falena® (Mikai) devices are currently being conducted.

THE COMBINATION OF ISP AND ENDOSCOPIC DECOMPRESSION

Since ISP may reduce sciatica-type low back and leg pain by minimizing instability-related dynamic lateral recess and foraminal stenosis, the author's objective was to address axial and radicular pain with endoscopic transforaminal decompression in combination with a lumbar ISP through the same transforaminal access portal. The authors hypothesized that patients meeting the inclusion criteria should benefit from combining both procedures, making the surgical treatment more [8] reliable and more durable. The advantages of this combined approach are apparent: Patients are exposed to lower perioperative and long-term risks. The added stabilization and indirect decompression achieved by simultaneous placement of the ISP should diminish the reoperation rates.

SURGICAL TECHNIQUE

The employed endoscopes had working channels ranging from 2.7 mm to 4.0 mm. The additional access portal for the authors' cylindrical interspinous spacer was placed at 16 cm from the midline. The access trajectories and skin entry points have been published elsewhere [1 - 5]. A transforaminal discectomy was performed [9]. The discectomies were done endoscopically under mild sedation and local anesthesia in the prone position *via* the transforaminal access. Bony and soft tissue was removed if needed to complete the decompression. The surgical corridor to the interspinous interval was established from the access portal with progressively larger dilatators ranging from 8 mm to 14 mm under fluoroscopic control. The implant's size was maximized for a snug fit (Fig. **1**).

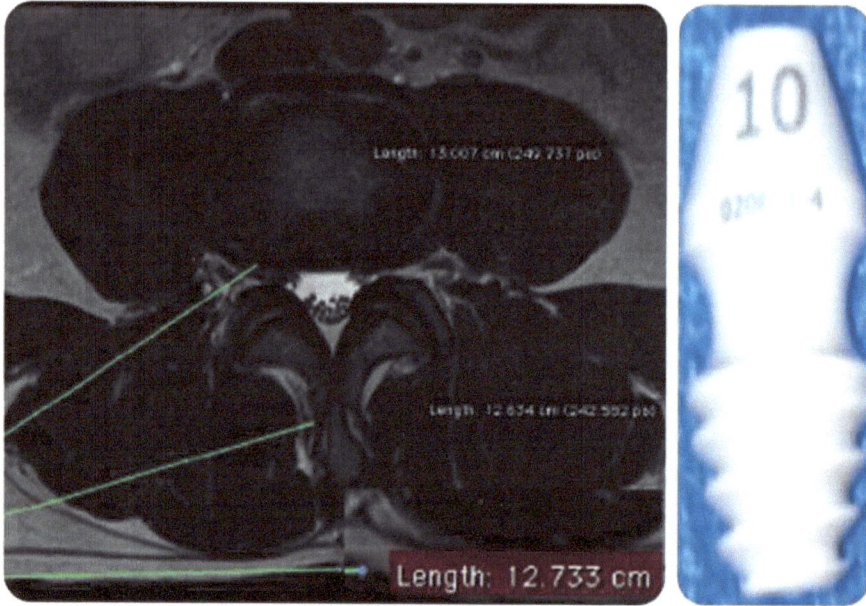

Fig. (1). Axial MRI scan of the L4/5 surgical level with extraforaminal disc herniation and facet arthropathy is shown on the left, and the interspinous process spacer on the right.

COHORT STUDY

Patients' demographic and diagnostic information was retrospectively recorded and analyzed. Primary outcome measures were the VAS score of axial back and radicular leg pain and the Oswestry Disability Index. The functional outcome measures were compared to the preoperative status at one month, six months, and 24 months. Moreover, the patients' general satisfaction with the combined endoscopic decompression and ISP procedure was assessed at a minimum follow-up of two years from the index procedure. The authors' study included a consecutive case study of 152 patients who underwent transforaminal endoscopic decompression with simultaneous ISP placement through the same incision over eight years from 2008 to 2016. There were 80 male and 72 female patients. Clinical data analysis was done on 142 patients two years postoperatively since ten patients were lost in follow-up. The patients' average age was 49 years ranging from 35 to 72. The In-Space was placed in the first 30 patients. The remaining 122 patients received a cylindrical threaded spacer from peak or titanium. Only patients with failed conservative care of a minimum of 3 months were enrolled in the study. The primary indication for surgery was sciatica-type leg- and back pain with or without an axial pain component due to facet arthropathy. We also included patients with axial and radicular pain. In the authors' opinion, the ideal patient should be a candidate for both the transforaminal decompression and the ISP procedure (Table **2**) [10].

Table 2. Indications for combined endoscopic transforaminal decompression and simultaneous ISP placement through the same incision.

Indication	Endoscopic Transforaminal Decompression
-	extruded disc herniation contained disc herniation axial pain, radicular pain, foraminal and extraforaminal stenosis
-	Simultaneous ISP Placement Through Same Incision
-	neurogenic claudication due to central and foraminal stenosis, grade 1 degenerative spondylolisthesis lateral recess stenosis degenerative disc disease (DDD) facet syndrome, disc herniation prevention and treatment for adjacent segment disease DDD with reducible grade 1 retrolisthesis on the x-rays prevention of future reherniation after massive reherniation

RESULTS

In the 152 patients, 214 ISPs were placed as part of their transforaminal decompression surgery, which was performed for axial in 68 patients for radicular claudication pain due to foraminal and canal stenosis. Another 84 patients underwent the combined procedure primarily for axial back pain (Fig. **2**). At the final follow-up, the postoperative VAS reduction was 6.4 points for axial back pain and 5.7 for radicular leg pain. The two-year follow-up postoperative ODI reduction was 42.2. According to the modified Macnab criteria, the vast majority of patients (90%) were satisfied with their clinical results and reported excellent and good outcomes (Fig. **2**).

The authors' series included 14 patients who experienced a complication. Of these, seven required revision surgery. In one patient, the ISP migrated out of the interspinous interval and had to be removed. Another patient was hurt in a car accident, and the dislodge ISP was removed during conversion to an open laminectomy. Two additional patients with spondylolisthesis experienced a spinous process fracture. Therefore, these two patients were revised with an open revision laminectomy and fusion. Another patient with an L5 spinous process fracture was successful treated with Percudyn screws. Conversion to open surgery was necessary for one patient where the L5 spinous process resorbed postoperatively. Consequently, the L4/5 and L5/S1 ISPs failed and, thus, prompted revision surgery due to recurrence of symptoms. One revision surgery was done by replacing the dislodged ISP with a DIAM spacer. Of the other seven patients with adverse events, three were noted to have asymptomatic partial dislodgement of the ISP that ultimately was inconsequential. The remaining patients had superficial wound infections that eventually did not affect their long-term outcomes.

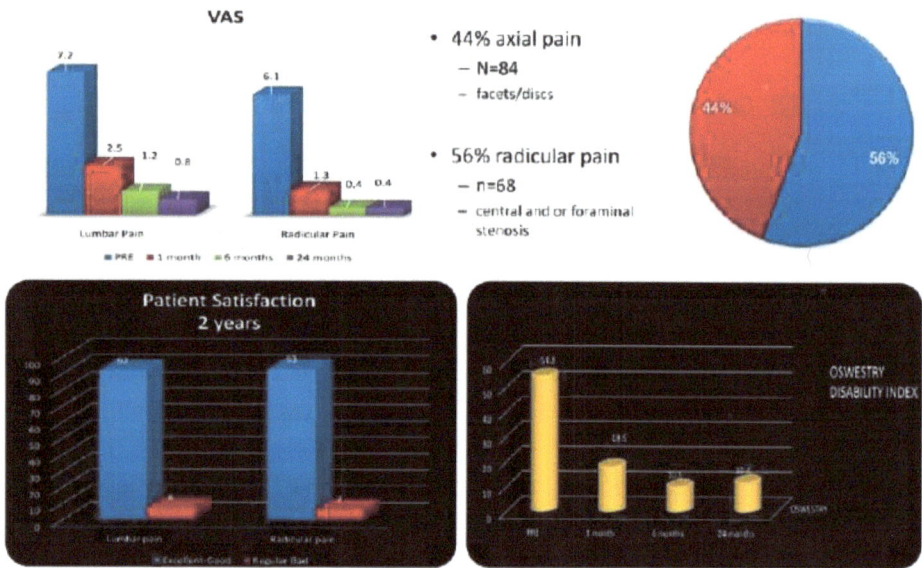

Fig. (2). Clinical outcomes with the endoscopic foraminal decompression and simultaneous ISP placement.

DISCUSSION

The simultaneous ISP implantation during routine transforaminal endoscopy improved clinical outcomes, likely because of the ISP' stabilizing and distracting effect. There were adverse implant-related problems, such as dislocation or migration of the ISP device within the minimum two-year follow-up period. The idea of adding a stabilization procedure to endoscopically decompressed lumbar spinal motion segments to improve the reliability and durability of the procedure is not new. It is based on preventing post-decompression instability. One of the main limitations of this retrospective case series, is the lack of a control group study. However, our study included many patients and therefore has merit in the proposed discussion of combining ISP with endoscopic decompression surgery.

The ISP has the potential to stabilize the posterior spinal column and fits within the framework of simplified outpatient spinal surgery concepts. It can be applied to patients whose medical comorbidities may not permit an open lumbar decompression surgery or who do not want it.

Technically, the operation is not necessarily tricky but can be challenging at the L5/S1 level. A high-riding iliac crest can obliterate access to the L5/S1 interspinous process interval. Lateral bending of the lumbar spine during the positioning of the patient on the operating room table may alleviate this problem. While placing the ISP at the L5/S1 level may be possible by performing a choreographed entry maneuver with the inserter handle being moved around the iliac crest, removing the inserter may not be as easy without dislodging the implant. In some patients, the S1 spinous process may be tiny, thus, making the operation impossible. Another concern with the L5/S1 level is regarding the large interlaminar window. The authors recommend considering an interlaminar window larger than 12 mm as a relative contraindication to the procedure as the implant may dislodge into the spinal canal [12].

While the authors of this study have demonstrated that it is feasible to combine the endoscopic transforaminal decompression and ISP stabilization procedure, the indications and contraindications should be studied further in the short- and long term. The long-term reoperation rates with the ISP have been reported as a negative factor [35, 36]. A recent systematic review shows that a common mode of failure of IPSs is the loss of distraction due to implant erosion through the adjacent spinous processes or mechanical failure resulting in loosening [35]. True implant failure occurred in only 4 cases in the authors' study, suggesting an added benefit to combining the PTED with the ISP procedure, perhaps making both methods more reliable.

CONCLUSION

The authors concluded that the combination of percutaneous transforaminal endoscopic decompression and interspinous devices could be a valuable adjunct to the transforaminal decompression employing the endoscopic platform. Successful outcomes may be achieved in patients suffering from axial back and radicular leg pain caused by a herniated disc and foraminal or lateral recess stenosis in the absence of high-grade spondylolisthesis or deformity. On the contrary, as demonstrated in our patients, it may be particularly beneficial in patients with low-grade spondylolisthesis. There does not seem to be a high complication rate associated with combining these two procedures when performed at a high-skill level by well-trained surgeons [14, 15].

CONSENT FOR PUBLICATION

Not applicable.

CONFLICT OF INTEREST

The authors declare no conflict of interest, financial or otherwise.

ACKNOWLEDGEMENT

Declared none.

REFERENCES

[1]   Yeung AT. Endoscopic decompression, foraminal-plasty and dorsal rhizotomy for foraminal stenosis and lumbar spondylosis: a hybrid procedure in lieu of fusion. J Neurol Disord 2016; 4(8): 322.
[http://dx.doi.org/10.4172/2329-6895.1000322]

[2]   Yeung A, Yeung CA. Endoscopic identification and treating the pain generators in the lumbar spine that escape detection by traditional imaging studies. J Spine 2017; 6(2): 369.
[http://dx.doi.org/10.4172/2165-7939.1000369]

[3]   Yeung AT, Gore S. *In-vivo* endoscopic visualization of patho-anatomy in symptomatic degenerative conditions of the lumbar spine ii: intradiscal, foraminal, and central canal decompression. Surg Technol Int 2011; 21: 299-319.
[PMID: 22505004]

[4]   Yeung AT. *In-vivo* endoscopic visualization of pain generators in the lumbar spine. J Spine 2017; 6(4): 385.
[http://dx.doi.org/10.4172/2165-7939.1000385]

[5]   Yeung AT. The yeung percutaneous endoscopic lumbar decompressive technique (YESSTM). J Spine 2018; 7(1): 408.
[http://dx.doi.org/10.4172/2165-7939.1000408]

[6]   Luk KD, Chow DH, Holmes A. Vertical instability in spondylolisthesis: a traction radiographic assessment technique and the principle of management. Spine 2003; 28(8): 819-27.
[http://dx.doi.org/10.1097/01.BRS.0000058941.55208.14] [PMID: 12698127]

[7]   Gohil I, Vilensky JA, Weber EC. Vacuum phenomenon: Clinical relevance. Clin Anat 2014; 27(3): 455-62.
[http://dx.doi.org/10.1002/ca.22334] [PMID: 24288359]

[8]   Coulier B. The spectrum of vacuum phenomenon and gas in spine. JBR-BTR 2004; 87(1): 9-16.
[PMID: 15055327]

[9]   Balkissoon AR. Radiologic interpretation of vacuum phenomena. Crit Rev Diagn Imaging 1996; 37(5): 435-60.
[PMID: 8922894]

[10]   Serhan H, Mhatre D, Defossez H, Bono CM. Motion-preserving technologies for degenerative lumbar spine: The past, present, and future horizons. SAS J 2011; 5(3): 75-89.
[http://dx.doi.org/10.1016/j.esas.2011.05.001] [PMID: 25802672]

[11]   Gala RJ, Russo GS, Whang PG. Interspinous implants to treat spinal stenosis. Curr Rev Musculoskelet Med 2017; 10(2): 182-8.
[http://dx.doi.org/10.1007/s12178-017-9413-8] [PMID: 28324328]

[12]   Kim DH, Albert TJ. Interspinous process spacers. J Am Acad Orthop Surg 2007; 15(4): 200-7.

[http://dx.doi.org/10.5435/00124635-200704000-00003] [PMID: 17426291]

[13]   Sobottke R, Röllinghoff M, Siewe J, *et al*. Clinical outcomes and quality of life 1 year after open microsurgical decompression or implantation of an interspinous stand-alone spacer. Minim Invasive Neurosurg 2010; 53(4): 179-83.
[http://dx.doi.org/10.1055/s-0030-1263108] [PMID: 21132610]

[14]   Postacchini R, Ferrari E, Cinotti G, Menchetti PP, Postacchini F. Aperius interspinous implant *versus* open surgical decompression in lumbar spinal stenosis. Spine J 2011; 11(10): 933-9.
[http://dx.doi.org/10.1016/j.spinee.2011.08.419] [PMID: 22005077]

[15]   Kabir SM, Gupta SR, Casey AT. Lumbar interspinous spacers: a systematic review of clinical and biomechanical evidence. Spine 2010; 35(25): E1499-506.
[http://dx.doi.org/10.1097/BRS.0b013e3181e9af93] [PMID: 21102279]

[16]   Retrospective evaluation of performance of coflex® interlaminer technology *versus* decompression with or without fusion. clinicaltrails.gov Identifier, NCT03041896, sponsor: Paradigm Spine, Recruitment Status : Completed, First Posted : February 3, 2017, Last Update Posted 2018.https://clinicaltrials.gov/ct2/show/NCT03041896?term=NCT03041896&rank=1

[17]   Clinical Trial Comparing Decompression With and Without Coflex™ Interlaminar Technology Treating Lumbar Spinal Stenosis. ClinicalTrails.gov Identifier, NCT01316211, Verified February 2017 by Paradigm Spine. Recruitment status was: Active, not recruiting, First Posted 2017.https://clinicaltrials.gov/ct2/show/NCT01316211?term=NCT01316211&rank=1

[18]   Post-Approval 'Real Conditions of Use' Study (PAS003). A 2 and 5 Year Comparative Evaluation of Clinical Outcomes in the Treatment of Degenerative Spinal Stenosis With Concomitant Low Back Pain by Decompression With and Without Additional Stabilization Using the Coflex®. ClinicalTrials.gov Identifier: NCT02555280, Recruitment Status : Recruiting, First Posted 2019.https://clinicaltrials.gov/ct2/show/NCT02555280?term=NCT02555280&rank=1

[19]   The Coflex®COMMUNITY Study: An Observational Study of Coflex® Interlaminar Technology. ClinicalTrials.gov Identifier: NCT02457468, Recruitment Status: Recruiting, First Posted : May 29, 2015, Last Update Posted 2019. https://clinicaltrials.gov/ct2/show/NCT02457468?term=NCT-02457468&rank=1

[20]   Paolo DP, Gisberto E, Antonella V, *et al*. Biomechanichs of interspinous devices. BioMed Res Int 2014; 14: 1-7.

[21]   Patel VV, Whang PG, Haley TR, *et al*. Superion interspinous process spacer for intermittent neurogenic claudication secondary to moderate lumbar spinal stenosis: two-year results from a randomized controlled FDA-IDE pivotal trial. Spine 2015; 40(5): 275-82.
[http://dx.doi.org/10.1097/BRS.0000000000000735] [PMID: 25494323]

[22]   Patel VV, Nunley PD, Whang PG, *et al*. Superion(®) interspinous spacer for treatment of moderate degenerative lumbar spinal stenosis: durable three-year results of a randomized controlled trial. J Pain Res 2015; 8: 657-62.
[PMID: 26491369]

[23]   U.S. Food and Drug Administration. Summary of safety and effectiveness data: coflex Interlaminar Technology 2012. http://www.accessdata.fda.gov/cdrh_docs/pdf11/P110008b.pdf

[24]   Davis RJ, Errico TJ, Bae H, Auerbach JD. Decompression and Coflex interlaminar stabilization compared with decompression and instrumented spinal fusion for spinal stenosis and low-grade degenerative spondylolisthesis: two-year results from the prospective, randomized, multicenter, Food and Drug Administration Investigational Device Exemption trial. Spine 2013; 38(18): 1529-39.
[http://dx.doi.org/10.1097/BRS.0b013e31829a6d0a] [PMID: 23680830]

[25]   Davis R, Auerbach JD, Bae H, Errico TJ. Can low-grade spondylolisthesis be effectively treated by either coflex interlaminar stabilization or laminectomy and posterior spinal fusion? Two-year clinical and radiographic results from the randomized, prospective, multicenter US investigational device exemption trial: clinical article. J Neurosurg Spine 2013; 19(2): 174-84.

[http://dx.doi.org/10.3171/2013.4.SPINE12636] [PMID: 23725394]

[26]   Moojen WA, Arts MP, Jacobs WC, *et al.* Interspinous process device *versus* standard conventional surgical decompression for lumbar spinal stenosis: randomized controlled trial. BMJ 2013; 347(nov14 5): f6415.
[http://dx.doi.org/10.1136/bmj.f6415] [PMID: 24231273]

[27]   Moojen WA, Arts MP, Jacobs WC, *et al.* IPD without bony decompression *versus* conventional surgical decompression for lumbar spinal stenosis: 2-year results of a double-blind randomized controlled trial. Eur Spine J 2015; 24(10): 2295-305.
[http://dx.doi.org/10.1007/s00586-014-3748-2] [PMID: 25586759]

[28]   Bae HW, Lauryssen C, Maislin G, Leary S, Musacchio MJ Jr. Therapeutic sustainability and durability of coflex interlaminar stabilization after decompression for lumbar spinal stenosis: a four year assessment. Int J Spine Surg 2015; 9: 15.
[http://dx.doi.org/10.14444/2015] [PMID: 26056630]

[29]   Bae HW, Davis RJ, Lauryssen C, Leary S, Maislin G, Musacchio MJ Jr. Three-year follow-up of the prospective, randomized, controlled trial of Coflex interlaminar stabilization vs instrumented fusion in patients with lumbar stenosis. Neurosurgery 2016; 79(2): 169-81.
[http://dx.doi.org/10.1227/NEU.0000000000001237] [PMID: 27050538]

[30]   Musacchio MJ, Lauryssen C, Davis RJ, *et al.* Evaluation of decompression and interlaminar stabilization compared with decompression and fusion for the treatment of lumbar spinal stenosis: 5-year follow-up of a prospective, randomized, controlled trial. Int J Spine Surg 2016; 10: 6.
[http://dx.doi.org/10.14444/3006] [PMID: 26913226]

[31]   Tian NF, Wu AM, Wu LJ, *et al.* Incidence of heterotopic ossification after implantation of interspinous process devices. Neurosurg Focus 2013; 35(2): E3.
[http://dx.doi.org/10.3171/2013.3.FOCUS12406] [PMID: 23905954]

[32]   Röder C, Baumgärtner B, Berlemann U, Aghayev E. Superior outcomes of decompression with an interlaminar dynamic device *versus* decompression alone in patients with lumbar spinal stenosis and back pain: a cross registry study. Eur Spine J 2015; 24(10): 2228-35.
[http://dx.doi.org/10.1007/s00586-015-4124-6] [PMID: 26187621]

[33]   Richter A, Schütz C, Hauck M, Halm H. Does an interspinous device (Coflex) improve the outcome of decompressive surgery in lumbar spinal stenosis? One-year follow up of a prospective case control study of 60 patients. Eur Spine J 2010; 19(2): 283-9.
[http://dx.doi.org/10.1007/s00586-009-1229-9] [PMID: 19967546]

[34]   Richter A, Halm HF, Hauck M, Quante M. Two-year follow-up after decompressive surgery with and without implantation of an interspinous device for lumbar spinal stenosis: a prospective controlled study. J Spinal Disord Tech 2014; 27(6): 336-41.
[http://dx.doi.org/10.1097/BSD.0b013e31825f7203] [PMID: 22643187]

[35]   Epstein NE. A review of interspinous fusion devices: High complication, reoperation rates, and costs with poor outcomes. Surg Neurol Int 2012; 3:7.
[http://dx.doi.org/10.4103/2152-7806.92172]

[36]   Smith ZA. Interspinous process device *versus* standard conventional surgical decompression for lumbar spinal stenosis results in increased reoperation rates and costs without improving patient outcomes. Evid Based Med 2014; 19:136.
[http://dx.doi.org/10.1136/eb-2013-101689]

CHAPTER 13

Awake Endoscopic Transforaminal Lumbar Interbody Fusion

Ibrahim Hussain[1,*] and **Michael Y. Wang**[1]

[1] *Department of Neurological Surgery, University of Miami, Miami, FL 33136, USA*

Abstract: The transforaminal interbody fusion (TLIF) is a time-tested procedure for treating various lumbar degenerative pathologies. This approach leverages an access route through Kambin's triangle that typically requires a partial or total facetectomy for access to the disc space and neural decompression. Since its first published description in the early 1980s, the procedure has undergone extensive refinements concomitant with technology and technique advancements. Traditional open TLIF is effective but associated with adverse perioperative effects due to the amount of muscle dissection necessary for exposure, including increased blood loss, hospital length of stay, and extended recovery times. The transition to more minimally invasive, paramedian approaches has sought to reduce the burden of these consequences. Spinal endoscopy has witnessed a resurgence over the past decade paralleled by advancements in higher resolution optical systems along with more robust and enduring endoscopic instrumentation. This development, combined with increased awareness of healthcare economic costs, problems with narcotic dependency surrounding open spine surgery, and admission restrictions to hospitals during pandemic times, has fueled a push for "ultra" minimally invasive variants of the traditional TLIF. Patients, payors, and hospitals alike expect shorter inpatient stays, earlier mobilization and discharge from the hospital, as well as narcotic independence faster than ever before. To this end, awake endoscopic TLIF has recently been described with efficacious results to comply with these broader factors. In this chapter, the authors explain their awake endoscopic TLIF step-by-step and demonstrate the clinical advantages and the noninferiority data to traditional MIS TLIF based on their clinical series's one-year outcomes data.

Keywords: Endoscopic interbody fusion, Posterior supplemental fixation, Transforaminal lumbar interbody fusion.

* **Corresponding author Ibrahim Hussain:** Department of Neurological Surgery, University of Miami, Miller School of Medicine, 1095 NW 14TH TER RM 2-06, Miami, FL 33136, USA; Tel: (908) 922-7635; E-mail: ixh212@med.miami.edu

INTRODUCTION

The transforaminal route for accessing the lumbar intervertebral disc was initially performed by Parviz Kambin in 1973, generating the anatomically-geometric structure referred to as "Kambin's triangle." Initial descriptions of his approach were for purposes of percutaneous discectomy, whereby a working cannula was inserted through the "safe" zone of Kambin's triangle for aspiration of nucleus pulposus [1, 2]. Almost a decade later, Jürgen Harms described a similar approach for interbody fusion, leveraging a total facetectomy and hemilaminectomy to provide a safe corridor for discectomy and graft insertion. Controversy in the literature persists regarding Kambin's triangle's actual borders and its application to spinal interbody grafting procedures, for which it was not described initially [3]. Modern-day descriptions have adopted a prism morphology to this space, with different angles of the approach based on the intended goal of surgery (Fig. 1) [4].

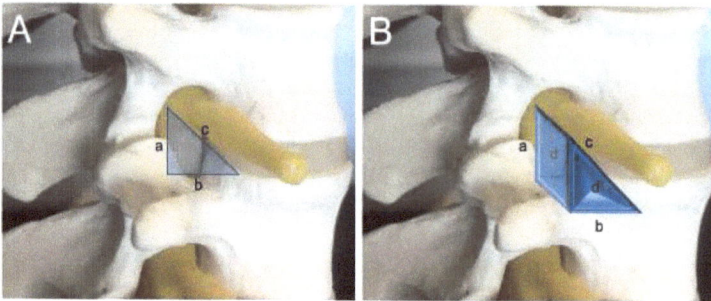

Fig. (1). Kambin's triangle *versus* Kambin's prism. **A)** In Kambin's original description, a two-dimensional triangle denoted the key anatomic landmarks. However, "a" was not assigned a specific structure, though implied the superior articulating process of the inferior vertebrae. "b" and "c" denoted the superior endplate of the inferior vertebra and the exiting nerve root (*i.e.* the "hypotenuse). **B)** In converting Kambin's triangle to a 3-dimensional prism, as described by Tumialán et al. [3], an additional structure can be included. This is "d" which denotes the thecal sac/traversing nerve root. The other structures (a-c) remain the same.

Since Harms' first description of the transforaminal interbody fusion (TLIF), the procedure has undergone revolutionary advancements yielding increasingly minimally-invasive alternatives. These advances have been generated concomitant with retractor technology developments (*i.e.*, tubular, specular), microscopy, and extended microsurgical instrumentation. These approaches allow a paramedian approach through the natural Wiltse plane to access the facet joint and, ultimately, the disc space [4]. Preservation of the posterior tension band while minimizing subperiosteal muscle dissection has demonstrated clear, durable advantages over the traditional midline approach. Numerous studies have shown that minimally-invasive surgery (MIS) TLIF results in lower blood loss, shorter hospital stay, faster recovery times, and less postoperative narcotic use while maintaining comparable clinical outcomes and fusion rates with conventional open TLIF [5 - 12]. Furthermore, comparative cost-effectiveness studies have demonstrated that MIS TLIF is superior to open TLIF with regards to hospital perspective costs (mean difference of $2,680 per surgery) and societal perspective costs attributed to lower absenteeism [12 - 21].

Endoscopic TLIF presents the newest iteration of an MIS-approach for TLIF. Reports of using an endoscope for spinal surgery were described as early as 1977 by Apuzzo et al. using the Hopkins rod lens system [22]. By the late 1990s, with growing interest and technology in MIS-approaches, endoscopic-assistance for performing TLIF in conjunction with tubular retractors was described by Foley and Fessler [23, 24]. These procedures typically used the endoscope as a visualization tool that could be substituted with the surgical microscope. Other technological barriers prevented wide-spread adoption at the time, in addition to a lack of billing codes and surgeon preferences. However, over the last two decades, enormous strides have been made in refining the endoscopic technology available in North America and its adaptation for performing a discectomy and interbody fusion. These include narrower rigid endoscopes, light-emitting diode (LED) illumination sources, ultra-high-definition optical displays, radiofrequency electrode probes for cauterization, disc preparation instruments, and expandable interbody grafts.

Endoscopic TLIF represents a facet of another increasingly recognized movement in MIS of "enhanced" or "fast-track" surgery [25 - 27]. These protocols employ multidisciplinary strategies to minimize complications and create a seamless patient experience that mitigates the burden of surgery and anesthesia. To this end, "awake" endoscopic TLIF was first described by the senior author in 2016 to reduce the extended stay, side-effects, and systemic limitations of general anesthesia, narcotic consumption, and overall healthcare costs with MIS TLIF [28 - 30]. In this chapter, we review the key technical steps of the "awake" endoscopic TLIF and up-to-date clinical outcomes.

ANESTHESIA & ENHANCED RECOVERY AFTER SURGERY (ERAS)

The ERAS pathway adopted for MIS endoscopic TLIF revolves around six core tenets. First, awake surgery is performed under monitored anesthesia care (MAC) rather than general endotracheal intubation. Typically, patients are pre-medicated with 1-2 mg of midazolam before coming to the operating room. After that, sedation maintenance is via a combination of propofol, ketamine, and dexmedetomidine infusions that are titrated until moderate (conscious) sedation is achieved [28]. At this stage, patients, remain asleep but are easily arousable. Supplemental oxygenations are provided by nasal cannular or face mask. Deep sedation (where the patient only responds to painful stimulation) is avoided since patient cooperation and feedback are required if the dorsal root ganglia (DRG) is stimulated during the procedure, signaling to the surgeon to alter maneuvers. This patient feedback is especially pertinent since continuous electromyography is not utilized as a surrogate for exiting nerve stimulation, though this method has also been described [22]. Based on patient risk factors, 1 g of intravenous acetaminophen and 2-4 mg of ondansetron are administered for analgesia and antiemesis, respectively. Steroids and narcotics are not given before or during the procedure (Table **1**).

Table 1. Perioperative Anesthetic and Medication Considerations for Awake Endoscopic TLIF.

Preoperative	Intraoperative*	Postoperative
1-2 mg midazolam	Dexmedetomidine	Acetaminophen (standing)
1 g IV acetaminophen	Propofol	Oxycodone/hydromorphone PRN
2-4 mg ondansetron	Ketamine	Diazepam (or other muscle relaxer) PRN
Prophylactic antibiotics	Phenylephrine or nicardipine for SBP control PRN	Gabapentin/pregabalin

*Intraoperative medications are given either as continuous infusions that are titrated or PRN pushes
Abbreviations: IV=intravenous; SBP=systolic blood pressure; PRN= pro re nata (as needed).

The second tenet is endoscopic-technology for visualization and performing discectomy through as minimally-invasive of an approach as possible. Third, osteobiologics are used for the augmentation of arthrodesis. Unlike in open surgery, the posterior facet complexes and transverse processes are not decorticated and packed with bone graft. The discectomy may not be as complete as accomplished through a series of traditional large curettes and shavers. Therefore, we use recombinant human bone morphogenetic protein-2 (rh-BM--2), packed into the disc space and demineralized bone allograft matrix for packing the interbody graft. Expandable cage technology inserted through the narrow 8 mm portal introduced under endoscopic and fluoroscopic guidance is the fourth tenet. Fifth, percutaneous pedicle screw instrumentation can be placed through limited 1 cm transmuscular incisions and linked with rods passed submuscular to avoid large fascial openings and extensive muscle dissection. The sixth and final tenet is the use of long-acting sodium-channel blockers in the form of liposomal bupivacaine, which can be administered before initial incision under ultrasonic guidance as a thoracolumbar interfacial plane (TLIP) block and along with the facet join and trajectory of percutaneous pedicle screws [30 - 32]. These concepts are summarized in Table **2**.

Table 2. ERAS Components of Awake Endoscopic TLIF.

Component	Methodology/Device
Awake surgery	MAC for moderate sedation, no endotracheal intubation
MIS discectomy/decompression	Transforaminal endoscopy through 8mm working cannula
Osteobiologics	Rh-BMP-2, demineralized bone matrix allograft
Expandable interbody	Mesh graft that is inserted flat then filled with bone graft
Percutaneous pedicle screw stabilization	Single step pedicle screw device with built in K-wire or traditional fenestrated screws with K-wires using fluoroscopic or 3D navigation. Submuscular rods passed. Minimal fascial opening and muscle dissection
Long acting Na-channel blockers	Liposomal bupivacaine injected as part of preoperative TLIP block and around the facet joints and trajectory of percutaneous pedicle screws

Abbreviations: 3D=3-dimensional MAC=monitored anesthesia care; MIS=minimally invasive surgery; Na=sodium; TLIP= Thoracolumbar interfascial plane; Rh-BMP-2= recombinant human bone morphogenetic protein-2.

INDICATIONS

The indications for endoscopic TLIF need to consider patient symptomatology and anatomy. Traditional open and MIS TLIF require partial or complete facetectomy for direct neural decompression plus stabilization with pedicle screw instrumentation. However, there are other considerations when performing endoscopic TLIF. First, complete decompression via total facetectomy and laminectomy is not typically performed. While feasible via endoscopic approaches, these procedures require longer operative times for facetectomy using currently available drills and a separate interlaminar approach for hemi- or ipsi-contralateral laminectomy. Therefore, those patients with severe central canal stenosis in whom laminectomy is required are not appropriate for this particular approach. This procedure is dependent on indirect decompression of central and contralateral foraminal stenosis by restoring disc height and reducing spondylolisthesis degree. Furthermore, in patients with kyphotic disc angles, in whom segmental lordosis is required, are also not appropriate for this approach. While expandable, lordotic TLIF interbody cages are commonly used in MIS TLIF, their application via the 8mm cannula used for endoscopic access is not available at the moment.

ROOM SET UP & PATIENT POSITIONING

A schematic of the optimal room set up is demonstrated in Fig. (**2**). The patient is brought to the operating room and positioned prone on a flat Jackson table with a Wilson frame. The Wilson frame's padded arches are released from their frame, which places the patient in the least kyphotic position while maintaining comfort. Furthermore, the "give" of the Wilson frame in this setup mitigates that amount of force absorbed by the patient when malleting instruments later in the procedure. Single plane anteroposterior (AP) X-rays with a single C-arm machine is utilized for initial anatomic planning. It is imperative to obtain adequate imaging and orientation before beginning the procedure. The superior endplate of the caudal level of interest should appear as a single line. The pedicles should have a clear ovoid-shape, and the spinous process should be aligned in the middle of the vertebral body (the so-called "owl-face" morphology.

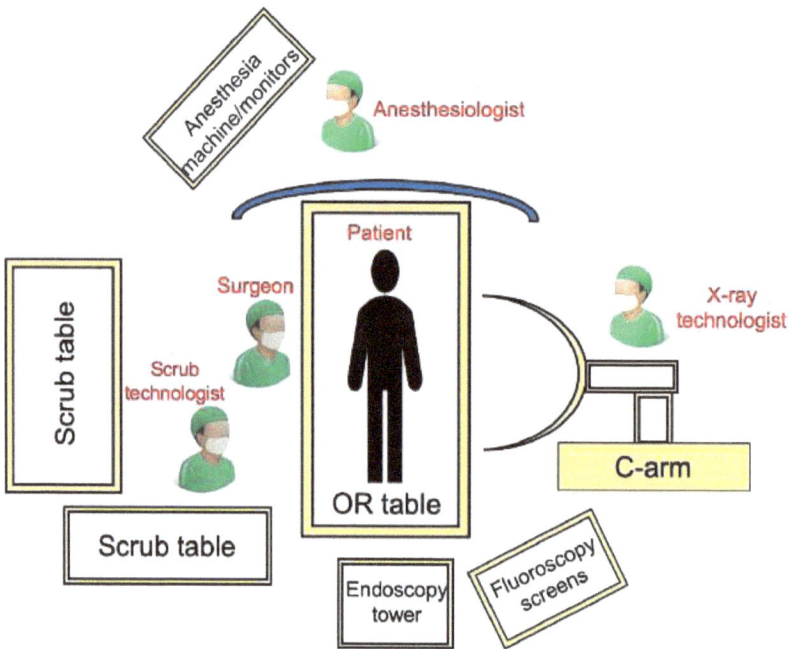

Fig. (2). Schematic of room setup for awake endoscopic TLIF with approach from the left side. The surgeon always works opposite the C-arm, and monitors for the endoscopy and fluoroscopy screens are positioned to maximize ergonomic comfort and line of sight for the surgeon.

The distance from midline where the incision is made varies from patient to patient but typically ranges from 8-10 cm. Considerations for this include patient habitus, angle of trajectory, and the ultimate goal for positioning the interbody graft. Starting more laterally allows for better access to the disc itself and contralateral disc material and increases the risk of dorsal root ganglia (DRG) injury.

APPROACH

Once the entry site is determined, 1% lidocaine with epinephrine infiltration is performed in the planned incision region. Infiltration is first performed superficially along the skin for analgesia and vasoconstriction, then carried deep along the endoscope's trajectory to the paraspinal musculature. Next, an 18-gauge spinal needle is inserted and under AP fluoroscopy aimed towards the facet joint, used to target the superior articulating process of the caudal level [33]. Once docked on the superior articulating process of the facet joint, further infiltration with 1% lidocaine with epinephrine can be performed to further anesthetize and vasoconstrict the neurovascular structures around the joint. The needle is carefully "walked" down (ventrally) the SAP until it drops off into the disc space, characterized by a loss of resistance. AP fluoroscopy will demonstrate this as the needle passing the lateral border of the pedicle. Care should be taken not to advance the needle past the pedicle wall's medial border until the needle position is confirmed on lateral X-ray. On the lateral shot, the needle should be traversing the foramen in the caudal most position possible within the foramen and into the disc space, which minimizes the risk of injury to the exiting nerve root, which is located in the cranial aspect of the foramen.

A nitinol wire was inserted into the spinal needle, and the spinal needle was removed. A transverse incision is made lateral and medial to the needle with an 11-blade scalpel just through the dermis – a deeper fascial incision is not required. Then successive dilators are used to expand this corridor up to 6mm. Resistance will be encountered when the dilator rests on the annulus of the disc. Gentle downward pressure or malleting of the dilator is required to penetrate and dilate the annulus. After the last dilator is inserted, the beveled working cannular is inserted with the beveled opening facing the cranial to avoid exiting nerve root injury upon entry. Once the working cannula is safe with the disc, the bevel is turned 90 degrees clockwise (facing medially). At this point, the endoscope is brought in for the discectomy.

DISCECTOMY

The annular defect and disc material should be immediately apparent once the endoscope is introduced into the working channel (Fig. **3A**). Using a series of instruments, the discectomy is performed. The discectomy begins by first establishing the centrum of the discectomy, which essentially will define the corridor for the interbody graft position. Subsequent instruments will essentially dilate and expand the discectomy around this central tract. This portion is initially accomplished with a combination of Kerrison rongeurs and straight and angled pituitary rongeurs (Fig. **3B**). The technique for this step is unlike that of the traditional discectomy procedure. Small, quick bites are taken to begin dismantling the nucleus pulposus. The endoscopic system's continuous irrigation will usually wash most of these little bits away as the surgeon works. The surgeon should avoid taking large bites and persistently removing the instrument from the endoscope for cleaning, which only adds time to the discectomy and is inefficient for the purpose required. The discectomy is carried roughly to the midline on AP views and the disc space's front on lateral views. Care should be taken not to penetrate the anterior longitudinal ligament (ALL), resulting in vascular injury and potential interbody graft migration into the retroperitoneum. Inspection of the exiting nerve root can be intermittently checked by turning the working cannular 90 degrees counterclockwise (bevel open cranially; Fig. **3C**). Typically, small vessels and perineural fat will be indicated when the nerve is nearby. A bipolar cautery ball-tipped curved probe is used for hemostasis and shrinking back fat tissue, as well as a blunt dissector.

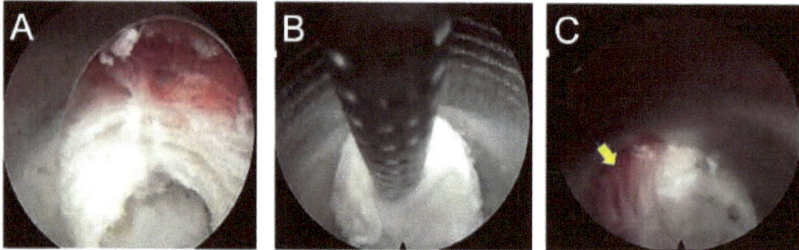

Fig. (3). Endoscopic discectomy. **A)** Straight and curved (pictured) pituitary rongeurs are used to create the initial centrum of disc removal. **B)** Pulling back the working cannula demonstrates the edge of the annulus with the defect. This annulotomy can be widened with Kerrison rongeurs and cauterization as needed. **C)** turning the working cannular counter clockwise so that the beveled opening faces cranially allows for visualization of the exiting nerve root (arrow).

Larger dilators are placed to expand the working corridor to 8 mm. The discectomy is then further carried out using a series of drills, brushes, and shavers to expose the endplates and prep the disc space for interbody graft placement. At our institution, we use the Food and Drug Administrations (FDA)-approved OptiMesh Expandable Interbody Fusion System (Spineology, St, Paul, MN). A working cannula is then impacted into the disc space with a built depth gauge resting on the patient's body and preventing plunging with subsequent instruments. Subsequent disc removal is accomplished with larger pituitary rongeurs, hand drill, fan-blade shaver, backbiting rongeur, and straight/angled wire brushes on a power drill. These instruments are manually turned in all directions to maximize disc removal (Fig. **4**).

An expandable balloon with opaque dye is then assessed in the disc space under fluoroscopy. This step is essential in demonstrating which area of the disc has not been adequately removed. Based on this information, the endoscope is then reinserted. Further discectomy with the straight and angled pituitary rongeurs under direct visualization is performed. If necessary, the second round of disc preparation under fluoroscopy with the series of instruments mentioned previously. This step is critical to preventing delayed pseudarthrosis and interbody graft migration, as was observed in our early experience [34, 35].

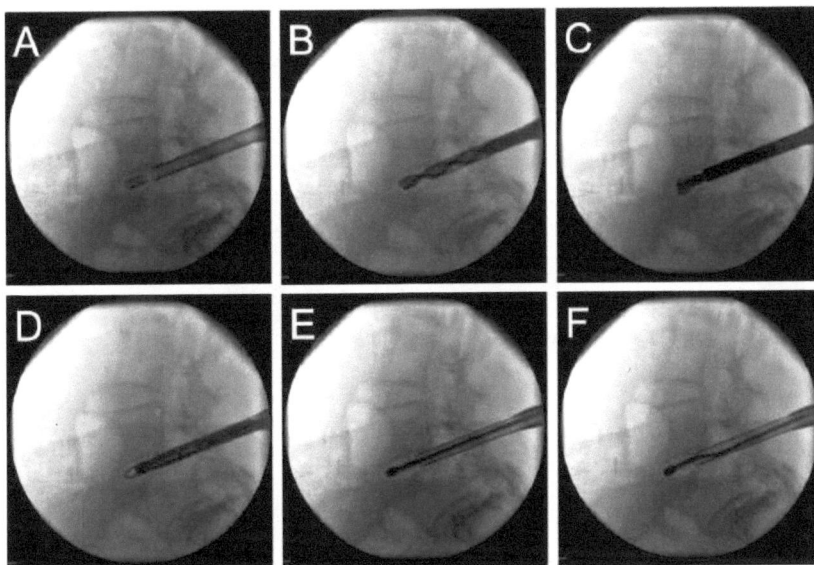

Fig. (4). Workflow and instruments for disc preparation through the endoscopic working cannula. **A)** The initial working cannula is passed over a dilator tube and positioned shallow in the disc space. Placing the 8 mm working cannula here allows the subsequent instruments to clean out as much disc material as possible. **B)** Hand twist drill to widen the centrum of the disc. **C)** "Butterfly" fan-shaver, which can be manually adjusted to dilate and retract the fan blades. This maneuver allows the instrument to scrape along the endplates based on the height of the disc space. **D)** Backbiting rongeur, which can be rotated in multiple directions to maximize further disc removal. **E)** and **F)** straight and angled wire brushes clear away any remaining disc material, and further prepare the endplates for graft implantation.

INTERBODY GRAFT INSERTION

Once adequate disc preparation has been accomplished, an extra-small kit of rh-BMP-2 is inserted for fusion enhancement (2.1 mg, off-label FDA use). Inserting this sponge is different from traditional open or MIS TLIF, given the endoscopic approach's closed-pressure system. First, a straight suction tubing is used to suck up any remaining blood or water in the disc space. The BMP sponge is carefully and slowly inserted through the working cannula and pushed to its lowest depth with a plunger. Inserting the sponge too quickly can cause it to bunch up at a proximal location or to rip apart, leaving pieces close to the neural elements, which can cause long-term complications with heterotopic bone compression. Once the sponge is in an optimal location at the front of the disc space, the deflated mesh interbody graft is inserted, and the place is confirmed with an X-ray. A series of pre-filled tubes with demineralized bone matrix allograft is then impacted in different directions within the mesh to allow for a homogenous expansion of the expandable device in three dimensions. The mesh graft is crimped shut, and any carrier matrix in the exiting nerve's vicinity is thoroughly rinsed out. Final AP and lateral fluoroscopy are taken to confirm implant location and increase in disc height.

PEDICLE SCREW STABILIZATION

Pedicle screw stabilization is performed in conjunction with all endoscopic transforaminal interbody grafts. Multiple systems are available to accomplish this in a minimally invasive fashion. We typically use a single-step pedicle screw system with integrated K-wire and self-tapping, fluted-tip screws (Viper Prime, DePuy-Synthes, Raynham, MA). However, other cannulated, K-wire based systems can be used, and screws can be placed with fluoroscopy or 3D navigation based on available resources and surgeon preference (Fig. **5**).

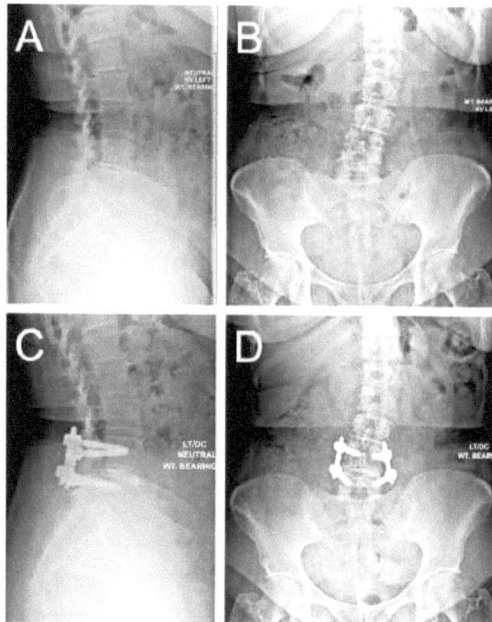

Fig. (5). Preoperative **A)** lateral and **B)** AP radiographs compared with postoperative **C)** lateral and **D)** AP radiographs following awake endoscopic TLIF. Note the increase in foraminal height with reduction of the Grade 1 spondylolisthesis. A cannulated percutaneous pedicle screw system was used for non-segmental posterior supplemental fixation.

CLINICAL SERIES & OUTCOMES

To date, the senior author has performed over 300 awake endoscopic TLIFs. Of the first 100 consecutive cases with a minimum of 1-year follow-up [34], the majority (N=84) have been single-level, with the remaining being 2-level surgeries (Table **3**).

Table 3. Clinical and outcomes data for first 100 patients undergoing awake endoscopic TLIF with 1-year follow-up.

Variable	Value (+/- SD or %)
Age (mean)	66.0 +/- 11.0
Sex	44 male/56 female
OR Time (minutes)	84.5 +/- 21.7 (one-level) 128.1 +/- 48.6 (two-level)
Level Treated **Total** **L1/2** **L2/3** **L3/4** **L4/5** **L5/S1**	116 2 2 22 89 1
Hospital length of stay (mean)	1.4 +/- 1.0
Conversion to GETA	4 (4%)
Surgical Complications **Total** **Graft Migration** **Endplate Fracture** **Osteomyelitis**	4 (4%) 2 (2%) 1 (1%) 1 (1%)
Change in ODI Score	-12.3

Abbreviations: GETA=General endotracheal anesthesia; ODI=Oswestry Disability Index.
Adapted from Kolcun et al. Neurosurg Focus. 2019 Apr 1;46(4):E14.

The cohort's mean age was 66 years old with mean operative times of 85 and 128 minutes for one- and two-level surgeries, respectively. Mean intraoperative blood loss ranged from 65-74 mL, and length of stay was 1.4 days. Mean Oswestry Disability Index (ODI) scores decreased from 29.6 to 17.2 during the study period. In four cases, conversion to general endotracheal intubation had to be performed (emesis, epistaxis, and anxiety). These incidents ultimately influenced the perioperative medication regimen, including anxiolytics, antiemetics, and strict blood pressure control. Other surgical complications include two cases of graft migration, one case of osteomyelitis, and one case of endplate fracture. Three of these four complications occurred in the first fifty cases. Another study from our group focusing on the economics of the procedure further demonstrated that the ERAS applications of endoscopic TLIFs result in an average of $3,444 of acute care hospitalization savings when compared with traditional MIS TLIF [29].

DISCUSSION

Bringing awake endoscopic TLIF to fruition required a significant collaborative effort between neurosurgical and anesthesia teams well before the first case was performed. Our anesthetic protocol has evolved as more cases were performed and complications were encountered. At our institution, we perform these cases with the same anesthesiologist who was instrumental in the development of this protocol. The attending or an experienced trainee provides second-to-second attention to these patients throughout the procedure. Apnea, epistaxis, nausea, anxiety, and patient movement must be immediately addressed for the safety of the patient as well as for the efficiency of the procedure. In a similar vein, another component of this procedure that has only increased the efficiency and safety can be attributed to dedicated staff including scrub and radiology technicians. While logistical constraints may not allow this at many large university medical centers, we cannot underscore the importance of this. Ultimately, there are three different components of the procedure that each require their own instrumentation and equipment which are complicated in their own respect. From the endoscopic equipment, to the disc prep instruments and interbody grafts, and finally the percutaneous pedicle screw stabilization system, over 20 advanced instruments are required to complete the surgery which must be provided to the surgeon in rapid succession during the case. Our workflow has gotten to the point now where instruments are simply handed in the expected order and do not even need to be called out by the surgeon. Similarly, time is not wasted trying to figure out the right angles of the C-arm machine to line up the endplates and pedicles, as the radiology technician has significant experience to make corrections on their own without requiring extensive feedback.

In an effort to minimize the number of instruments required to complete the procedure, the percutaneous pedicle screw instrumentation portion provides the best opportunity. As mentioned previously, we typically use a single step pedicle screw stabilization system that allows screws to be placed in one shot without having to switch out instruments for Jamshidi needles, K-wires, and taps. We typically place these screws with AP fluoroscopy with a final depth check using lateral shots. This allows for extremely efficient and accurate screw placement but comes with a caveat. These devices do not leave room for error, especially when small pedicles are being cannulated. Due to the cutting flute nature of the screws, placing them in the wrong trajectory makes it extremely difficult to place a screw in a new trajectory without falling into the old track or damaging the pedicle to the point that screw purchase is compromised. Bail out solutions include upsizing the diameter of the screws or reverting back to traditional techniques with Jamshidi and K-wires which is not always successful. It is imperative that every attempt is made to place the screw correctly the first time when using these devices, otherwise, their inherent efficiency can cause issues that add unanticipated time to the surgery.

In terms of levels that can be optimally treated with the endoscopic TLIF, the L5-S1 level still presents a challenge. Approach-related constraints of the iliac crest can make this disc access from the usual paraspinal transforaminal approach very difficult. Even when the disc space can be accessed, the trajectory of the approach more closely resembles an approach with a cranial-caudal angulation which is suboptimal for a contralateral discectomy and places a greater risk of iatrogenic injury to the DRG and the endplates during disc preparation. Patients with transitional anatomy are more amenable to this approach at L5-S1, considering this more closely resembles the L4-5 level. The transiliac approach for the L5-S1 disc space has been described by other groups [36 - 39] as an alternative option, which involves reaming through the ilium posterior to the sacral ala and cephalad to the S1 pedicle. However, these reports have been limited to decompression procedures and not specifically for interbody graft placement.

As mentioned previously, complications are inevitable with any new procedure in the spine field. Interbody graft migration was noted in early experience which was due to inadequate disc preparation. We evolved our protocol to include going back into the disc space with the endoscope after the first round of fluoroscopy-guided disc preparation to remove the further disc in the contralateral or anterior space. The prevents the graft from asymmetric filling and ensures that the BMP sponge and graft itself can be placed as anterior as possible in the disc space to prevent nerve irritation. Further complications are likely to be uncovered with longer term follow-up and larger studies. We have performed this procedure in patients with lumbar degenerative scoliosis, grade II spondylolisthesis, osteoporosis, near collapsed disc spaces, early adjacent level disc degeneration, and high-grade foraminal stenosis. Studies are ongoing to evaluate the long-term success and failure of patients in these cohorts who undergo awake endoscopic TLIF.

CONCLUSION

Awake endoscopic TLIF is the most recent advancement in the realm of "ultra" MIS surgery. When employed with the principles of ERAS, the excellent patient reported outcomes can be achieved due to the lack of general endotracheal intubation, less muscle dissection, less narcotic dependency, and faster operative times. Long-term radiographic, clinical, and economic outcomes are ongoing with comparison with conventional open and MIS TLIF.

CONSENT FOR PUBLICATION

Not applicable.

CONFLICT OF INTEREST

The authors declare no conflict of interest, financial or otherwise.

ACKNOWLEDGEMENT

Declared none.

REFERENCES

[1]   Kambin P, Sampson S. Posterolateral percutaneous suction-excision of herniated lumbar intervertebral discs. Report of interim results. Clin Orthop Relat Res 1986; (207): 37-43.
[PMID: 3720102]

[2]   Kambin P, Brager MD. Percutaneous posterolateral discectomy. Anatomy and mechanism. Clin Orthop Relat Res 1987; (223): 145-54.
[PMID: 3652568]

[3]   Tumialán LM, Madhavan K, Godzik J, Wang MY. The history of and controversy over kambin's triangle: a historical analysis of the lumbar transforaminal corridor for endoscopic and surgical approaches. World Neurosurg 2019; 123: 402-8.
[http://dx.doi.org/10.1016/j.wneu.2018.10.221] [PMID: 30415041]

[4]   Wiltse LL, Bateman JG, Hutchinson RH, Nelson WE. The paraspinal sacrospinalis-splitting approach to the lumbar spine. J Bone Joint Surg Am 1968; 50(5): 919-26.
[http://dx.doi.org/10.2106/00004623-196850050-00004] [PMID: 5676831]

[5]   Jin-Tao Q, Yu T, Mei W, *et al.* Comparison of MIS vs. open PLIF/TLIF with regard to clinical improvement, fusion rate, and incidence of major complication: a meta-analysis. Eur Spine J 2015; 24(5): 1058-65.
[http://dx.doi.org/10.1007/s00586-015-3890-5] [PMID: 25820353]

[6]   Khan NR, Clark AJ, Lee SL, Venable GT, Rossi NB, Foley KT. Surgical outcomes for minimally invasive *vs* open transforaminal lumbar interbody fusion: an updated systematic review and meta-analysis. Neurosurgery 2015; 77(6): 847-74.
[http://dx.doi.org/10.1227/NEU.0000000000000913] [PMID: 26214320]

[7]   Adogwa O, Parker SL, Bydon A, Cheng J, McGirt MJ. Comparative effectiveness of minimally invasive *versus* open transforaminal lumbar interbody fusion: 2-year assessment of narcotic use, return to work, disability, and quality of life. J Spinal Disord Tech 2011; 24(8): 479-84.
[http://dx.doi.org/10.1097/BSD.0b013e3182055cac] [PMID: 21336176]

[8]   Gu G, Zhang H, Fan G, *et al.* Comparison of minimally invasive *versus* open transforaminal lumbar interbody fusion in two-level degenerative lumbar disease. Int Orthop 2014; 38(4): 817-24.
[http://dx.doi.org/10.1007/s00264-013-2169-x] [PMID: 24240484]

[9]   Guan J, Bisson EF, Dailey AT, Hood RS, Schmidt MH. Comparison of clinical outcomes in the national neurosurgery quality and outcomes database for open *versus* minimally invasive transforaminal lumbar interbody fusion. Spine 2016; 41(7): E416-21.
[http://dx.doi.org/10.1097/BRS.0000000000001259] [PMID: 26536435]

[10]   Lim JK, Kim SM. Radiographic results of Minimally Invasive (MIS) Lumbar Interbody Fusion (LIF) compared with conventional lumbar interbody fusion. Korean J Spine 2013; 10(2): 65-71.
[http://dx.doi.org/10.14245/kjs.2013.10.2.65] [PMID: 24757461]

[11]   Seng C, Siddiqui MA, Wong KP, *et al.* Five-year outcomes of minimally invasive *versus* open transforaminal lumbar interbody fusion: a matched-pair comparison study. Spine 2013; 38(23): 2049-55.
[http://dx.doi.org/10.1097/BRS.0b013e3182a8212d] [PMID: 23963015]

[12]   Wong AP, Smith ZA, Stadler JA III, *et al.* Minimally invasive transforaminal lumbar interbody fusion (MI-TLIF): surgical technique, long-term 4-year prospective outcomes, and complications compared with an open TLIF cohort. Neurosurg Clin N Am 2014; 25(2): 279-304.
[http://dx.doi.org/10.1016/j.nec.2013.12.007] [PMID: 24703447]

[13]   Djurasovic M, Gum JL, Crawford CH, *et al.* Cost-effectiveness of minimally invasive midline lumbar interbody fusion *versus* traditional open transforaminal lumbar interbody fusion. J Neurosurg Spine 2019; 1-5.
[PMID: 31518977]

[14]   Droeghaag R, Hermans SMM, Caelers IJMH, Evers SMAA, van Hemert WLW, van Santbrink H. Cost-effectiveness of open transforaminal lumbar interbody fusion (OTLIF) *versus* minimally invasive transforaminal lumbar interbody fusion (MITLIF): a systematic review and meta-analysis. Spine J 2021; 21(6): 945-54.
[http://dx.doi.org/10.1016/j.spinee.2021.01.018] [PMID: 33493680]

[15]   Parker SL, Adogwa O, Bydon A, Cheng J, McGirt MJ. Cost-effectiveness of minimally invasive *versus* open transforaminal lumbar interbody fusion for degenerative spondylolisthesis associated low-back and leg pain over two years. World Neurosurg 2012; 78(1-2): 178-84.
[http://dx.doi.org/10.1016/j.wneu.2011.09.013] [PMID: 22120269]

[16]   Parker SL, Mendenhall SK, Shau DN, *et al.* Minimally invasive *versus* open transforaminal lumbar interbody fusion for degenerative spondylolisthesis: comparative effectiveness and cost-utility analysis. World Neurosurg 2014; 82(1-2): 230-8.
[http://dx.doi.org/10.1016/j.wneu.2013.01.041] [PMID: 23321379]

[17]   Pelton MA, Phillips FM, Singh K. A comparison of perioperative costs and outcomes in patients with and without workers' compensation claims treated with minimally invasive or open transforaminal lumbar interbody fusion. Spine 2012; 37(22): 1914-9.
[http://dx.doi.org/10.1097/BRS.0b013e318257d490] [PMID: 22487713]

[18]   Rampersaud YR, Gray R, Lewis SJ, Massicotte EM, Fehlings MG. Cost-utility analysis of posterior minimally invasive fusion compared with conventional open fusion for lumbar spondylolisthesis. SAS J 2011; 5(2): 29-35.
[http://dx.doi.org/10.1016/j.esas.2011.02.001] [PMID: 25802665]

[19]   Singh K, Nandyala SV, Marquez-Lara A, *et al.* A perioperative cost analysis comparing single-level minimally invasive and open transforaminal lumbar interbody fusion. Spine J 2014; 14(8): 1694-701.
[http://dx.doi.org/10.1016/j.spinee.2013.10.053] [PMID: 24252237]

[20]   Sulaiman WA, Singh M. Minimally invasive *versus* open transforaminal lumbar interbody fusion for degenerative spondylolisthesis grades 1-2: patient-reported clinical outcomes and cost-utility analysis. Ochsner J 2014; 14(1): 32-7.
[PMID: 24688330]

[21]   Ver MLP, Gum JL, Crawford CH, *et al.* Index episode-of-care propensity-matched comparison of transforaminal lumbar interbody fusion (TLIF) techniques: open traditional TLIF *versus* midline lumbar interbody fusion (MIDLIF) *versus* robot-assisted MIDLIF. J Neurosurg Spine 2020; 1-7.
[http://dx.doi.org/10.3171/2019.9.SPINE1932] [PMID: 31978884]

[22]   Apuzzo ML, Heifetz MD, Weiss MH, Kurze T. Neurosurgical endoscopy using the side-viewing telescope. J Neurosurg 1977; 46(3): 398-400.
[http://dx.doi.org/10.3171/jns.1977.46.3.0398] [PMID: 839267]

[23]   Foley KT, Smith MM, Rampersaud YR. Microendoscopic approach to far-lateral lumbar disc herniation. Neurosurg Focus 1999; 7(5): e5.

[http://dx.doi.org/10.3171/foc.1999.7.5.8] [PMID: 16918212]

[24]   Fessler RG, Khoo LT. Minimally invasive cervical microendoscopic foraminotomy: an initial clinical experience. Neurosurgery 2002; 51(5) (Suppl.): S37-45.
[http://dx.doi.org/10.1097/00006123-200211002-00006] [PMID: 12234428]

[25]   Delaney CP, Fazio VW, Senagore AJ, Robinson B, Halverson AL, Remzi FH. 'Fast track' postoperative management protocol for patients with high co-morbidity undergoing complex abdominal and pelvic colorectal surgery. Br J Surg 2001; 88(11): 1533-8.
[http://dx.doi.org/10.1046/j.0007-1323.2001.01905.x] [PMID: 11683754]

[26]   Development of an Enhanced Recovery After Surgery (ERAS) approach for lumbar spinal fusion. J Neurosurg Spine 2017; 26(4): 411-8.
[http://dx.doi.org/10.3171/2016.9.SPINE16375] [PMID: 28009223]

[27]   Wainwright TW, Immins T, Middleton RG. Enhanced recovery after surgery (ERAS) and its applicability for major spine surgery. Best Pract Res Clin Anaesthesiol 2016; 30(1): 91-102.
[http://dx.doi.org/10.1016/j.bpa.2015.11.001] [PMID: 27036606]

[28]   Wang MY, Grossman J. Endoscopic minimally invasive transforaminal interbody fusion without general anesthesia: initial clinical experience with 1-year follow-up. Neurosurg Focus 2016; 40(2): E13.
[http://dx.doi.org/10.3171/2015.11.FOCUS15435] [PMID: 26828882]

[29]   Wang MY, Chang HK, Grossman J. Reduced Acute Care Costs With the ERAS® Minimally Invasive Transforaminal Lumbar Interbody Fusion Compared With Conventional Minimally Invasive Transforaminal Lumbar Interbody Fusion. Neurosurgery 2018; 83(4): 827-34.
[http://dx.doi.org/10.1093/neuros/nyx400] [PMID: 28945854]

[30]   Brusko GD, Kolcun JPG, Heger JA, *et al.* Reductions in length of stay, narcotics use, and pain following implementation of an enhanced recovery after surgery program for 1- to 3-level lumbar fusion surgery. Neurosurg Focus 2019; 46(4): E4.
[http://dx.doi.org/10.3171/2019.1.FOCUS18692] [PMID: 30933921]

[31]   Roh MS, Kucher OA, Shick KM, Knolhoff DR, McGarvey JS, Peterson SC. Intramuscular Liposomal Bupivacaine Decreases Length of Stay and Opioid Usage Following Lumbar Spinal Fusion. Clin Spine Surg 2020; 33(8): E359-63.
[http://dx.doi.org/10.1097/BSD.0000000000001006] [PMID: 32427717]

[32]   Tomov M, Tou K, Winkel R, *et al.* Does Subcutaneous Infiltration of Liposomal Bupivacaine Following Single-Level Transforaminal Lumbar Interbody Fusion Surgery Improve Immediate Postoperative Pain Control? Asian Spine J 2018; 12(1): 85-93.
[http://dx.doi.org/10.4184/asj.2018.12.1.85] [PMID: 29503687]

[33]   Basil GW, Wang MY. Technical considerations of endoscopic kambin's triangle lumbar interbody fusion. World Neurosurg 2021; 145: 670-81.
[http://dx.doi.org/10.1016/j.wneu.2020.05.118] [PMID: 32485242]

[34]   Kolcun JPG, Brusko GD, Basil GW, Epstein R, Wang MY. Endoscopic transforaminal lumbar interbody fusion without general anesthesia: operative and clinical outcomes in 100 consecutive patients with a minimum 1-year follow-up. Neurosurg Focus 2019; 46(4): E14.
[http://dx.doi.org/10.3171/2018.12.FOCUS18701] [PMID: 30933915]

[35]   Kolcun JPG, Brusko GD, Wang MY. Endoscopic transforaminal lumbar interbody fusion without general anesthesia: technical innovations and outcomes. Ann Transl Med 2019; 7 (Suppl. 5): S167.
[http://dx.doi.org/10.21037/atm.2019.07.92] [PMID: 31624733]

[36]   Bai J, Zhang W, Wang Y, *et al.* Application of transiliac approach to intervertebral endoscopic discectomy in L5/S1 intervertebral disc herniation. Eur J Med Res 2017; 22(1): 14.
[http://dx.doi.org/10.1186/s40001-017-0254-0] [PMID: 28376859]

[37]   Choi G, Kim JS, Lokhande P, Lee SH. Percutaneous endoscopic lumbar discectomy by transiliac

approach: a case report. Spine 2009; 34(12): E443-6.
[http://dx.doi.org/10.1097/BRS.0b013e31817c4f39] [PMID: 19454997]

[38] Osman SG, Sherlekar S, Malik A, *et al.* Endoscopic trans-iliac approach to L5-S1 disc and foramen - a report on clinical experience. Int J Spine Surg 2014; 8: 8.
[http://dx.doi.org/10.14444/1020] [PMID: 25694926]

[39] Patgaonkar P, Datar G, Agrawal U, *et al.* Suprailiac *versus* transiliac approach in transforaminal endoscopic discectomy at L5-S1: a new surgical classification of L5-iliac crest relationship and guidelines for approach. J Spine Surg 2020; 6 (Suppl. 1): S145-54.
[http://dx.doi.org/10.21037/jss.2019.09.14] [PMID: 32195423]

CHAPTER 14

Endoscopic Transforaminal Lewlif™ Interbody Fusion with a Standalone Expandable Interbody Fusion Cage

Kai-Uwe Lewandrowski[1,2,3,*] and **Jorge Felipe Ramírez León**[4]

[1] *Center for Advanced Spine Care of Southern Arizona and Surgical Institute of Tucson, Tucson, AZ, USA*

[2] *Departmemt of Orthopaedics, Fundación Universitaria Sanitas, Bogotá, D.C., Colombia, USA*

[3] *Visiting Professor Department of Neurosurgery in the Video-Endoscopic Postgraduate Program at the Universidade Federal do Estado do Rio de Janeiro — UNIRIO, Rio de Janeiro, Brazil*

[4] *Centro de Columna – Cirugía Mínima Invasiva. Bogotá, D.C., Colombia, Clínica Reina Sofía – Clínica Colsanitas. Bogotá, D.C., Colombia, Fundación Universitaria Sanitas. Bogotá, D.C., Colombia, USA*

Abstract: Endoscopic spinal fusion is on the horizon. Many surgeons have offered various endoscopically assisted decompression and fusion surgeries that consist of an interbody device and posterior supplemental screws. Stabilization of the spine *via* an anterior column fusion implant has excellent advantages of improving the fusion rate *via* bone graft containment. It can enhance spinal alignment and assist in direct and indirect decompression of neural elements *via* restoring normal lumbar curvature and neuroforaminal height. However, further use of posterior supplemental fixation has the disadvantage of adding to the operation's complexity in blood loss, time, equipment needs, and complications. Therefore, a simplified standalone anterior interbody fusion procedure to be carried out through the transforaminal approach *via* a small posterolateral skin incision was of interest to the authors of this chapter, who are introducing the complete endoscopic implantation of a threaded expandable cylindrical fusion cage. This fusion system was developed to mitigate subsidence and migration problems seen with non-threaded lumbar interbody fusion cages, many of which require posterior pedicle screw fixation. This chapter describes step-by-step transforaminal decompression fusion technique suitable for an outpatient ambulatory surgery center setting.

Keywords: Anterior column stabilization, Endoscopy, Interbody fusion.

* Corresponding author Kai-Uwe Lewandrowski: Center for Advanced Spine Care of Southern Arizona and Surgical Institute of Tucson, Tucson, AZ, USA, Department of Orthopaedic Surgery, UNIRIO, Rio de Janeiro, Brazil and Department of Orthoapedic Surgery, Fundación Universitaria Sanitas, Bogotá, D.C., Colombia, USA; Tel: +1 520 204-1495; Fax: +1 623 218-1215; E-mail: business@tucsonspine.com

INTRODUCTION

Endoscopic surgery is increasingly favored by patients and surgeons alike for its simplicity in execution and low burden in postoperative recovery [1, 2]. Negligible blood loss, minimal incisional pain, fast mobilization, and a lower incidence of peri- and long-term postoperative problems are the primary motivators [3, 4]. However, the limits of the procedure seem to be at the decompression level. More complex clinical indications requiring the deployment of implants typically often cannot be completed through the small endoscopic access portals. Some authors have circumvented the problem with hybrid endoscopically assisted instrumented fusion procedures. Standalone endoscopic interbody fusion through the same small access portal without additional portals or enlarging the incisions is a novelty and became possible with the advent of expandable cages. The FDA approval of a cylindrical threaded expandable device designed for standalone interbody fusion without additional use of posterior supplemental fixation has provided both the technological and regulatory basis for a pure endoscopic interbody fusion procedure [5 - 7].

MIS lumbar interbody fusion cages stabilize the spine while restoring neuroforaminal height and fusion [8]. They may restore spinal curvature and aid indirect decompression of painful neural elements. Static interbody fusion cages have been around for more than two decades, and their clinical track record is well documented. Endplate decortication is ideally done by maintaining the integrity of the subchondral bone. Posterior pedicle screw fixation may improve stability and minimize the observed cage migration and subsidence problems [9 - 11] Pedicle screw fixation may add to operative time, increase blood loss, and lead to a higher complication rate [12 - 14], Propagation of adjacent segment disease is another concern [15]. A standalone endoscopic transforaminal decompression and fusion procedure would capitalize on time-proven benefits of minimal muscle dissection and access-related problems by employing advanced endoscopes and standard neurosurgical and motorized decompression instruments (Fig. **1**). With the advent of advanced foraminoplasty techniques, a combination of "outside-in" and "inside-out" techniques became feasible, allowing direct visualization of the epidural and intradiscal space during the same surgery.

Ideally, the implant has a large chamber for a bone graft. Moreover, openings allow the graft to fuse between the adjacent endplates, which can easily be monitored radiographically. In skilled hands, endplate preserving decortication techniques coupled with gentle advancement of a threaded device over a guidewire into the intervertebral disc space could be added without complicating the routine transforaminal endoscopic decompression surgery too much. Such an implant should be adjustable by a turning motion where clockwise rotation advances the threaded implant. The devices' counterclockwise turning retrieves it without losing the purchase. The expansion of the cage *in situ* distracts the adjacent endplates, thereby indirectly stabilizing the surgical motion segment *via* ligamentotaxis without the need for pedicle screws (Fig. **2**).

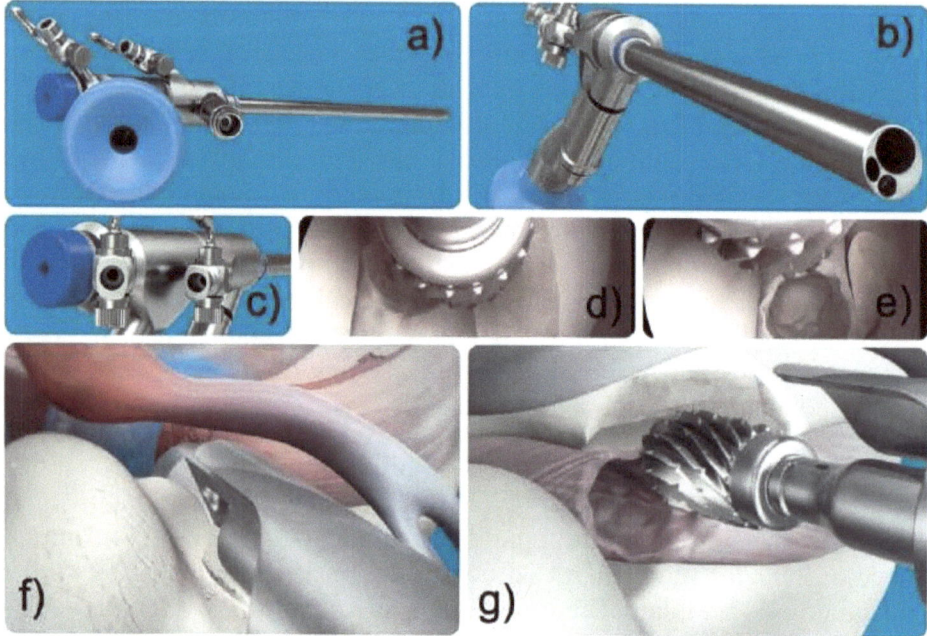

Fig. (1). Example of a modern foraminoscope (**a-b**) with a 4.1 mm inner working channel and integrated suction and irrigation channel (**c**) introduction of standard 4.0 mm diameter neurosurgical decompression tools becomes feasible. A motorized burr is employed to drill down osteophytes of the hypertrophic ring apophysis to prepare the cage's introitus (**d**). The same burr may also be used to prepare entry into the disc space and prepare the endplates (**e**). Kerrison rongers may be employed to perform the foraminoplasty by resecting parts of the superior (**f**) and inferior articular process (**g**). The bladed tip of the beveled endoscopic working cannula is strategically positioned to retract the exiting nerve root (g).

PATIENT SELECTION CRITERIA

The authors began endoscopic spinal fusion in 2016 by building on the existing outpatient spinal surgery program. The main indication for this procedure is end-stage degenerative disc disease with associated grade I spondylolisthesis causing unrelenting radiculopathy and claudication symptoms unresponsive to conservative care supported by advanced imaging demonstrating foraminal or lateral recess stenosis. Patients with higher anterolisthesis or severe central stenosis defined as less than 100 mm^2 cross-sectional canal area [16], extreme facet hypertrophy, infection, and metastatic disease were excluded.

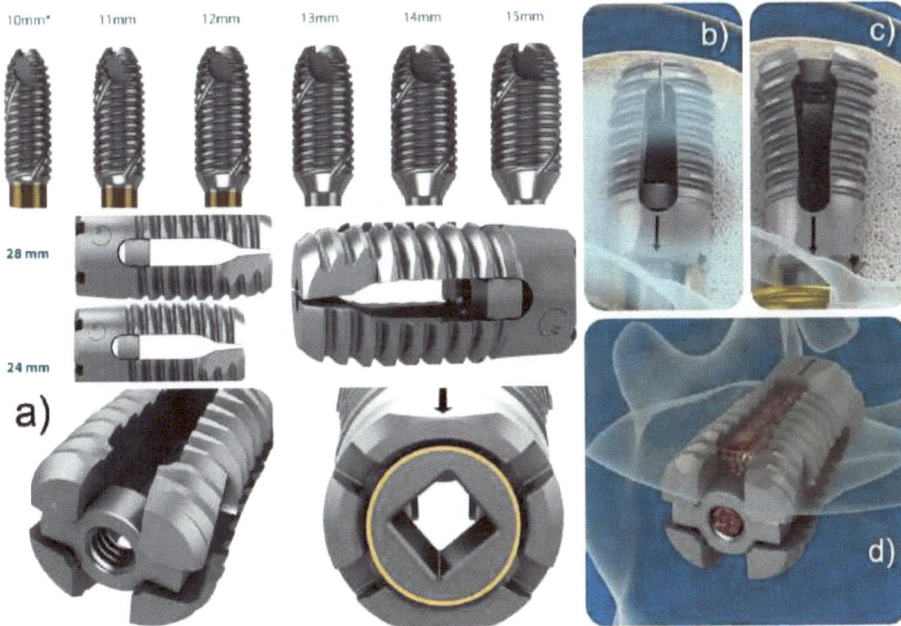

Fig. (2). Images of the available tap and expandable cage sizes ranging from 10 to 15 mm in diameter **(a)** . The surgeon can choose between a 24 mm or 28 mm long cage. The center expansion block is advanced to the tapered tip **(b-c)**, thereby opening the bone graft chamber **(d)**, which can be closed with an end cap (a).

SURGICAL TECHNIQUES

The endoscopic transforaminal approach accesses the epidural space *via* foraminoplasty and the "outside-in" approach was defined as a LEWLIF™ (USPTO Serial Number 88338772, Registration Number, 5867644). The procedure is indicated for advanced lumbar disc degeneration, spinal stenosis, and instability using a single oblique threaded expandable cage. The decompression is started at the inferior pedicle by placing the working sheath inferiorly in the neuroforamen. The bladed tip of the beveled working cannula can be strategically positioned to retract the exiting nerve root. As described below, the net effect is a foraminoplasty. The inside-out technique is employed during the intradiscal portion of the procedure when preparing the endplates and completing the discectomy. While theoretically feasible under local anesthesia and sedation, surgeons should expect more stimulation and need for intraoperative pain control during the fusion portion of the surgery, particularly though during the implantation and *in situ* expansion of the implant. Therefore, the authors recommend following the balanced anesthesia protocol outlined in volume 1 of this Bentham series on spinal endoscopy – a combination of propofol, fentanyl in conjunction with a laryngeal mask or endotracheal ventilation. This balanced anesthesia protocol could be considered a step-down version of the traditional general anesthesia protocol. Patients undergoing open lumbar fusion surgery are typically subjected to more prolonged mechanical ventilation with inhalation gas, muscle relaxants, and larger doses of narcotics. The adjunctive local anesthesia use with 0.25% bupivacaine will further decrease the need for pharmacologically assisted anesthesia and facilitate a rapid wake-up. The endoscopic transforaminal approach to the lumbar has been described elsewhere and in detail throughout this text [17 - 26]. The entry points are as follows: L3/4 - 7 - 9 cm, L4/5 - 8 - 10 cm, and L5/S1 - 10-12 cm lateral to the midline. The targeted neuroforamen was accessed as follows:

1. Needle Placement: The foraminal safe zone is first cannulated with an 18-G 8-inch long spinal needle aimed at the inferior pedicle followed by insertion of a guidewire (Fig. **3**) [27 - 29].

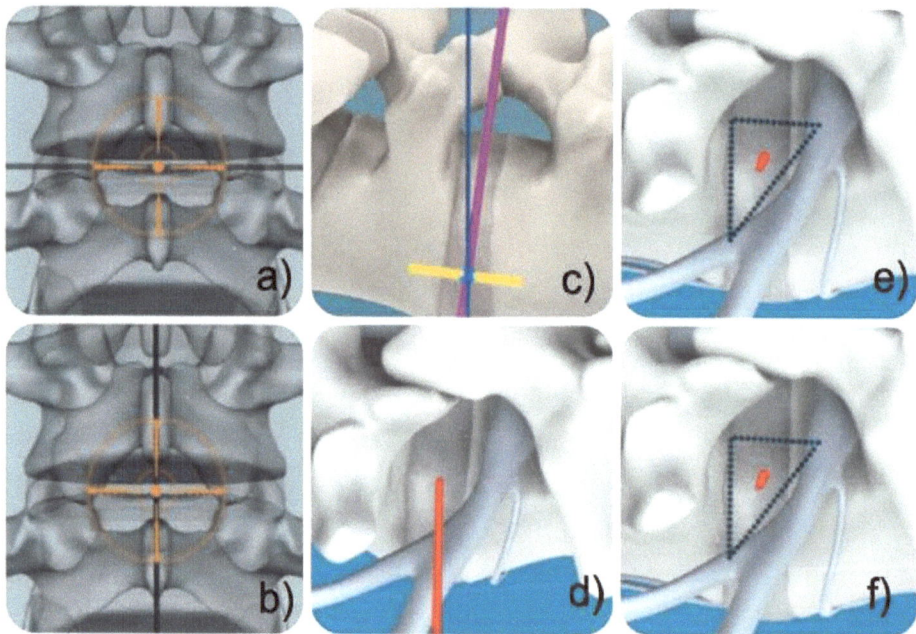

Fig. (3). Schematic depiction of the fluoroscopically aided identification of the target level in the anterior-posterior plane outline a line parallel to the surgical disc space (**a**) and the interspinous process line (**b**). In the lateral plane, the endoscopic working cannula should be lined up parallel to the disc space (**c**). The intersecting lines best suggest the optimum skin entry point to get a straight shot at the triangular safe zone (**e-f**).

2. Placement of Working Cannula: An initial foraminoplasty is performed with power drills, and trephines of increasing diameters. Serial dilation is employed to place the working cannula onto the surgical facet joint complex's lateral aspect. Occasionally, an endoscopic chisel can come in handy to facilitate the resection of

larger bone pieces from hypertrophied facet joints. The endochisel is particularly useful when transecting the tip of the supraarticular process (SAP). Cannulated reamers with an outer diameter of 7 and 9 mm can also be placed over a nitinol guidewire with and without a protective working cannula. The smaller 7 mm reamer can be placed through the standard 8.9 mm working cannula for the authors' foraminoscope (Fig. **1**).

3. <u>Foraminoplasty & SAP Resection</u>: The foraminoplasty is now taken to the lateral recess until the traversing nerve root is visualized. The above-mentioned Endoscopic osteotomes, power drills, and Kerrison rongeurs are very useful in completing this task. Ideally, the SAP is resected at its base with the pedicle. Regardless of which instrument, the entire decompression procedure was performed under direct visualization. Local bone graft should be harvested mainly from the SAP resection to be used in interbody fusion (Fig. **4**).

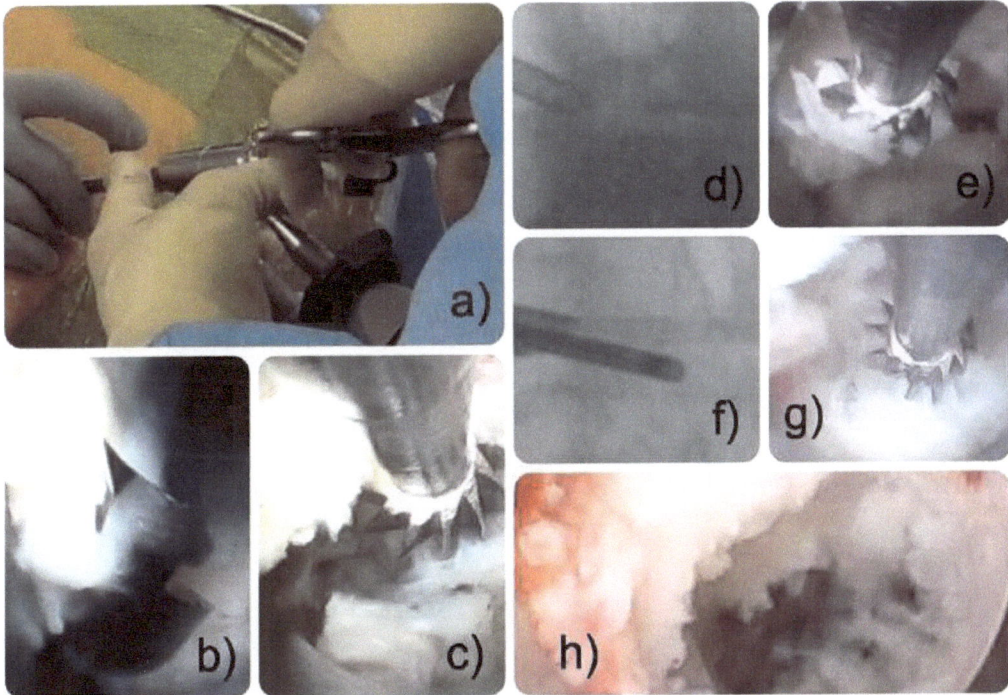

Fig. (4). Intraoperative fluoroscopic and endoscopic views of the transforaminal access to the lumbar facet joint complex are shown **(a)**. Drills and rongeurs are used to remove portions of the hypertrophic facet joint complex **(b-d)** aiming to enter the facet joint by placing the working cannular right into the joint space **(e)**. The safe zone between the traversing and exiting nerve root is widely exposed. The drill and a rongeur can be used to enter the disc space **(f, g)**, which is then cleaned under direct visualization **(h)**.

4. Partial Pediculolectomy: Upon completion of the foraminoplasty, partial resection of the inferior pedicle may be necessary to gain intervertebral disc space access. Additional, resection of the ring apophysis, particularly in cases of advanced vertical collapse of the disc space, may be necessary to get the tapered cage started. A trajectory parallel to the disc space should now be taken to facilitate parallel alignment of the cage within the vertebral interspace. Decompression below the traversing nerve root may require removal of bone from the inferior ring-apophysis below the traversing nerve root. If needed to get the implant started, bony resection of the distal endplate and pedicle are preferred to such maneuvers at the superior vertebral body's rostral endplate to minimize subsidence and traction injury to the exiting nerve root. Surgeons should be vigilant of any extruded disc fragments when completing the discectomy. Typically, there is some bleeding from epidural veins or the bony decompression sites. Some of it may be controllable with the radiofrequency probe (Ellman®; Ellman International LLC, USA).

5. Discectomy & Interspace Preparation: Propagation of implant subsidence is of concern during this step. After annulotomy and discectomy, cannulated paddle shavers are inserted over a 1 mm nitinol guidewire and rotated carefully clockwise while maintaining parallel alignment with the interspace to avoid violation of the subchondral bone during the decortication. The endoscope is inserted periodically to assure that any disc tissue that could impede interbody fusion is removed (Fig. **5a-b**).

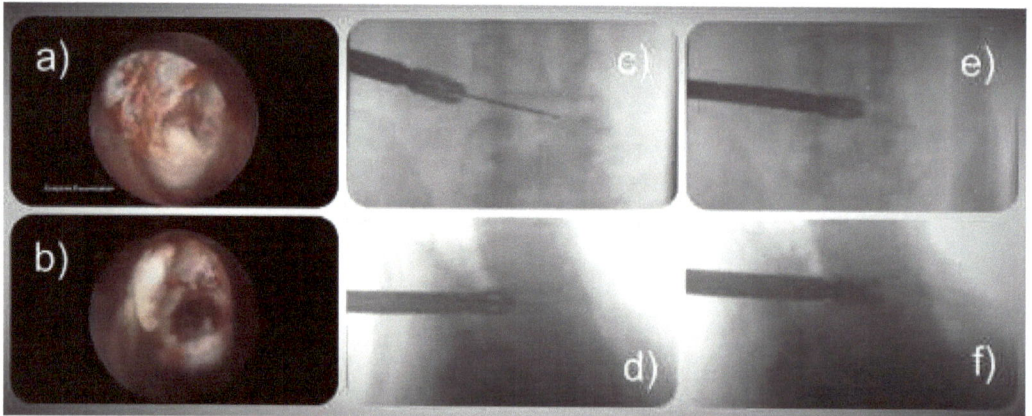

Fig. (5). Endoscopic endplate preparation (**a**), and the intervertebral disc space (**b**). The VariLift®-L implant is inserted *via* a nitinol guide wire obliquely into the midportion of the intervertebral disc space as shown here in the anteroposterior (**c** and **e**), and the lateral (**d** and **f**) fluoroscopic projection.

6. Sizing & Taping: The implant (VariLift®-L) comes in sizes starting at 10 mm to 15 mm initial insertion diameter, which will expand another one mm after expansion. The initial outer diameter of the cannulated conical tap is 4 mm smaller at the tip. Final sizing is best determined initially with a snug feel of the paddle shavers followed by taps, which in its final size should securely capture both adjacent endplates. These steps of the procedure are highly skill-dependent. Under-sizing and over distraction should be avoided as both scenarios can lead to implant failure either by rapid expulsion or subsidence. The orientation of the obliquely placed cage is typically dictated by the transforaminal attack angles between 40 to 60 degrees in the axial plane. Ideally, the cage crosses the midline and reaches the opposite medial interpedicular line in the anterior-posterior fluoroscopic projection (Fig. **5c-f**). Cage insertion at L5/S1 can be challenging in patients with high iliac crest and sacralized L5 vertebral bodies. Other obstacles, including a sizeable sacral alar and a laterally hypertrophic facet joint, may have to be dealt with.

7. Cage Insertion & Expansion: The cage is mounted on a cannulated inserter and guided into the interspace *via* the same one-mm nitinol guidewire by turning it clockwise. The ideal position of this single oblique device is in the midline position in the anterior-posterior fluoroscopic plane and as much anteriorly as possible and anterior to the posterior vertebral line in the lateral fluoroscopic view. The final implant position should be inspected endoscopically and directly visualized on the video screen to ensure it is 3 mm recessed below the annulus. In the lateral projection, the cage should be placed such that both openings of the bone graft chamber can be seen without obstruction. Only then should the central expansion screw be advanced all the way forward in a clockwise motion to expand the cage (Fig. **6a**).

8. Bone Grafting: The cages design captures some local bone grafts during the clockwise rotation. However, the authors recommend inserting additional bone grafts through the inserter into the cage's central chamber. Ideally, bone graft extrudes into the interspace *via* the implant's fenestrations. The local bone graft from the facetectomy should be inserted anteriorly and opposite from the intended cage position through the endoscope under direct visualization (Fig. **6b**). The final step involves the placement of the end cap and the removal of the inserter.

The steps outlined above increase the neuroforaminal volume and maximize the cage's introitus through the triangular safe zone formed by traversing and exiting the nerve root and the pedicle below. These maneuvers should be performed under direct endoscopic visualization to safely retract the neural elements throughout the surgery and ensure the completion of the discectomy and endplate integrity during their decortication.

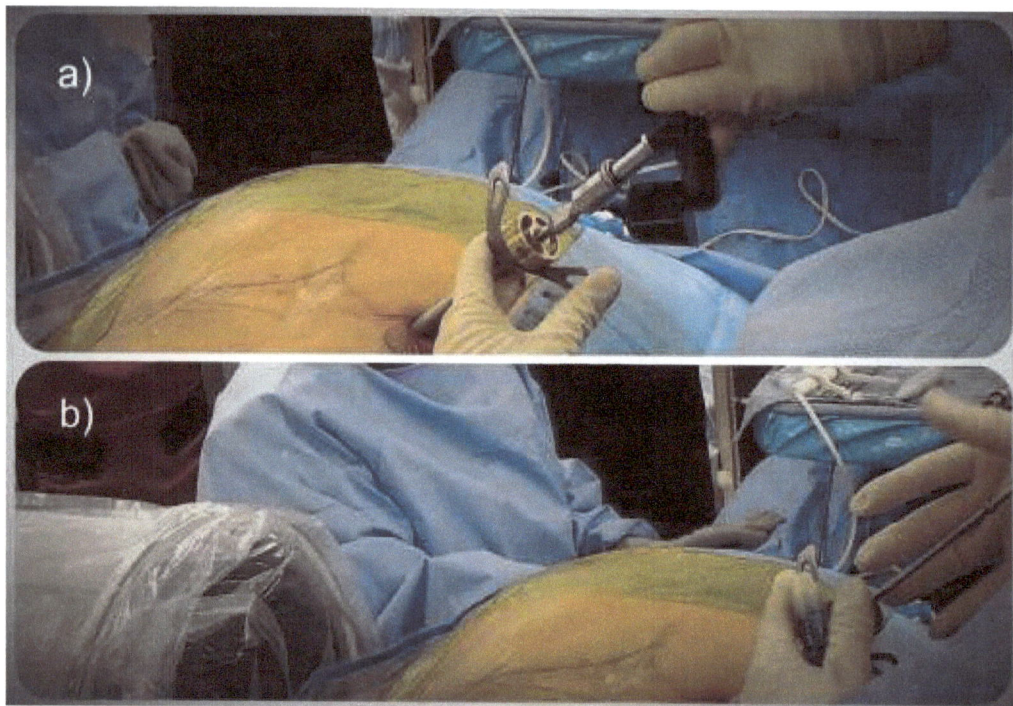

Fig. (6). The VariLift®-L implant is expanded by turning the center expansion set screw clockwise *via* the inserter's central working channel (**a**). The bone graft is extruded through the lateral cage fenestrations into the intervertebral disc space.

CASE SERIES

The authors' case series included a total of 48 patients of ages of 32 to 88 years and a mean of 64.9 years, consisting of 29 females and 19 males. Study patients underwent standalone endoscopically assisted LEWLIF™ procedure using the VariLift-L interbody fusion system (Wenzel Spine, Austin, TX, USA) employing the inclusion/exclusion criteria and techniques outlined earlier in this chapter [30]. Patients came back to the clinic for periodic follow-up examinations. Radiographic assessment of fusion could be done on each study patient at two years from the index operation. Clinical outcomes were assessed with the modified Macnab criteria [31, 32]. The indication for surgery was spondylolisthesis in 44 of the 48 patients. An exemplary case is shown in Figs. (**7 - 9**). Two additional patients suffered severe central and lateral recess stenosis, and another two had stenosis related to adjacent segment disease.

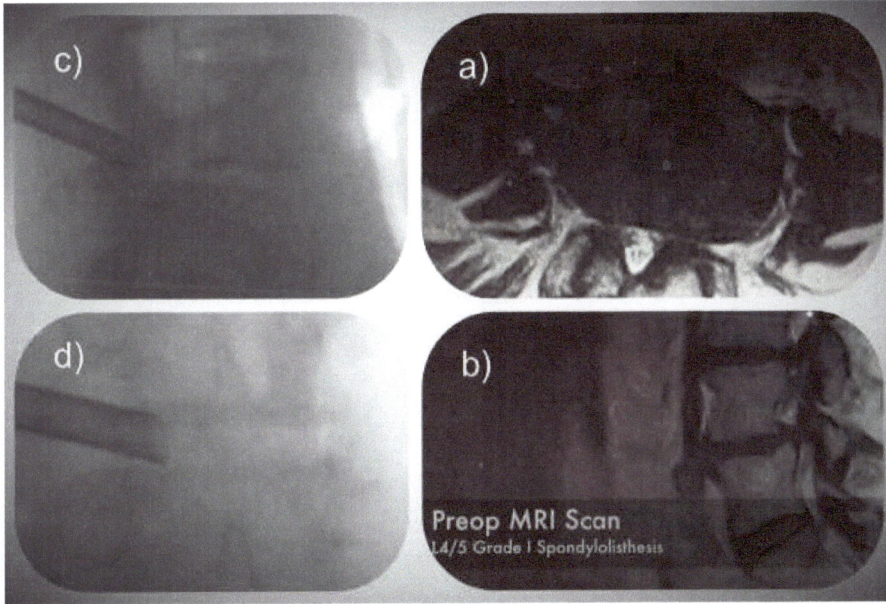

Fig. (7). Preoperative axial (**a**), and sagittal (**b**) MRI scan at L4/5 and lateral recess and foraminal stenosis. A transforaminal working cannula was placed at the lateral recess as shown in the lateral (**c**), and in the anterior-posterior (**a**) projection.

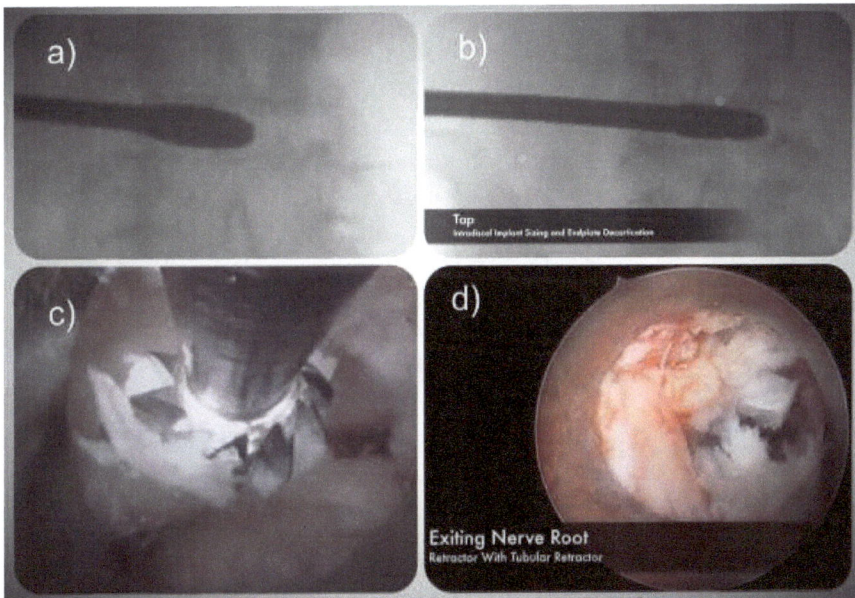

Fig. (8). Shown is an anterior posterior fluoroscopy view (**a**) of a paddle shaver placed through the transfoaminal approach to decorticate the endplates, followed by a threaded tap (**b**) The decompression was carried out by accessing the facet joint and resection of the superior articular process revealing the exiting and traversing nerve root.

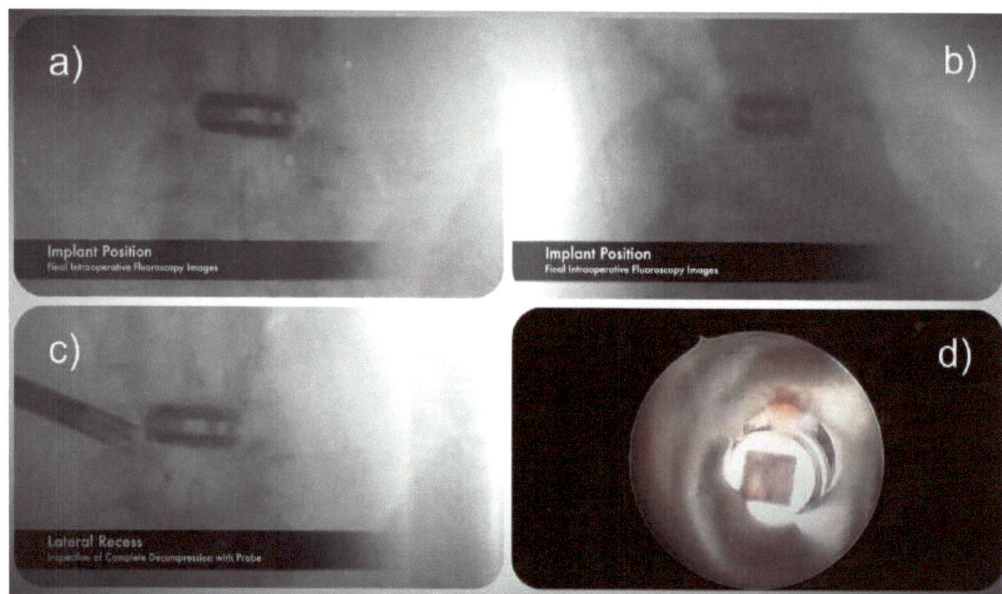

Fig. (9). The final implant position is shown in the PA **(a)** and **(b)** lateral view. The lateral recess decompression is complete as shown by the probe passing around the L5 pedicle **(c)**. The bone graft is contained with an end cap.

Analysis of level distribution showed that the indication for LEWLIF™ surgery was established and most frequently performed at the L4/5 in 37, at L3/4 in 3 patients, and L5/S1 in another ten patients at the L5/S1 level. Macnab outcomes were excellent in 29, good in 13 patients at final follow-up. Only four patients had fair, and two had poor results—twenty-nine of the 48 DRG irritations resolved with transforaminal epidural steroid injections (TESI). Only 12 of the 29 patients opted for TESI. Eleven of the 48 patients had single-level unilateral endoscopic transforaminal decompression procedures at adjacent symptomatic levels within the first six postoperative months. Three patients underwent combination-level surgery. Four patients had problems at the index level, including removal of a dislodged cage in one patient. Another patient had complex open revision surgery for an L5 vertebral body fracture. One patient had an asymptomatic cage fracture.

DISCUSSION

Standalone posterior lumbar interbody fusion (PLIF) has been reported with two smaller cylindrical cages during PLIF or one larger obliquely placed cage [5, 6]. Advances in endoscopic instrumentation and optics broadened the surgical indications with spinal endoscopy beyond herniated disc and spinal stenosis. The authors' study shows that a percutaneous endoscopically assisted transforaminal decompression, and fusion surgery with the expandable standalone VariLift®-L interbody fusion system is feasible employing the LEWLIF™ techniques [30]. The inside-out approach lends itself beautifully for the visualized discectomy and endplate preparation [19, 33 - 35]. The key steps to facilitate this true endoscopic fusion procedure are the foraminoplasty with resection of the superior articular process, any lateral overhang of a hypertrophic facet joint, and the endoscopically visualized preparation of the intersomatic space. Occasionally, a partial pediculolectomy and resection of osteophytes of the ring apophysis may be required to facilitate the entry of the cylindrical threaded cage. Interspace paddle shavers allow for endplate sparing decortication maneuvers, discectomy, distraction, mobilization, and sizing of the final goal implant. The authors recommend a snug fit of the last tap. Undersizing may lead to cage dislodgement and should be avoided. In the authors ' opinion, oversizing the implant by one mm is ideal in some cases where indirect decompression of the opposite lateral recess and neuroforamen is desired.

CONCLUSION

The application of the authors' LEWLIF™ technique and study show that a standalone endoscopic decompression and interbody fusion is feasible but should be carefully planned concerning optimal access, location of the compressive pathology, and the size of the implant. The importance of such planning has been stressed by Lee *et al.* [36]. Radiographic classification systems aiding in the preoperative decision-making found to correlate with clinical outcomes may also be helpful [33 - 36]. Understanding the applied endoscopic anatomy of the lumbar spine and gaining access to the intervertebral disc space requires experience and should not be attempted by the novice surgeon unless the learning curve has been mastered.

CONSENT FOR PUBLICATION

Not applicable.

CONFLICT OF INTEREST

The authors declare no conflict of interest, financial or otherwise.

ACKNOWLEDGEMENT

Declared none.

REFERENCES

[1]   Xie L, Wu WJ, Liang Y. Comparison between minimally invasive transforaminal lumbar interbody fusion and conventional open transforaminal lumbar interbody fusion. Chin Med J (Engl) 2016; 129(16): 1969-86.

[http://dx.doi.org/10.4103/0366-6999.187847] [PMID: 27503024]

[2]   Goldstein CL, Phillips FM, Rampersaud YR. Comparative effectiveness and economic evaluations of open *versus* minimally invasive posterior or transforaminal lumbar interbody fusion. Spine 2016; 41 (Suppl. 8): 1.
[http://dx.doi.org/10.1097/BRS.0000000000001462] [PMID: 26825793]

[3]   Virdee JS, Nadig A, Anagnostopoulos G, George KJ. Comparison of peri-operative and 12-month lifestyle outcomes in minimally invasive transforaminal lumbar interbody fusion *versus* conventional lumbar fusion. Br J Neurosurg 2017; 31(2): 167-71.
[http://dx.doi.org/10.1080/02688697.2016.1199790] [PMID: 27331649]

[4]   Phan K, Rao PJ, Kam AC, Mobbs RJ. Minimally invasive *versus* open transforaminal lumbar interbody fusion for treatment of degenerative lumbar disease: systematic review and meta-analysis. Eur Spine J 2015; 24(5): 1017-30.
[http://dx.doi.org/10.1007/s00586-015-3903-4] [PMID: 25813010]

[5]   Barrett-Tuck R, Del Monaco D, Block JE. One and two level posterior lumbar interbody fusion (PLIF) using an expandable, stand-alone, interbody fusion device: a VariLift® case series. J Spine Surg 2017; 3(1): 9-15.
[http://dx.doi.org/10.21037/jss.2017.02.05] [PMID: 28435912]

[6]   Emstad E, Del Monaco DC, Fielding LC, Block JE. The VariLift(®) Interbody Fusion System: expandable, standalone interbody fusion. Med Devices (Auckl) 2015; 8: 219-30.
[PMID: 26060414]

[7]   Neely WF, Fichtel F, del Monaco DC, Block JE. Treatment of Symptomatic Lumbar Disc Degeneration with the VariLift-L Interbody Fusion System: Retrospective Review of 470 Cases. Int J Spine Surg 2016; 10: 15.
[http://dx.doi.org/10.14444/3015] [PMID: 27441173]

[8]   Blumenthal SL, Ohnmeiss DD. Intervertebral cages for degenerative spinal diseases. Spine J 2003; 3(4): 301-9.
[http://dx.doi.org/10.1016/S1529-9430(03)00004-4] [PMID: 14589191]

[9]   Chen L, Yang H, Tang T. Cage migration in spondylolisthesis treated with posterior lumbar interbody fusion using BAK cages. Spine 2005; 30(19): 2171-5.
[http://dx.doi.org/10.1097/01.brs.0000180402.50500.5b] [PMID: 16205342]

[10]   Choi JY, Sung KH. Subsidence after anterior lumbar interbody fusion using paired stand-alone rectangular cages. Eur Spine J 2006; 15(1): 16-22.
[http://dx.doi.org/10.1007/s00586-004-0817-y] [PMID: 15843972]

[11]   Zdeblick TA, Phillips FM. Interbody cage devices. Spine 2003; 28(15) (Suppl.): S2-7.
[http://dx.doi.org/10.1097/01.BRS.0000076841.93570.78] [PMID: 12897467]

[12]   Babu R, Park JG, Mehta AI, *et al.* Comparison of superior-level facet joint violations during open and percutaneous pedicle screw placement. Neurosurgery 2012; 71(5): 962-70.
[http://dx.doi.org/10.1227/NEU.0b013e31826a88c8] [PMID: 22843132]

[13]   Zhang Q, Xu YF, Tian W, *et al.* Comparison of Superior-Level Facet Joint Violations Between Robot-Assisted Percutaneous Pedicle Screw Placement and Conventional Open Fluoroscopic-Guided Pedicle Screw Placement. Orthop Surg 2019; 11(5): 850-6.
[http://dx.doi.org/10.1111/os.12534] [PMID: 31663290]

[14]   Patel RD, Graziano GP, Vanderhave KL, Patel AA, Gerling MC. Facet violation with the placement of percutaneous pedicle screws. Spine 2011; 36(26): E1749-52.
[http://dx.doi.org/10.1097/BRS.0b013e318221a800] [PMID: 21587106]

[15]   Lee CS, Hwang CJ, Lee SW, *et al.* Risk factors for adjacent segment disease after lumbar fusion. Eur Spine J 2009; 18(11): 1637-43.
[http://dx.doi.org/10.1007/s00586-009-1060-3] [PMID: 19533182]

[16]   Sengupta DK, Herkowitz HN. Lumbar spinal stenosis. Orthop Clin North Am 2003; 34(2): 281-95.
[http://dx.doi.org/10.1016/S0030-5898(02)00069-X] [PMID: 12914268]

[17]   Lewandrowski KU, Yeung A. Lumbar endoscopic bony and soft tissue decompression with the hybridized inside-out approach: a review and technical note. Neurospine 2020; 17 (Suppl. 1): S34-43.
[http://dx.doi.org/10.14245/ns.2040160.080] [PMID: 32746516]

[18]   Tsou PM, Alan Yeung C, Yeung AT. Posterolateral transforaminal selective endoscopic discectomy and thermal annuloplasty for chronic lumbar discogenic pain: a minimal access visualized intradiscal surgical procedure. Spine J 2004; 4(5): 564-73.
[http://dx.doi.org/10.1016/j.spinee.2004.01.014] [PMID: 15363430]

[19]   Yeung A, Lewandrowski KU. Five-year clinical outcomes with endoscopic transforaminal foraminoplasty for symptomatic degenerative conditions of the lumbar spine: a comparative study of *inside-outversusoutside-in* techniques. J Spine Surg 2020; 6(S1) (Suppl. 1): S66-83.
[http://dx.doi.org/10.21037/jss.2019.06.08] [PMID: 32195417]

[20]   Yeung A, Lewandrowski KU. Early and staged endoscopic management of common pain generators in the spine. J Spine Surg 2020; 6(S1) (Suppl. 1): S1-5.
[http://dx.doi.org/10.21037/jss.2019.09.03] [PMID: 32195407]

[21]   Yeung AT, Roberts A, Shin P, Rivers E, Paterson A, Paterson A. Suggestions for a practical and progressive approach to endoscopic spine surgery training and privileges. J Spine 2018; 7(2)
[http://dx.doi.org/10.4172/2165-7939.1000414]

[22]   Yeung A, Roberts A, Zhu L, Qi L, Zhang J, Lewandrowski KU. Treatment of soft tissue and bony spinal stenosis by a visualized endoscopic transforaminal technique under local anesthesia. Neurospine 2019; 16(1): 52-62.
[http://dx.doi.org/10.14245/ns.1938038.019] [PMID: 30943707]

[23]   Yeung AT, Tsou PM. Posterolateral endoscopic excision for lumbar disc herniation: Surgical technique, outcome, and complications in 307 consecutive cases. Spine 2002; 27(7): 722-31.
[http://dx.doi.org/10.1097/00007632-200204010-00009] [PMID: 11923665]

[24]   Yeung AT, Yeung CA. Advances in endoscopic disc and spine surgery: foraminal approach. Surg Technol Int 2003; 11: 255-63.
[PMID: 12931309]

[25]   Yeung AT, Yeung CA. *In-vivo* endoscopic visualization of patho-anatomy in painful degenerative conditions of the lumbar spine. Surg Technol Int 2006; 15: 243-56.
[PMID: 17029183]

[26]   Yeung AT, Yeung CA. Minimally invasive techniques for the management of lumbar disc herniation. Orthop Clin North Am 2007; 38(3): 363-72.
[http://dx.doi.org/10.1016/j.ocl.2007.04.005] [PMID: 17629984]

[27]   Kambin P, Nixon J, Chait A, Schaffer JL. Annular Protrusion. Spine 1988; 13(6): 671-5.
[http://dx.doi.org/10.1097/00007632-198813060-00013] [PMID: 2972071]

[28]   Kambin P, Sampson S. Posterolateral percutaneous suction-excision of herniated lumbar intervertebral discs. Report of interim results. Clin Orthop Relat Res 1986; (207): 37-43.
[PMID: 3720102]

[29]   Kambin P, Schaffer JL. Percutaneous lumbar discectomy. Review of 100 patients and current practice. Clin Orthop Relat Res 1989; 238(238): 24-34.
[http://dx.doi.org/10.1097/00003086-198901000-00004] [PMID: 2910608]

[30]   León JFR, Ardila ÁS, Rugeles Ortíz JG, *et al.* Standalone lordotic endoscopic wedge lumbar interbody fusion (LEW-LIF™) with a threaded cylindrical peek cage: report of two cases. J Spine Surg 2020; 6(S1) (Suppl. 1): S275-85.
[http://dx.doi.org/10.21037/jss.2019.06.09] [PMID: 32195434]

[31] Macnab I. Negative disc exploration. An analysis of the causes of nerve-root involvement in sixty-eight patients. J Bone Joint Surg Am 1971; 53(5): 891-903.
[http://dx.doi.org/10.2106/00004623-197153050-00004] [PMID: 4326746]

[32] Macnab I. The surgery of lumbar disc degeneration. Surg Annu 1976; 8: 447-80.
[PMID: 936011]

[33] Lewandrowski KU. The strategies behind "inside-out" and "outside-in" endoscopy of the lumbar spine: treating the pain generator. J Spine Surg 2020; 6(S1) (Suppl. 1): S35-9.
[http://dx.doi.org/10.21037/jss.2019.06.06] [PMID: 32195412]

[34] Lewandrowski KU, León JFR, Yeung A. Use of "inside-out" technique for direct visualization of a vacuum vertically unstable intervertebral disc during routine lumbar endoscopic transforaminal decompression—a correlative study of clinical outcomes and the prognostic value of lumbar radiographs. Int J Spine Surg 2019; 13(5): 399-414.
[http://dx.doi.org/10.14444/6055] [PMID: 31741829]

[35] Lim KT, Meceda EJA, Park CK. Inside-out approach of lumbar endoscopic unilateral laminotomy for bilateral decompression: a detailed technical description, rationale and outcomes. Neurospine 2020; 17 (Suppl. 1): S88-98.
[http://dx.doi.org/10.14245/ns.2040196.098] [PMID: 32746522]

[36] Lee S, Kim SK, Lee SH, *et al.* Percutaneous endoscopic lumbar discectomy for migrated disc herniation: classification of disc migration and surgical approaches. Eur Spine J 2007; 16(3): 431-7.
[http://dx.doi.org/10.1007/s00586-006-0219-4] [PMID: 16972067]

CHAPTER 15

Endoscopic Intravertebral Canal Decompression after Spinal Fracture

Xifeng Zhang[1,2,*], **Lei-Ming Zhang**[3] and **Jiang Letao**[4]

[1] *Department of Orthopedics, First Medical Center, PLA General Hospital, Beijing 100853, China*

[2] *Department of Orthopedics, Beijing Yuho Rehabilitation Hospital, Beijing 100853, China*

[3] *Department of Neurosurgery, Sixth Medical Center, PLA General Hospital, Beijing 100048, China*

[4] *Department of Orthopedics, Affiliated Hospital of Yangzhou University, Yangzhou 225001, China*

Abstract: Spinal endoscopy allows creating access to areas of the spine that are ordinarily difficult to reach, thereby reducing the collateral damage from extensive exposure to treat common degenerative or traumatic conditions of the spine. In this chapter, the authors present a case of endoscopic spinal canal decompression in a patient who sustained a burst fracture near the thoracolumbar junction. The endoscopic decompression technique was employed, which resulted in removing bone fragments, causing compression of the neural elements. The burst fracture was then stabilized with a percutaneous short pedicle screw construct. The patient did well with the hybridized endoscopic and minimally invasive decompression and stabilization technique. The authors are making a case for considering the endoscopic spinal surgery platform other than the traditionally accepted indications in the interest to diminish further blood loss, pain, and complication rates associated with spinal fracture surgeries.

Keywords: Endoscopic decompression, Hybridized endoscopic and minimally invasive technique, Percutaneous short pedicle screw construct, Thoracolumbar fracture.

INTRODUCTION

High energy trauma to the spine frequently causes fractures across the thoracolumbar junction [1]. Depending on the posterior-longitudinal ligament complex's integrity, the extent of canal compromise by posteriorly displaced bone fragments, and neurological deficits, surgery may be recommended to stabilize

---

* **Corresponding author Xifeng Zhang:** Department of Orthopedics, First Medical Center, PLA General Hospital, Beijing 100853, China and Department of Orthopedics, Beijing Yuho Rehabilitation Hospital, Beijing, 100853, China; Tel: (908) 922-7635; E-mail: xifengzhang301@outlook.com

Kai-Uwe Lewandrowski, Jorge Felipe Ramírez León, Anthony Yeung, Gun Choi, Stefan Hellinger and Álvaro Dowling (Eds.)

the spine and recover neurological function [2]. If the latter category of patients is left untreated, quality of life is typically severely impacted [2]. Burst fractures make up about 20% of all fractures of the thoracolumbar spine [3]. Several classification systems have been published delineating surgical indications *versus* non-operative treatment with braces [4]. Minimally invasive techniques have been tried to diminish blood loss further, reduce operation time while accomplishing canal decompression, and improving sagittal alignment [5 - 10]. Short pedicle screw constructs are center stage in the surgical stabilization of thoracolumbar fractures to avoid anterior column insufficiency with instability and kyphosis if left untreated [10 - 12]. However, posterior surgery alone is often insufficient to adequately decompress the spinal canal [13] - a notion of particular importance in patients with neurological deficits. Therefore, the authors of this chapter present a novel application of the endoscopic spinal surgery technique where they employ the endoscope to access the middle column to remove bone fragments from the spinal canal before internal fixation with the minimally invasive placement of percutaneous short pedicle screw constructs.

CASE DETAILS

We report on a 29-year-old male patient with a chief complaint of right-sided flank and back pain. The patient could not walk for one week after trauma and experienced severe pain after falling downstairs one week ago. After the initial bed rest, the pain was not resolved and instead became gradually severe and rendering the patient unable to walk. The symptoms worsened after sitting for a long time. Squatting and other daily activities also agravated his symptoms. The pain was so intense that the patient was unable to work and had difficulty with urination. He presented to our healthcare facility with symptoms consistent with conus medullaris syndrome. Before admission to our facility, the patient was treated with mannitol and steroid therapy in an outside hospital without much relief. On admission, physical examination showed tenderness over the T12, L1, L2 spinous process tenderness. There was preserved motor strength in the right lower extremity muscles assessed at 5/5. In the left lower limb, motor strength was severely diminished with no voluntary movement. The examination of this patient's incomplete spinal cord injury further revealed intact sensation pain, temperature, light touch, and deep sensation in both lower limbs was normal. The bilateral knee tendon and achilles tendon reflexes were also present. There were no upper motor neuron signs with absent clonus and without other pathological reflexes. The bilateral straight leg elevation test was negative, and he had a staggering gait. X-rays of the lumbar spine suggested L1 and L2 compression fractures (Fig. **1**). CT and MRI (not shown in this chapter) of the lumbar spine showed L1 and L2 compression fractures, with bone fragments occupying space in the spinal canal most consistent with a burst fracture of the L1 vertebral body

(Fig. **2**). The thoracolumbar injury classification and severity score (TLICS) [10] was 7 points, and therefore the indication for surgery was established. The patient decided to undergo surgical treatment. Percutaneous pedicle screw internal fixation was performed first to stabilize the spine and see whether the bone fragment would reduce as a result of the short pedicle screw construct [10]. A postoperative CT scan proved otherwise. Therefore, the authors performed a bilateral endoscopic transforaminal decompression of the spinal canal by removing several large bone fragments in piecemeal (Figs. **2** and **3**).

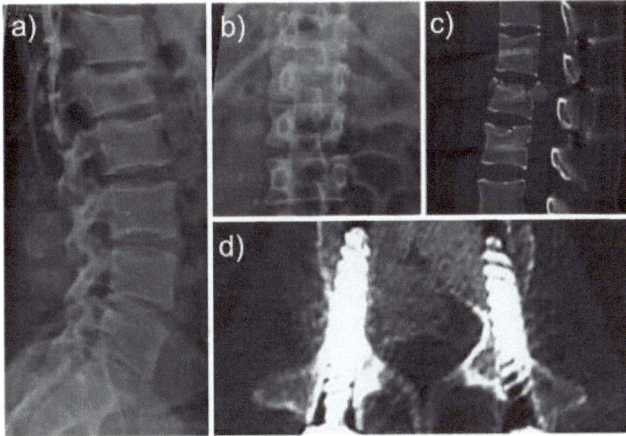

Fig. (1). Lateral (**a**) and anteroposterior (**b**) x-rays of the lumbar spine vertebrae showing L1 (burst) and L2 (compression) vertebral fracture are shown. The patient underwent percutaneous short pedicle screw fixation which did not reduce the posterior wall fragments. Postoperative CT scan of the lumbar spine showed large bone fragments to remain in the spinal canal typical of a burst fracture.

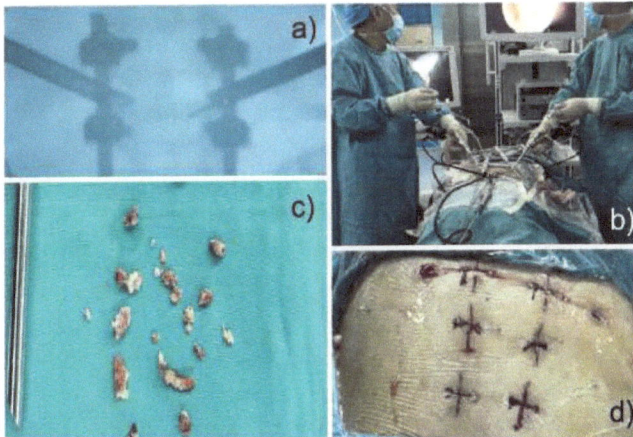

Fig. (2). The patient's canal compromise seen on postoperative CT scan (Fig. **1**) after initial percutaneous short pedicle screw construct prompted the surgeons to perform a bilateral (**a**) T12/L1 endoscopic transforaminal decompression (**b**) of the bone fragments anterior to dural sac. Several large bone fragments were removed endoscopically (**c**) through the bilateral paraspinal incisions (**d**).

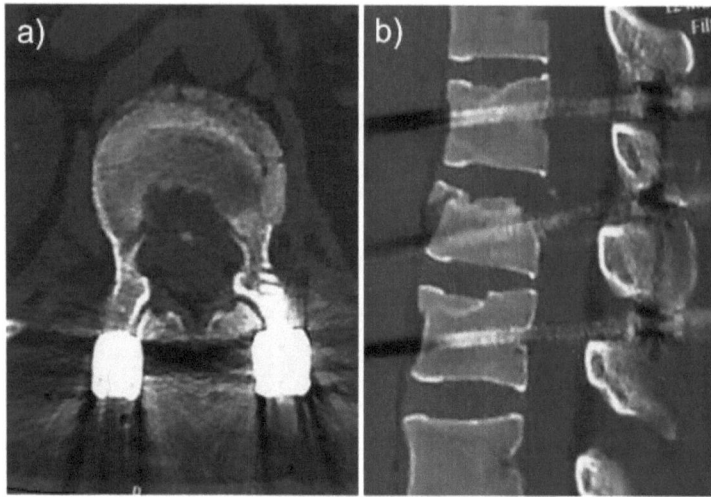

Fig. (3). The postoperative axial (**a**) and sagittal (**b**) CT scan after the T12/L1 transforaminal endoscopic decompression of the spinal canal anterior to the thecal sac at the fracture level showed adequate decompression. The patient's neurological function improved immediately after the endoscopic decompression. No incidental durotomy was encountered during the endoscopic decompression, which was performed after the initial percutaneous short pedicle screw construct placement.

SURGICAL STEPS

The surgical team decided first to perform percutaneous stabilization with a short pedicle screw construct for internal fixation. Postoperative CT scanning was anticipated to see whether the posteriorly displaced bone fragments of the failed posterior wall of the L1 vertebral body would spontaneously reduce to the point where further surgery was not needed. Besides, the surgeons would take the patient's neurological function into account. Improvement of neurological symptoms would not call for additional surgery. For the pedicle screw fixation, 1% lidocaine was injected around the paraspinal tissues from T12 to L2 for local anesthesia. The short pedicle screw construct was assembled by placing the pedicle screws percutaneously under fluoroscopic guidance. The patient's surgery under local anesthesia with some sedation allowed the surgeons to communicate with the patient to ensure that his neurological function would not deteriorate during surgery. After this first operation, a CT scan of the thoracolumbar spine was performed to ascertain whether the bone fragments were reduced. Unfortunately, they did not, and the patient's neurological deficits had not worsened but also not improved (Fig. **1**). Therefore, the authors opted for an additional minimally invasive surgery directed at the decompression of the bony fragments anterior to the dural sac at the L1 fracture level – a bilateral transforaminal endoscopic decompression (Figs. **2** and **3**). The endoscopic procedure was performed in a staged manner at a different time, again under local anesthesia with 1% lidocaine. Two 18G spinal needleswere advanced into the

T12/L1 neuroforamina bilaterally for the transforaminal approach. Guidewires were placed through the spinal needles, which were then used to advance an endoscopic 6 mm working cannula on both sides after serial dilation. Two surgeons worked with two separate endoscopic systems on both sides of the patient simultaneously by initially advancing the spiinal endoscope towards the fracture fragments (Fig. **2**). A spinal endoscopic burr was used to remove the fracture fragments from both sides. Additionally, bone fragments were removed with rongeurs. A postoperative CT following this endoscopic canal decompression showed that the fracture fragments in the spinal canal were removed in their entirety (Fig. **3**).

DISCUSSION

Unstable burst fractures are mainly manifested as injuries of the spine's anterior and middle column, often accompanied by fracture fragments protruding into the spinal canal [10]. Neurological deficits are observed in about 20%-40% of injuries [14, 18]. For such patients, adequate decompression and stabilization are necessary [2]. Traditional open spinal decompression and internal fixation for unstable compression fractures can achieve satisfactory clinical results. Still, there are many complications, which have directed widespread attention to less aggressive spinal surgery techniques [5, 7, 8, 10, 12, 15 - 17, 19]. With the development of minimally invasive spinal surgery techniques (MIS), decompression can be achieved through small incisions, either with microsurgical dissection with the use of MIS retractors via the translaminar route and with the aid of an operating microscope or with endoscopic working channels which can be placed through the transforaminal access corridor to reach the undersurface of the anterior dural sac. These MIS procedures can be combined with percutaneous internal fixation for the treatment of unstable spinal fractures. The indication for surgery can be established with the TLICS scoring system [10], which typically indicates surgery when there is nerve damage or incomplete neurological deficit. Every attempt has to be made to improve the patient's long-term functioning and quality of life.

In this context, consideration of MIS techniques is highly relevant as the collateral damage from open surgery and the associated blood loss, increased postoperative pain, and longer recovery- and return to work times are of relevance to younger patients, who are most affected by this sometimes devastating injury of the spine. Shorter recovery times and earlier return to work may be accomplished with MIS spinal surgery techniques. The endoscopic procedure can be considered an ultra-minimally invasive technique where the collateral tissue damage is minimal. The burden related to anesthesia is also less because it can be carried out under local anesthesia. Awake patient gives the surgeon the additional advantage of communicating with the patient to ensure that no other neurological function is lost during surgery. In the illustrative case provided by the authors showcases their endoscopic decompression technique, the motor strength was preserved, and the patient, in fact, recovered the function in the left lower extremity, which was impaired as a result of the incomplete spinal cord injury so close to the conus medullaris. At the end of the surgery, the awake patient demonstrated a normal straight leg elevation test without any pain on the left leg's full elevation. Conus medullaris injury or ongoing irritation by the large bony fragment causing severe canal stenosis at the fracture level was suspected of causing the patient difficulty in urination. Therefore, the authors chose the two-stage endoscopic decompression and percutaneous fixation with a short pedicle screw construct – the standard of care in most developed countries for this type of injury [10]. Ultimately, the authors were proven right because the patient's neurological function nearly returned to normal with an almost regular gait pattern after full recovery.

CONCLUSION

Unstable spinal fractures may require decompression of the anterior spinal canal directly under the dural sac, where retropulsed bony fragments often cause acute canal stenosis. The indication for surgery is readily made if the patient has neurological deficits, and advanced imaging studies of the spine suggest instability. The authors' illustrative case demonstrates the utility of the spinal endoscope to assist in decompressing these types of fractures. They recommend that every endoscopic spine surgeon consider implementing the endoscope into their surgical armamentarium whenever surgical treatment of spine fractures becomes necessary.

CONSENT FOR PUBLICATION

Not applicable.

CONFLICT OF INTEREST

The authors declare no conflict of interest, financial or otherwise.

ACKNOWLEDGEMENT

Declared none.

REFERENCES

[1]　Deqing L, Kejian L, Teng L, *et al.* Does the fracture fragment at the anterior column in thoracolumbar burst fractures get enough attention? Medicine (Baltimore) 2017; 96: e5936.
[http://dx.doi.org/10.1097/MD.0000000000005936]

[2]   Piccone L, Cipolloni V, Nasto LA, *et al.* Thoracolumbar burst fractures associated with incomplete neurological deficit in patients under the age of 40: Is the posterior approach enough? Surgical treatment and results in a case series of 10 patients with a minimum follow-up of 2 years. Injury 2020; 51(2): 312-6.
[http://dx.doi.org/10.1016/j.injury.2019.12.031] [PMID: 31917009]

[3]   Moon YJ, Lee KB. Relationship Between Clinical Outcomes and Spontaneous Canal Remodeling in Thoracolumbar Burst Fracture. World Neurosurg 2016; 89(89): 58-64.
[http://dx.doi.org/10.1016/j.wneu.2016.02.010] [PMID: 26872515]

[4]   Ankomah F, Ikpeze T, Mesfin A. The Top 50 Most-Cited Articles on Thoracolumbar Fractures. World Neurosurg 2018; 118(118): e699-706.
[http://dx.doi.org/10.1016/j.wneu.2018.07.022] [PMID: 30010075]

[5]   Schnake KJ, Scheyerer MJ, Spiegl UJA, *et al.* [Minimally invasive stabilization of thoracolumbar osteoporotic fractures]. Unfallchirurg 2020; 123(10): 764-73.
[http://dx.doi.org/10.1007/s00113-020-00835-1] [PMID: 32613278]

[6]   Pannu CD, Farooque K, Sharma V, Singal D. Minimally invasive spine surgeries for treatment of thoracolumbar fractures of spine: A systematic review. J Clin Orthop Trauma 2019; 10(10) (Suppl. 1): S147-55.
[http://dx.doi.org/10.1016/j.jcot.2019.04.012] [PMID: 31695274]

[7]   Defino HLA, Costa HRT, Nunes AA, *et al.* Open *versus* minimally invasive percutaneous surgery for surgical treatment of thoracolumbar spine fractures- a multicenter randomized controlled trial: study protocol. BMC Musculoskelet Disord 2019; 20: 397.
[http://dx.doi.org/10.1186/s12891-019-2763-1]

[8]   Pishnamaz M, Schemmann U, Herren C, *et al.* Muscular changes after minimally invasive *versus* open spinal stabilization of thoracolumbar fractures: A literature review. J Musculoskelet Neuronal Interact 2018; 18(1): 62-70.
[PMID: 29504580]

[9]   Ganse B, Pishnamaz M, Kobbe P, *et al.* Microcirculation in open vs. minimally invasive dorsal stabilization of thoracolumbar fractures. PLoS One 2017; 12: e0188115.
[http://dx.doi.org/10.1371/journal.pone.0188115]

[10]   Wood KB, Li W, Lebl DR, Ploumis A. Management of thoracolumbar spine fractures. Spine J 2014; 14(1): 145-64.
[http://dx.doi.org/10.1016/j.spinee.2012.10.041] [PMID: 24332321]

[11]   Wang H, Mo Z, Han J, *et al.* Extent and location of fixation affects the biomechanical stability of short- or long-segment pedicle screw technique with screwing of fractured vertebra for the treatment of thoracolumbar burst fractures: An observational study using finite element analysis. Medicine (Baltimore) 2018; 97: e11244.
[http://dx.doi.org/10.1097/MD.0000000000011244]

[12]   Sahai N, Faloon MJ, Dunn CJ, *et al.* Short-Segment Fixation With Percutaneous Pedicle Screws in the Treatment of Unstable Thoracolumbar Vertebral Body Fractures. Orthopedics 2018; 41(6): e802-6.
[http://dx.doi.org/10.3928/01477447-20180912-05] [PMID: 30222793]

[13]   Liao JC, Chen WP, Wang H. Treatment of thoracolumbar burst fractures by short-segment pedicle screw fixation using a combination of two additional pedicle screws and vertebroplasty at the level of the fracture: a finite element analysis. BMC Musculoskelet Disord 2017; 18: 262.
[http://dx.doi.org/10.1186/s12891-017-1623-0]

[14]   Korovessis P, Repantis T, Petsinis G, Iliopoulos P, Hadjipavlou A. Direct reduction of thoracolumbar burst fractures by means of balloon kyphoplasty with calcium phosphate and stabilization with pedicle-screw instrumentation and fusion. Spine 2008; 33(4): E100-8.
[http://dx.doi.org/10.1097/BRS.0b013e3181646b07] [PMID: 18277858]

[15]   Uchida K, Kobayashi S, Matsuzaki M, *et al*. Anterior *versus* posterior surgery for osteoporotic vertebral collapse with neurological deficit in the thoracolumbar spine. Eur Spine J 2006; 15(12): 1759-67.
[http://dx.doi.org/10.1007/s00586-006-0106-z] [PMID: 16676156]

[16]   Knop C, Fabian HF, Bastian L, Blauth M. Late results of thoracolumbar fractures after posterior instrumentation and transpedicular bone grafting. Spine 2001; 26(1): 88-99.
[http://dx.doi.org/10.1097/00007632-200101010-00016] [PMID: 11148651]

[17]   Lee JY, Vaccaro AR, Lim MR, *et al*. Thoracolumbar injury classification and severity score: a new paradigm for the treatment of thoracolumbar spine trauma. J Orthop Sci 2005; 10(6): 671-5.
[http://dx.doi.org/10.1007/s00776-005-0956-y] [PMID: 16307197]

[18]   Lewandrowski K, McLain RF. Thoracolumbar fractures: evaluation, classification and treatment The adult and pediatric spine Philadelphia. Lippincott Williams & Wilkins 2004; pp. 817-43.

[19]   Ntilikina Y, Bahlau D, Garnon J, *et al*. Open *versus* percutaneous instrumentation in thoracolumbar fractures: magnetic resonance imaging comparison of paravertebral muscles after implant removal. J Neurosurg Spine 2017; 27(2): 235-41.
[http://dx.doi.org/10.3171/2017.1.SPINE16886] [PMID: 28598294]

CHAPTER 16

Treatment of Lumbar Tuberculosis with Spinal Endoscopy

Xifeng Zhang[1,2,*], Du Jianwei[3] and Bu Rongqiang[2]

[1] *Department of Orthopedics, First Medical Center, PLA General Hospital, Beijing 100853, China*

[2] *Department of Orthopedics, Beijing Yuho Rehabilitation Hospital, Beijing 100853, China*

[3] *Department of Orthopedics, Affiliated Hospital of Yangzhou University, Yangzhou 225001, China*

Abstract: The authors present a case of a 25-year old female patient who presented to their facility with a chief complaint of low back pain and discomfort for the previous two months. The symptoms gradually worsened. The patient denied any fever, night sweats, and other aches. Symptoms worsened when standing up. They were also aggravated by changing the body position. In particular, bending forward was restricted. There was no radiating pain in the lower extremities. An MRI of the lumbar spine revealed a lesion raising suspicions of tuberculosis of the spine, which was later confirmed with biopsy and cultures. The patient was placed on oral multi anti-tuberculosis antibiotic treatment but responded poorly to this treatment without much clinical improvement. Therefore, endoscopic access was chosen to debride and irrigate the paraspinal tuberculous abscess, which successfully treated the infection. The authors report the case details to illustrate that a combination of antibiotic treatment and endoscopic debridement may resolve the lumbar spine's complicated infection adequately. Minimally invasive endoscopic irrigation and lavage of paraspinal tuberculous abscesses can be considered an alternative to open surgery.

Keywords: Endoscopy, Irrigation & debridement, Lumbar spine, Tuberculosis.

INTRODUCTION

Tuberculosis (TB) of the spine is a disease of young adults and children. While TB should always be considered in the differential diagnosis of spinal infections in less developed countries, it is also on the rise in developed countries. Imaging studies typically show the destruction of the intervertebral disk space and the

---

* **Corresponding author Xifeng Zhang:** Department of Orthopedics, First Medical Center, PLA General Hospital, Beijing 100853, China and Department of Orthopedics, Beijing Yuho Rehabilitation Hospital, Beijing, 100853, China; Tel: (908) 922-7635; E-mail: xifengzhang301@outlook.com

Kai-Uwe Lewandrowski, Jorge Felipe Ramírez León, Anthony Yeung, Gun Choi, Stefan Hellinger and Álvaro Dowling (Eds.)

adjacent vertebral bodies, producing a vertical collapse of the spinal motion segment.

The kyphotic deformity may also develop mainly if the infection occurs at the thoracolumbar junction. However, the thoracic spine is the most commonly affected area of the spine. The infectious process is often walled off or may form a phlegmon, which may appear as a 'cold' abscess. Patients often complain of pain around the infected area. Spinal instability may result in neurological deficits if not treated on time. MRI is the imaging modality of choice as x-rays and CT-scans are not as sensitive and better show the vertebral bodies' infectious involvement on either side of the infected intervertebral disc and their destruction. Image-based needle biopsy of the infected area is key to making a definitive diagnosis *via* histopathological analysis and cultures. The index of clinical suspicion should be higher in immunocompromised patients, and in particular in those with HIV. Once the diagnosis is confirmed, anti-tuberculosis medical management remains the first-line treatment of choice. Surgery is considered only in those patients in whom medical treatment with antibiotics is ineffective. The prognosis is typically favorable if discovered and treated early in the disease process before spinal deformity, and neurological deficits ensue.

CLINICAL CASE

Physical examination of our 25-year old female patient showed normal spinal physical curvature, but some slight limitation of forward bending movement, mild low and mild lower back tenderness with negative percussive pain. The skin sensation, range of motion, and strength in both lower limbs were nearly symmetrical and normal. She had a positive straight leg raise test at minimal leg elevation. The laboratory testing on admission showed an elevated C-reactive protein of 18.24 mg/L and an erythrocyte sedimentation rate of 35 mm/h. Advanced imaging showed a destructive process at the L3/4 disc space with an associated paraspinal abscess (Fig. **1**). After admission, initial treatment consisted of standard oral anti-tuberculosis treatment. An endoscopic debridement of the infected area at the L3/4 level was performed after the non-operative care with antibiotics had failed (Fig. **2**). The endoscopic access to the infected intervertebral disc space was also used to place an irrigation drainage catheter into the infected area. At the same time, CT-guided needle aspiration of the abscess in the psoas major muscle was performed (Fig. **3**). This catheter was also used to inject anti-tuberculous medication into the psoas abscess for another ten days at the patient's bedside. After discharge from the hospital, the patient continued the daily irrigation of the abscess area with local antibiotic treatment in a similar way. At the final follow-up, the patient was noticed to have recovered from the spinal infection (Fig. **4**).

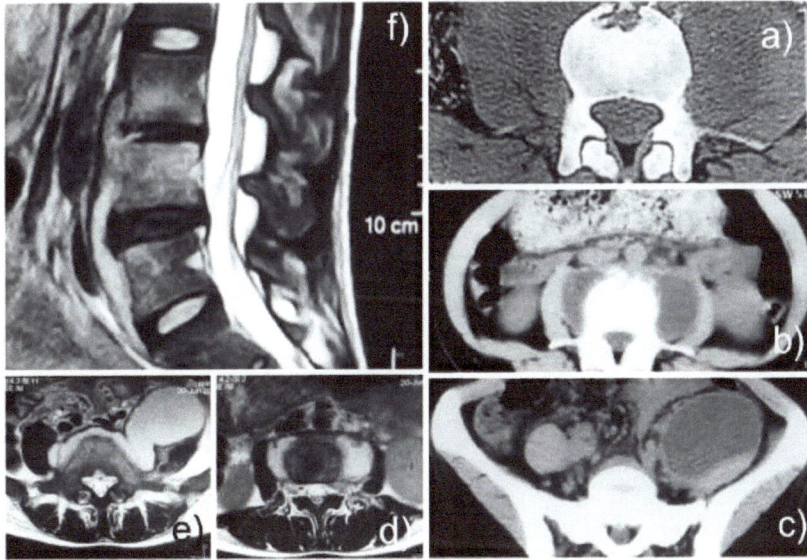

Fig. (1). The preoperative CT examination showed that the psoas major muscle was infected, and the vertebral bone was destroyed. Further investigation of preoperative MRI showed that the intervertebral space collapsed, the vertebral body destruction was relatively light, and the paravertebral infection abscess was huge.

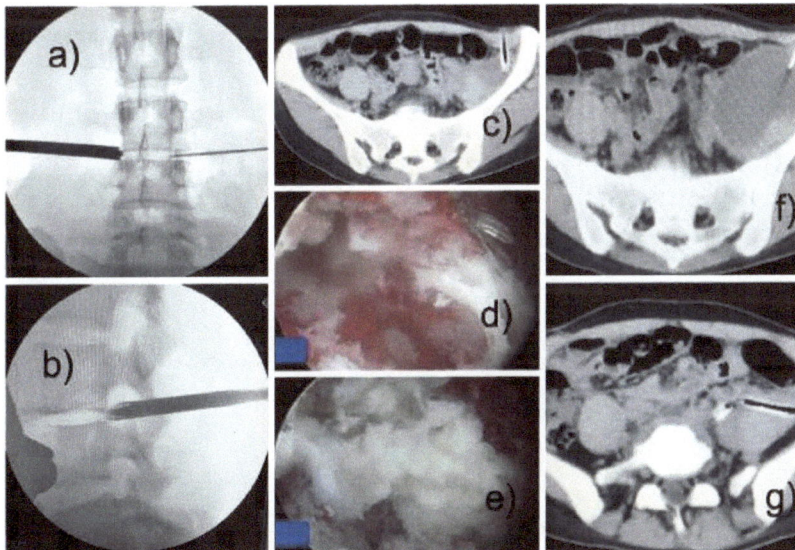

Fig. (2). Intraoperative puncture location (**a, b**), the side with severe symptoms are cleared under endoscopy. A double-lumen perfusion irrigation tube is placed (**c**), and an epidural tube is placed on the opposite side. Endoscopy shows the necrotic tissue in the intervertebral space and the situation after cleaning (**d, e**). Selecting the largest part of the iliac fossa abscess, a CT-guided puncture to the abscess anteriorly was performed by placing an indwelling a double-cavity perfusion irrigation tube for continuous irrigation and drainage.

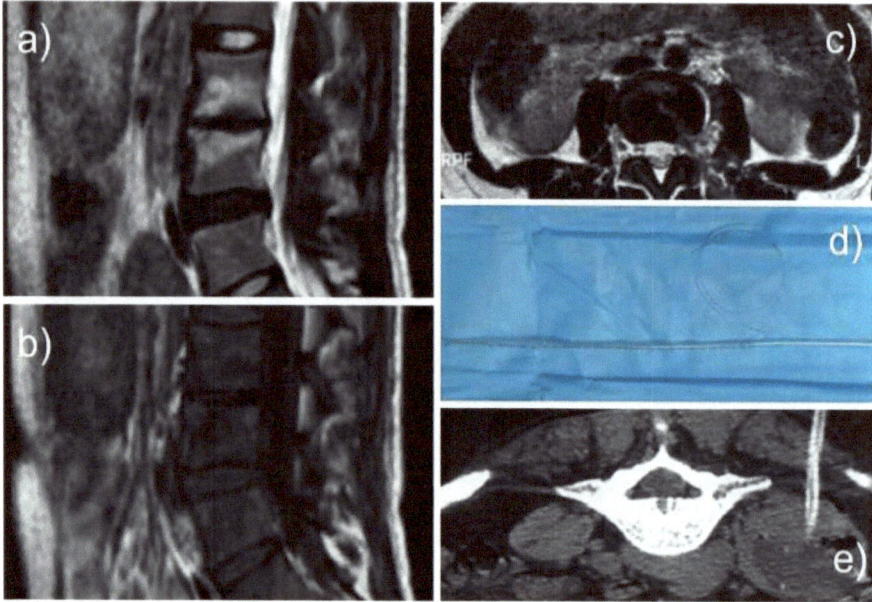

Fig. (3). Traces of puncture and catheterization were still visible after three months of postoperative reexamination (**a, b**), paravertebral abscess disappeared, and vertebral body destruction did not significantly aggravate (**c**). A self-made double-lumen perfusion irrigation tube was placed into the abscess (**d, e**).

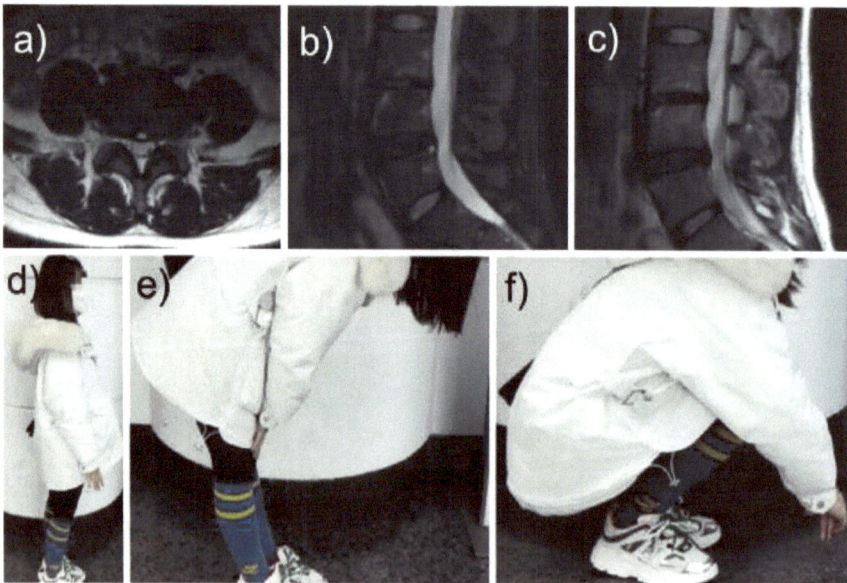

Fig. (4). After six months of reexamination, the condition was well controlled. The patients range of motion had significantly improved without pain.

SURGICAL CAVEATS

We chose an indwelling catheter, with a diameter of 0.3 mm, inserted with a stylet using a relatively hard 18F silicone tube. A double lumen epidural tube 25 cm in length that can be perfused and flushed was used during the debridement of our patient. A secondary abscess perfusion irrigation tube was placed in the bilateral psoas major abscess because it was greater than 2 cm. The psoas abscess was punctured vertically from the backside. The iliac fossa psoas muscle abscess was punctured obliquely from the medial aspect of the anterior superior iliac spine under CT-guidance. A 5mm skin incision was made, and the dilation tube and multi-stage working sleeve were placed in sequence. The perfusion irrigation tube was inserted from the working sleeve, and sutured and fixed. The patient was on oral isoniazid 0.1 gram once a day. The abscess cavity was flushed with isoniazid 0.3g + 500 ml normal saline under continuous perfusion and flushing with a daily total flushing volume of approximately 1000-2000 ml until the irrigation fluid returned clear without any necrotic tissue or pus.

DISCUSSION

Spinal tuberculosis can seriously affect the patients' quality of life [1, 2]. In recent years, minimally invasive methods for treating spinal tuberculosis have been developed. The clinical treatment effect has been continually improved, and new concepts have been presented [2]. Endoscopic spinal surgery has increasingly been accepted as a minimally invasive treatment for common spinal conditions. The authors illustrate its use in the case of spinal tuberculosis.

Spinal tuberculosis is essentially an infectiouos and inflammatory disease, different from tumor lesions, deformities, degenerative diseases, or fractures. Anti-tuberculosis drugs are still the key and effective method for the treatment of spinal tuberculosis [3]. Surgery should follow the principles of minimal trauma and the most straightforward method [2, 4, 5]. Patients with relatively minor damage to the vertebral body and without apparent spinal instability who underwent ineffective conservative drug treatment, endoscopically assisted irrigation and debridement of an infectious lesion are an appropriate alternative to aggressive surgical debridement. Endoscopic placement of a double-lumen irrigation and drainage tubing for continued flushing of the infectious lesion may help treat the abscess cavity, particularly if the irrigation fluid is enhanced with anti-tuberculotic drugs. The operation time is short, the trauma and the amount of bleeding is minimal, and the procedure hardly burdens the patient. Endoscopic irrigation and debridement may be an acceptable alternative for patients with medical comorbidities who cannot tolerate aggressive surgeries or anesthesia. First, the endoscopic debridement should focus on removing the necrotic and inflammatory tissue, which should quickly reduce the symptoms of local inflammatory pain, and at the same time, can avoid the sizeable surgical trauma caused by open surgery. Continous postoperative irrigation can also reduce the chance of necrotic tissue, blocking the irrigation catheter. It may also shorten the irrigation time. After the initial debridement, the authors recommend treating the lesion with the anti-tuberculotic drugs for another three months.

Bone destruction affects the stability of the spine. In severe cases, noticeable kyphosis may occur. For pain caused by instability, relative immobilization can be achieved through bed rest. There is no internal fixation for minimally invasive treatment of spinal tuberculosis with spinal endoscopy. Postoperative kyphosis may increase slightly in patients, but most of them are within the acceptable range. For severe deformities, corrective stabilizing surgery should be performed after the spinal infection is well controlled [2, 6]. For patients whose vertebral body is damaged more than 1/3, the pain caused by vertebral body instability is often severe and rarely tolerated without treatment. Particularly if spinal cord compression ensues which could affect postoperative nerve function recovery [2, 4, 5]. Spinal endoscopy, combined with local irrigation, can effectively decompress the abscess and the anterior dural sac. During the endoscopic debridement the surgeon should avoid dura mater injury at all cost.

CONCLUSION

Endoscopic debridement and irrigation of tuberculous abscesses even with large cavities are feasible. As illustrated by our case, the infection may successfully be irradicated by initial endoscopic drainage and continuous postoperative irrigation and drainage for additional lavage and medical treatment. Infected patients have vertebral body destruction and relatively loose bone. Therefore, the operation must be gentle to avoid further damage to the vertebral body and prevent the spread of the infection into the abdominal organs or the retroperitoneal space. The endoscope should be primarily used to clean the primary lesion from necrotic inflammatory tissue within the intervertebral disc space and cavernous lesions in the vertebral bodies. The dead bone should be removed. During the postoperative catheter flushing period, the patient should remain on bedrest and postoperative laboratory studies including erythrocyte sedimentation rate, biochemical, and routine blood tests should be carried out.

CONSENT FOR PUBLICATION

Not applicable.

CONFLICT OF INTEREST

The authors declare no conflict of interest, financial or otherwise.

ACKNOWLEDGEMENT

Declared none.

REFERENCES

[1]   Moon MS. Tuberculosis of spine: current views in diagnosis and management. Asian Spine J 2014; 8(1): 97-111.
        [http://dx.doi.org/10.4184/asj.2014.8.1.97] [PMID: 24596613]

[2]   Jain AK. Tuberculosis of the spine: a fresh look at an old disease. J Bone Joint Surg Br 2010; 92: 905-13.

[3]   Bhojraj S, Nene A. Lumbar and lumbosacral tuberculous spondylodiscitis in adults. Redefining the indications for surgery. J Bone Joint Surg Br 2002; 84(4): 530-4.
        [http://dx.doi.org/10.1302/0301-620X.84B4.0840530] [PMID: 12043773]

[4]   Wu W, Lyu J, Liu X, *et al.* Surgical Treatment of Thoracic Spinal Tuberculosis: A Multicenter Retrospective Study. World Neurosurg 2018; 110: e842-50.
        [http://dx.doi.org/10.1016/j.wneu.2017.11.126] [PMID: 29208449]

[5]   Gan F, Jiang J, Xie Z, *et al.* Minimally invasive direct lateral interbody fusion in the treatment of the thoracic and lumbar spinal tuberculosisMini-DLIF for the thoracic and lumbar spinal tuberculosis. BMC Musculoskelet Disord 2018; 19(1): 283.
        [http://dx.doi.org/10.1186/s12891-018-2187-3] [PMID: 30086740]

[6]   Shi J, He J, Niu N, Yang Z, Yuan H, Ding H. [Application of small incision approach in anterior surgery of thoracic and lumbar spinal tuberculosis]. Zhongguo Xiu Fu Chong Jian Wai Ke Za Zhi 2019; 33(6): 698-706. [Application of small incision approach in anterior surgery of thoracic and lumbar spinal tuberculosis].
        [PMID: 31197996]

CHAPTER 17

Treatment of Degenerative Scoliosis with Percutaneous Spinal Endoscopy Assisted Interbody Fusion and Percutaneous Pedicle Screw Fixation

Xifeng Zhang[1,2,*], Du Jianwei[3], Lei-Ming Zhang[4] and Wang Yu[3]

[1] *Department of Orthopedics, First Medical Center, PLA General Hospital, Beijing 100853, China*

[2] *Department of Orthopedics, Beijing Yuho Rehabilitation Hospital, Beijing 100853, China*

[3] *Department of orthopedics, Affiliated Hospital of Yangzhou University, Yangzhou 225001, China*

[4] *Department of orthopedics, Sixth Medical Center, PLA General Hospital, Beijing 100048, China*

Abstract: Deformity correction is an integral part of spinal surgery. For patients with painful coronal and sagittal plane deformity, correction to restore lumbar lordosis and scoliosis is the surgical treatment goal. Traditional open spinal surgery techniques are associated with wound problems, long-recovery times, high blood loss, and many other disadvantages compared to their more modern minimally invasive counterparts. While the minimally invasive percutaneous placement of pedicle-screw-rod constructs has been tried, anterior column release and fusion techniques to facilitate deformity correction often require excessive surgical exposures to gain access to the anterior column. This chapter presents a percutaneous transforaminal endoscopic interbody decompression and fusion technique to release the anterior column and facilitate deformity correction with the posterior column pedicle screw constructs. When combined with percutaneous minimally invasive screw placement, the patient's overall burden by the long-segment spinal fusion procedure can be significantly lowered by simplifying the entire procedure and carrying it out through small percutaneous incisions. An illustrative case is presented to demonstrate the utility of endoscopically assisted interbody fusion in scoliosis patients.

Keywords: Coronal plane deformity correction, Endoscopic surgery, Interbody fusion, Long-segment, Percutaneous pedicle screws, Scoliosis.

* **Corresponding author Xifeng Zhang:** Department of Orthopedics, First Medical Center, PLA General Hospital, Beijing 100853, China and Department of Orthopedics, Beijing Yuho Rehabilitation Hospital, Beijing, 100853, China; Tel: (908) 922-7635; E-mail: xifengzhang301@outlook.com

Kai-Uwe Lewandrowski, Jorge Felipe Ramírez León, Anthony Yeung, Gun Choi, Stefan Hellinger and Álvaro Dowling (Eds.)

INTRODUCTION

Nowadays, surgical correction of adult degenerative scoliosis in patients with unrelenting symptoms who have been unresponsive to conservative care is commonplace [1 - 4]. Typically, the condition is slowly progressive, and many patients put up with the symptoms for many years before seeking medical attention and even before considering surgery [2]. Pain generators reside within the asymmetrically degenerated and vertically collapsed intervertebral disc space, the arthritic facet joints, which often show significant hypertrophy. The instability-induced degenerative process may lead to disc bulges and thickening of the ligamentum flavum [4]. Consequently, pain and weakness may develop due to these structural changes producing spinal stenosis in the central canal and foraminal nerve root entrapment. The latter may add a radicular pain component to the mechanical deformity-driven pain component. Reduced walking endurance and increasing difficulty with activities of daily living is the consequence. By nature of the coupled motion within the thoracolumbar spine dictated by the facet joint anatomy, the coronal plane deformity is associated with rotatory deformity, and lateral listhesis, which is least well tolerated by patients and often prompts surgery. The asymmetric multilevel vertical collapse of the intervertebral disc spaces may lead to progressive loss of lumbar lordosis potentiating the coronal and sagittal plane deformity and disruption of spinopelvic proportions [5]. Osteoporotic vertebral compression fractures may aggravate this situation.

Many patients with adult degenerative scoliosis are coming up for surgery at older ages [6, 7]. At that point, many of them suffer from medical comorbidities that may place them at a higher risk for surgery [8, 9]. Therefore, surgeons have been looking for ways on how to simplify surgical treatment for such patients. For example, a smaller subset of patients with symptomatic degenerative scoliosis who predominantly present with radicular pain stemming from single-level unilateral nerve root compression may be a candidate for a minimally invasive foraminal decompression to lower the perioperative risks with open multilevel surgeries [10]. In this chapter, the authors are presenting their way of simplifying the surgical treatment of patients who have symptomatic degenerative scoliosis by combining the endoscopically assisted interbody fusion procedure with a threaded and expandable interbody fusion cage with percutaneously placed pedicle screws connected to a long-rod construct to decompress neural elements while correcting the deformity. While the surgical indications for degenerative thoracolumbar scoliosis are subject to constant debate, the authors by no means intended to weigh in on that discussion. Instead, they merely intended to illustrate how to employ the endoscope during such complex spinal surgery so that the operation can be simplified to the patient's advantage.

CASE DETAILS

The patient of our illustrative case is a 56-year-old female with a chief complaint of low back pain for the last 20 years. Additionally, she complained of left lower extremity radicular pain that has been going on for the previous seven years but recently experienced worsening pain over the last 20 days. There was normal 5/5 motor strength with normal sensation to light touch, pinprick, and temperature on physical examination. Proprioception and lower extremity reflexes were also normal, and pathological upper motor neuron signs were absent. Advanced imaging studies, including an MRI scan of the thoracolumbar spine, revealed progressive degenerative changes with associated spinal stenosis at the L1/2, L2/3, L3/4, and L4/5 levels. Further radiographic and clinical evaluation at the First Affiliated Hospital of Harbin Medical University determined that the patient suffered from radicular and mechanical pain in the lumbar spine based on a 32° degenerative lumbar scoliosis with multilevel vertical collapse, a small rotatory component, and loss of lumbar lordosis with flattening of the thoracolumbar spine (Fig. **1**). Surgery with multilevel foraminal decompression with interbody fusion cages and a long-rod construct was suggested to the patient since she had failed multiple rounds of non-operative care measures and could no longer function with her daily activities. However, the patient was still deemed well balanced, so an osteotomy was not advised.

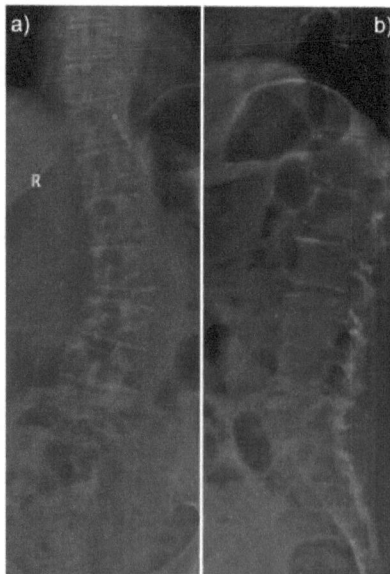

Fig. (1). Shown are anteroposterior (**a**) and lateral (**b**) views of the lumbar spine showing scoliosis with a measured Cobb angle of 32°. The patient's radiographic sagittal balance examination shows loss of normal lordosis with some lumbar spine flattening.

PREOPERATIVE PLANNING AND SURGICAL TECHNIQUES

The patient was to be positioned prone on a spinal frame initially under total intravenous anesthesia (TIVA). The surgical team developed the following plan. The intervertebral discs at L2/3, L3/4, L4/5, and L5/S1 would be removed in the first step. This maneuver would entail an anterolateral release of any tethering, decompression of foraminal and lateral recess stenosis, interbody fusion with iliac crest autologous bone graft, and placement of an expandable cylindrical threaded interbody fusion cage. In the second step, the posterolateral instrumented fusion needed to be carried out from T12 to S1 to correct the deformity and stabilize the spine with the placement of cannulated percutaneous pedicle screws. During the second portion of the surgery, the surgical team opted for general anesthesia as cooperation from the patient in their experience was not required and to preempt increased pain during the instrumented fusion surgery. The surgical team debated the inclusion of the L5/S1 level in the construct since it was deemed not to be involved in the patient's symptomatology; Finally, it was decided to be included based on the advanced degenerative changes to preempt the development of symptomatic adjacent segment disease in the early postoperative convalesce period, improve fusion, and avoid distal junctional failure (Fig. **2**). The L5/S1 motion segment was considered stiff due to the complete collapse. The patient was instructed that extension of the fusion to the ilium may be necessary if such a problem was to occur.

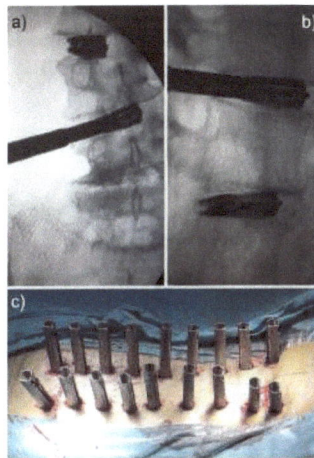

Fig. (2). Intraoperative anteroposterior (**a**) and lateral (**b**) views of the lumbar spine taken during the interbody release and reconstructive fusion procedure are shown. For optimum coronal plane correction, the surgical team opted for interbody fusion from L to S1. The endoscopic working cannula was placed into the triangular safe zone after foraminoplasty. The endoscopic release of anterolateral tethering of the spine and placement of the threaded titanium interbody fusion cages was done with the transforaminal approach at L2/3, L3/4, and L4/5, and with the interlaminar approach at L5/S1. A percutaneous long-segment cannulated pedicle screw construct was placed from T10 to S1 for posterior fixation.

Intraoperatively, the surgeons noted that the L3/4 interbody fusion cage was ideally placed slightly to the left. This was in part dictated by the facet joint anatomy, which requires little endoscopic resection, and by the endplate orientation produced by the scoliotic deformity. As a result, the patient experienced some postoperative numbness and dysesthesia in the L3 dermatome on the left side, which resolved spontaneously with supportive care. The final corrective result is shown in Fig. (**3**). The coronal plane deformity of the patient was nearly corrected to normal. Despite the minimally invasive nature of the scoliosis deformity correction surgery employed by the authors, the patient's postoperative hemoglobin was reduced to 7.7 g/dl underlining the aggressive nature of these types of surgeries even if minimally invasive techniques are employed.

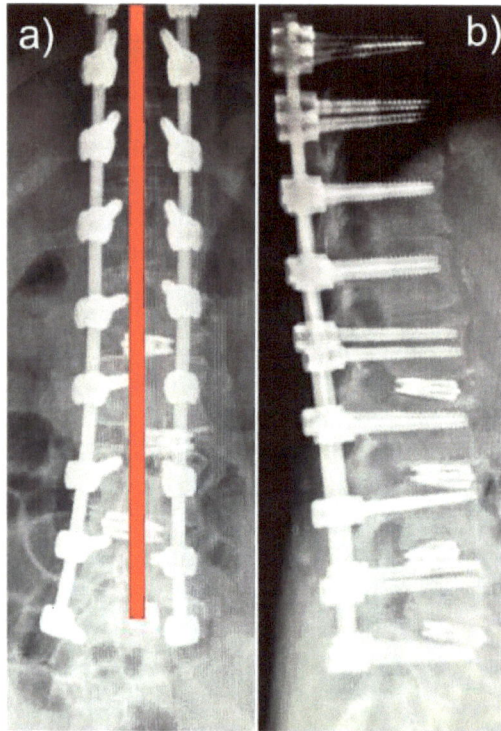

Fig. (3). Postoperative anteroposterior (**a**) and lateral (**b**) view of the lumbar spine following the percutaneous instrumented T10 to S1 long-segment fusion with cannulated pedicle screws and one contiguous long rod on both sides demonstrating correction of scoliosis are shown. The patient's radiographic sagittal balance examination appears unchanged from the preoperative lateral projection images. Note that the L3/4 endoscopic interbody fusion cage was intentionally placed slightly to the left on the curvature's convex side for maximum coronal plane correction.

It is apparent that these types of minimally invasive deformity correction surgeries using both percutaneous and endoscopic procedures are still time-consuming. The resultant operative time may be longer than with traditional open corrective surgery leading to a cumulative blood loss that may be significant. Alternatively, the low hemoglobin could have been dilutional with infusion of large amounts of intravenous fluids. Nonetheless, this patient's postoperative recovery was uneventful, with much less postsurgical wound pain as typically observed. There was no wound problem or infection.

DISCUSSION

Simplifying surgical care in patients with adult degenerative scoliosis has been advocated by many. Some authors advocated decompressive laminectomy or foraminotomy as a less aggressive surgical strategy. Clinical outcomes seem to be favorable as the patients primarily reflect on the operation's success with the radicular pain resolution while deliberately ignoring the overall sagittal imbalance, lateral listhesis, or scoliotic deformity. In the elderly, this treatment protocol is of a definitive advantage as they are not exposed to major surgery's surgical risks. The downside of this approach is that some patients may develop mechanical instability, which forms the basis for recurrent symptoms. Therefore, limited decompression and multilevel segment posterior spinal fusion with pedicle screw rod constructs has become a commonplace in the surgical treatment of patients suffering from symptomatic progressive or decompensated adult degenerative scoliosis. The minimally invasive versions of this corrective surgery are attractive as they in skilled hands may limit the patient's perioperative burden. However, this dynamic does not change the overall outlook on this operation's long-term risks, which include adjacent-segment disease, failed instrumentation, proximal or distal junctional failure with kyphotic deformity, particularly in osteoporotic patients, and infection. Therefore, the authors became interested in hybridizing the endoscopic spinal surgery techniques with other well-established minimally invasive procedures including the percutaneous placement of cannulated pedicle screws over multiple levels to assemble a long-segment fusion construct. As shown by the authors' illustrative case, this corrective deformity surgery's goals can still be achieved while avoiding the common problems associated with traditional open fusion surgeries, which are typically performed using a long midline incision. Wound breakdown is a definitive concern with open surgery but was not a problem in our patient. The postoperative dysesthesia was likely due to irritation of the dorsal root ganglion from the transforaminal insertion of the cylindrical threaded expandable interbody fusion cage - a well-recognized common and self-limiting problem.

Without attempting a complete discussion of the surgical indications for long-segment fusion in adult scoliosis patients, the authors are compelled to discuss a few highlights relevant to their patients' management and the consideration of spinal endoscopy in scoliosis surgery as a whole. The choice of long-segment fusion and fixation of the lower end vertebrae is controversial concerning whether the fixation should end at the S1 vertebral body or include the ilium. For Lenke-Silva type VI adult degenerative scoliosis, the effects of short-segment decompression/fusion and long-segment decompression/fusion and osteotomy are unclear [11]. Studies have shown comparable clinical outcomes in patients with Lenke-Silva type VI adult curves undergoing short-segment decompression fusion or long-segment decompression fusion with osteotomy [12]. Also, the choice of the distal fusion level is controversial. Whether or not a healthy L5-S1 motion segment should be included in the fusion is still controversial. In the case presented herein, the S1 vertebral body's fixation was performed to lower the risk of late S1 fracture due to kyphotic distal junctional failure at L5-S1.

CONCLUSION

As illustrated by the authors' case presentation, endoscopic spinal surgery techniques can be considered an adjunct to scoliosis correction surgery to further diminish the burden on the patient related to open exposures. These are typically required in traditional open spine surgery just to gain access to the deformed and tethered spinal motion segments. In skilled hands, the endoscopic approach may produce a similar benefit. However, this should be analyzed in more comprehensive clinical investigations.

CONSENT FOR PUBLICATION

Not applicable.

CONFLICT OF INTEREST

The authors declare no conflict of interest, financial or otherwise.

ACKNOWLEDGEMENT

Declared none.

REFERENCES

[1]　Aebi M. The adult scoliosis. Eur Spine J 2005; 14(10): 925-48.
[http://dx.doi.org/10.1007/s00586-005-1053-9] [PMID: 16328223]

[2]　Graham RB, Sugrue PA, Koski TR. Adult Degenerative Scoliosis. Clin Spine Surg 2016; 29(3): 95-107.
[http://dx.doi.org/10.1097/BSD.0000000000000367] [PMID: 26945131]

[3]   Wang G, Hu J, Liu X, Cao Y. Surgical treatments for degenerative lumbar scoliosis: a meta analysis. Eur Spine J 2015; 24(8): 1792-9.
[http://dx.doi.org/10.1007/s00586-015-3942-x] [PMID: 25900294]

[4]   Wolff S, Riouallon G. Scoliosis in adulthood: a constant evolution. Rev Prat 2016; 66(3): 298-302.
[PMID: 30512641]

[5]   Dangelmajer S, Zadnik PL, Rodriguez ST, Gokaslan ZL, Sciubba DM. Minimally invasive spine surgery for adult degenerative lumbar scoliosis. Neurosurg Focus 2014; 36(5): E7.
[http://dx.doi.org/10.3171/2014.3.FOCUS144] [PMID: 24785489]

[6]   Shaw R, Skovrlj B, Cho SK. Association between age and complications in adult scoliosis surgery: an analysis of the scoliosis research society morbidity and mortality database. Spine 2016; 41(6): 508-14.
[http://dx.doi.org/10.1097/BRS.0000000000001239] [PMID: 26693670]

[7]   Silva FE, Lenke LG. Adult degenerative scoliosis: evaluation and management. Neurosurg Focus 2010; 28(3): E1.
[http://dx.doi.org/10.3171/2010.1.FOCUS09271] [PMID: 20192655]

[8]   Riouallon G, Bouyer B, Wolff S. Risk of revision surgery for adult idiopathic scoliosis: a survival analysis of 517 cases over 25 years. Eur Spine J 2016; 25(8): 2527-34.
[http://dx.doi.org/10.1007/s00586-016-4505-5] [PMID: 26964785]

[9]   Yagi M, Michikawa T, Hosogane N, *et al.* Treatment for frailty does not improve complication rates in corrective surgery for adult spinal deformity. Spine 2019; 44(10): 723-31.
[http://dx.doi.org/10.1097/BRS.0000000000002929] [PMID: 30395095]

[10]   Benner B, Ehni G. Degenerative lumbar scoliosis. Spine 1979; 4(6): 548-52.
[http://dx.doi.org/10.1097/00007632-197911000-00018] [PMID: 515844]

[11]   Zhang HC, Yu HL, Yang HF, *et al.* Short-segment decompression/fusion *versus* long-segment decompression/fusion and osteotomy for Lenke-Silva type VI adult degenerative scoliosis. Chin Med J (Engl) 2019; 132(21): 2543-9.
[http://dx.doi.org/10.1097/CM9.0000000000000474] [PMID: 31652142]

[12]   Faldini C, Di Martino A, Borghi R, Perna F, Toscano A, Traina F. Long *vs.* short fusions for adult lumbar degenerative scoliosis: does balance matters? Eur Spine J 2015; 24 (Suppl. 7): 887-92.
[http://dx.doi.org/10.1007/s00586-015-4266-6] [PMID: 26441257]

CHAPTER 18

Treatment of Thoracic Meningioma with Spinal Canal Decompression under Spinal Endoscopy

Xifeng Zhang[1,2,*], **Lei-Ming Zhang**[3] and **Yang Liu**[4]

[1] *Department of Orthopedics, First Medical Center, PLA General Hospital, Beijing 100853, China*

[2] *Department of Orthopedics, Beijing Yuho Rehabilitation Hospital, Beijing 100853, China*

[3] *Department of Orthopedics, Sixth Medical Center, PLA General Hospital, Beijing 100048, China*

[4] *Department of Orthopedics, Affiliated Hospital of Yangzhou University, Yangzhou 225001, China*

Abstract: Extramedullary benign tumors of the spine may cause spinal cord compression. Patients may present with motor weakness and sensory loss in the extremities causing gait abnormalities. Surgical treatment is indicated when symptoms are no longer manageable. In this chapter, the authors present an 87-year-old female's case as an illustrative example of how the spinal endoscopy platform can be safely and effectively deployed in the treatment of such lesions. The example patient suffered from spinal cord compression from a large meningioma at the T7 level. The tumor was successfully removed *via* an endoscopic working cannula. The patient's symptoms improved, and a nine-month follow-up MRI scan showed adequate and maintained spinal cord decompression. This case example demonstrates that spinal endoscopy may be applied to an increasing number of surgical indications beyond the scope of degenerative disease. Further clinical investigation will need to show this technology's limits when treating benign tumors of the spine.

Keywords: Endoscopic decompression, Extramedullary benign tumors, Spinal cord compression.

INTRODUCTION

Meningiomas are mostly common intramedullary spinal tumors. Extramedullary spinal meningiomas have been reported to have four times higher recurrence rates [1] and to be locally more aggressive [2]. While extramedullary spinal meningiomas are rare, their intramedullary counterpart occurs in the thoracic

* **Corresponding author Xifeng Zhang:** Department of Orthopedics, First Medical Center, PLA General Hospital, Beijing 100853, China and Department of Orthopedics, Beijing Yuho Rehabilitation Hospital, Beijing, 100853, China; Tel: (908) 922-7635; E-mail: xifengzhang301@outlook.com

spine 80% of the time in individuals between the ages 50 to 60 and with women four times more often than men [3].

In comparison, extramedullary spinal meningiomas make up 3.3%–7.8% of all spinal meningiomas [4]. The age distribution of patients diagnosed with an extramedullary meningioma is much wider than with intramedullary meningiomas and ranges between 14 – 75 years with nearly half of the affected patients being younger than 30 years and the majority being women [5]. Extramedullary meningiomas occur mostly in the thoracic spine and cervical spine [6, 7]. In this chapter, the authors demonstrate their minimally invasive management style of extramedullary benign spinal tumors employing spinal endoscopy without attempting an in-depth discussion of their differential diagnosis, clinical outcomes, and management.

CASE DETAILS

The patient is an 87-year-old female with a chief complaint of unsteady gait for the last one and a half years, causing increasing numbness and clumsiness in both lower limbs for six months. Symptoms started without any provoking event. Proprioception was altered as the patient stated she felt that she was walking on cotton. There were no spontaneous twitches. There was no incontinence. The diagnosis and treatment were delayed. As symptoms worsened over the previous year before presentation to our clinic, the patient noted increasing coldness and swelling of both lower extremities and decreased sensation in the left lower extremity. The admission to our facility was prompted by the above symptoms gradually worsening. Our team's initial physical revealed staggering gait, loss of sensation below the groin on both sides, but a free normal movement with 5/5 motor strength and normal muscle tone of the bilateral lower extremities. Of the advanced imaging studies, the thoracic MRI scan showed an extramedullary round lesion at the T7 level well visualized on the T1- and short-echo T2-weighted image. The lesion measured approximately 8 x 11 x 15 mm with a clearly delineated margin, causing compression of the spinal cord (Fig. 1).

The patient became increasingly myelopathic with unmanageable symptoms leading up to the admission to our healthcare facility. Therefore, surgical decompression of the thoracic meningioma was indicated. The surgical team opted for an endoscopic decompression to minimize wound trauma and to simplify this patient's care. Therefore, a minimally invasive spinal endoscopic posterior laminectomy was contemplated to remove the tumor. The patient was positioned in a prone position on the spinal frame, and the surgery was performed under local anesthesia by infiltrating the surgical area with 1% lidocaine. Intraoperative fluoroscopy in multiple projections was used to accurately position the endoscopic working cannula after serial dilation over a guidewire, which had been placed over a spinal needle.

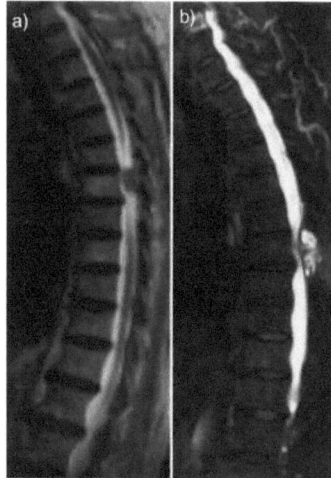

Fig. (1). An extramedullary round lesion at the T7 level well visualized on the T1-**(a)** and short-echo T2-weighted **(b)** image is shown. The lesion measured approximately 8 x 11 x 15 mm with a clearly delineated margin, causing the spinal cord's compression.

The surgical team was aware of the need for minimal manipulation of the spinal cord and careful drilling with the endoscopic power bur to remove the thoracic lamina at the T7 level to gain access to the spinal canal. Once access to the spinal canal was achieved, the meningioma was carefully dissected off the spinal cord without much difficulty. The stalk was identified and transected, allowing extirpation of the lesion in toto. Postoperatively, the patient was treated with supportive rehabilitation measures and improved significantly with near-complete gait some nine months postoperatively. No obvious postoperative complications were encountered. MRI imaging performed at that time showed adequate spinal cord decompression at the T7 level (Fig. **2**).

DISCUSSION

Meningiomas mostly originate from spinal cord arachnoid cells. The tumor grows slowly and often compresses the spinal cord, leading to spinal cord edema, nerve fiber degeneration, and ischemia, and eventually spinal cord damage. The clinical diagnosis is typically made on the MRI scan, determining the relationship between meningioma and surrounding tissues. The latter or the spinal cord are rarely invaded, making surgical extirpation of the lesion the treatment of choice. Meningiomas grow slowly, and clinically symptomatic recurrences are rare. The tumor is well visualized on routine T1- and T2 weighted MRI scans by demonstrating equal signal or slightly low signal intensity and uniform enhancement after contrast showing the tumor tissue's characteristic compactness. Sometimes extramedullary meningiomas are mistaken for metastases of another primary tumor with lymphoma, schwannoma, and cavernous angioma also being in the differential diagnosis [6]. Lymphoma should be expected with extramedullary lesions in the thoracic spine because they are somewhat difficult to distinguish from extramedullary meningioma [8]. Calcifications, on the other hand, are more suggestive of extramedullary meningioma [9].

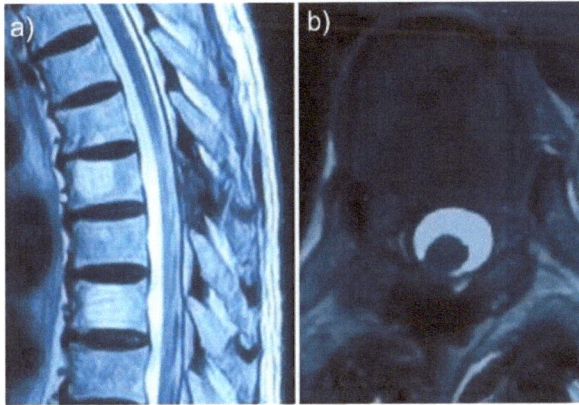

Fig. (2). Nine-months postoperative follow-up T2-weighted sagittal (**a**) and axial (**b**) MRI scans after the endoscopic resection of the T7 meningioma showed adequate decompression of the spinal cord at the T7 level. The patient's functioning had improved significantly.

The advantages of the traditional posterior total laminectomy combined with tumor resection are that the operation time is short, and the surgical decompression is more thorough than the broad exposure. The postoperative recovery is typically fast, and the clinical symptoms may improve significantly immediately after surgery. However, complications and wound problems are also more common. Another disadvantage is that the patient may develop postoperative instability, resulting in recurrent symptoms and the need for more surgery. With the development of minimally invasive techniques, clinicians are looking for ways to simplify the spine's surgical approach. Spinal endoscopy has been successfully employed in treating many common degenerative conditions in all areas of the spine. Our illustrative case report shows that it can also be applied to simple tumor resection.

Recurrence of the tumor is of concern since the probability of recurrence of extramedullary meningioma is four times higher than with intramedullary meningioma [8]. Long-term follow-up assessment in one study with 12 patients that open gross total resection resulted in no recurrence in four patients. However, out of the eight patients who underwent subtotal resection, one patient did have a recurrence 88 months after the index surgery [6]. Conceivable, better direct, and magnified videoendoscopic visualization under constant irrigation may allow the surgeon to perform a complete gross total resection, which was suggested to reduce the recurrence rate [10].

CONCLUSION

Surgical removal of meningioma has a high cure rate with few postoperative complications. The endoscopic spinal surgery platform should be considered an alternative to open laminectomy-type decompression surgeries for benign extramedullary tumors with well-delineated margins. As illustrated by our patient case example, the endoscopic decompression for these types of lesions can be safely carried out. Endoscopy is worthy of clinical application for their treatment. Other locally more aggressive and perhaps malignant lesions may be an absolute or relative contraindication to the endoscopic tumor removal. However, clinical studies will need to be performed to formally investigate what the technological limits of the technology in this arena are.

CONSENT FOR PUBLICATION

Not applicable.

CONFLICT OF INTEREST

The authors declare no conflict of interest, financial or otherwise.

ACKNOWLEDGEMENT

Declared none.

REFERENCES

[1]   Klekamp J, Samii M. Surgical results for spinal meningiomas. Surg Neurol 1999; 52(6): 552-62.
        [http://dx.doi.org/10.1016/S0090-3019(99)00153-6] [PMID: 10660020]

[2]   Messori A, Rychlicki F, Salvolini U. Spinal epidural en-plaque meningioma with an unusual pattern of calcification in a 14-year-old girl: case report and review of the literature. Neuroradiology 2002; 44(3): 256-60.
        [http://dx.doi.org/10.1007/s00234-001-0709-3] [PMID: 11942384]

[3]   Solero CL, Fornari M, Giombini S, *et al.* Spinal meningiomas: review of 174 operated cases. Neurosurgery 1989; 25(2): 153-60.
        [http://dx.doi.org/10.1227/00006123-198908000-00001] [PMID: 2671779]

[4]   Levy WJ Jr, Bay J, Dohn D. Spinal cord meningioma. J Neurosurg 1982; 57(6): 804-12.
        [http://dx.doi.org/10.3171/jns.1982.57.6.0804] [PMID: 7143063]

[5]   Frank BL, Harrop JS, Hanna A, Ratliff J. Cervical extradural meningioma: case report and literature review. J Spinal Cord Med 2008; 31(3): 302-5.
        [http://dx.doi.org/10.1080/10790268.2008.11760727] [PMID: 18795481]

[6]   Wu L, Yang T, Deng X, *et al.* Spinal extradural en plaque meningiomas: clinical features and long-

term outcomes of 12 cases. J Neurosurg Spine 2014; 21(6): 892-8.
[http://dx.doi.org/10.3171/2014.7.SPINE13819] [PMID: 25237843]

[7] Tuli J, Drzymalski DM, Lidov H, Tuli S. Extradural en-plaque spinal meningioma with intraneural invasion. World Neurosurg 2012; 77(1): 202.e5-202.e13.
[http://dx.doi.org/10.1016/j.wneu.2011.03.047] [PMID: 22405399]

[8] Cugati G, Singh M, Pande A, *et al.* Primary spinal epidural lymphomas. J Craniovertebr Junction Spine 2011; 2(1): 3-11.
[http://dx.doi.org/10.4103/0974-8237.85307] [PMID: 22013369]

[9] Yamada S, Kawai S, Yonezawa T, Masui K, Nishi N, Fujiwara K. Cervical extradural en-plaque meningioma. Neurol Med Chir (Tokyo) 2007; 47(1): 36-9.
[http://dx.doi.org/10.2176/nmc.47.36] [PMID: 17245014]

[10] Cohen-Gadol AA, Zikel OM, Koch CA, Scheithauer BW, Krauss WE. Spinal meningiomas in patients younger than 50 years of age: a 21-year experience. J Neurosurg 2003; 98(3) (Suppl.): 258-63.
[PMID: 12691381]

CHAPTER 19

Cervical Endoscopic Unilateral Laminotomy for Bilateral Decompression (CE-ULBD) – A Technical Perspective

Vincent Hagel[1,*] and **Kai-Uwe Lewandrowski**[2,3,4]

[1] Asklepios Hospital Lindau, Spine Center, Lindau, Germany

[2] Center for Advanced Spine Care of Southern Arizona and Surgical Institute of Tucson, Tucson AZ, USA

[3] Associate Professor of Orthopaedic Surgery, Universidad Colsanitas, Bogota, Colombia, USA

[4] Visiting Professor, Department Orthopaedic Surgery, UNIRIO, Rio de Janeiro, Brazil

Abstract: Cervical endoscopic unilateral laminotomy for bilateral decompression (CE-ULBD) is an applicable surgical method in cases of central canal stenosis, usually associated with myelopathy. Other authors have shown the feasibility, safety, and efficacy of this method. They could also demonstrate more favorable perioperative benchmark data of this procedure than anterior cervical discectomy and fusion (ACDF) in terms of duration of surgery, blood loss, and hospital stay. In this chapter, the authors focus on the technological advances making this surgery possible. Moreover, the authors review the relevant surgical anatomy to enable the aspiring endoscopic spine surgeon to safely and successfully perform the CE-ULBD procedure. Experience in advanced endoscopic surgery in other areas of the spine is recommended before imparting on the posterior endoscopic decompression of the stenotic central cervical spinal canal. The authors have implemented CE-ULBD in formalized and well-structured Endoscopic Spine Academy (Espinea®) training programs, intending to provide high educational standards to achieve favorable outcomes with the CE-ULBD procedure reproducibly.

Keywords: Cervical myelopathy, Cervical spinal canal stenosis, CE-ULBD, Laminotomy, Posterior cervical endoscopic decompression, Spinal cord compression.

---

* **Corresponding author Vincent Hagel:** Asklepios Hospital Lindau, Spine Center, Lindau, Germany; E-mail: vhagel@yahoo.de

INTRODUCTION

Degenerative cervical central canal stenosis is the most common cause of cervical myelopathy [1 - 11]. The progressive narrowing of the cervical spinal canal causes mechanical compression of the spinal cord. Hypoperfusion and segmental instability may add to the onset of symptoms, possibly causing rapid clinical deterioration [12]. Symptoms vary from fine motor deficits of the upper extremities, ataxia, hypesthesia of the lower extremities to bladder/bowel dysfunction [13, 14]. Several anatomical structures can cause central canal stenosis of the cervical spine. Typical reasons in the anterior spinal column are spondylotic changes leading to disc bulging [15] or ossification of the posterior longitudinal ligament [16]. In the posterior spinal column, medullary compression is mainly due to hypertrophic ligamentum flavum [5, 17, 18]. Compared to the lumbar spine, hypertrophy of the facet joint rarely contributes to stenosis [15]. The current literature remains unclear when surgically treating patients with a mild stenosis/myelopathy [11] and normal electrophysiological findings is indicated [15]. While these are individual decisions, in moderate and severe stenosis/myelopathy, there is no doubt about early surgical decompression being the treatment of choice [13, 19].

SURGICAL OPTIONS

Surgical options include a ventral or dorsal approach. While most surgeons are more familiar with and prefer a ventral approach [13, 19 - 21], there are circumstances where the posterior approach may be preferable [2, 21]. Several factors may dictate the approach of choice to the cervical spine. For example, the site of the maximum compression, the degree of stability, and the sagittal profile influences this decision-making [2]. A hypertrophic yellow ligament with or without associated kyphosis may dictate the posterior approach [15, 17]. In microsurgical techniques, posterior approaches to the cervical spine usually create significant destruction of the paravertebral musculature, generating prolonged neck pain, adding to kyphosis, or possibly evoking instability [22]. Endoscopic posterior approaches, on the other hand, seem to minimize these disadvantages [23 - 29]. However, few studies have compared the endoscopic approach to conventional open techniques to the cervical spine [30, 31]. Yet comparative studies from other spine areas suggest a reduced risk of postoperative kyphosis, instability, and infection [32 - 34]. The authors' preferred technique is the cervical endoscopic unilateral laminotomy for bilateral decompression (CE-ULBD) [30, 35].

PROCEDURAL STEPS

Choice of Endoscope

Different sized endoscopes can be used to perform a CE-ULBD. The most common ones have an overall diameter of 7.3 mm, or 10 mm (Fig. **1**). The smaller-sized endoscope provides more flexibility, thereby facilitating contralateral decompression. It also causes slightly less soft tissue trauma. On the other hand, a larger-diameter endoscope allows for introducing larger instruments and, consequently, more aggressive and perhaps faster decompression (Fig. **2**). Also, its working sleeve remains outside the canal throughout the procedure, leading to less risk of accidentally compressing the spinal cord.

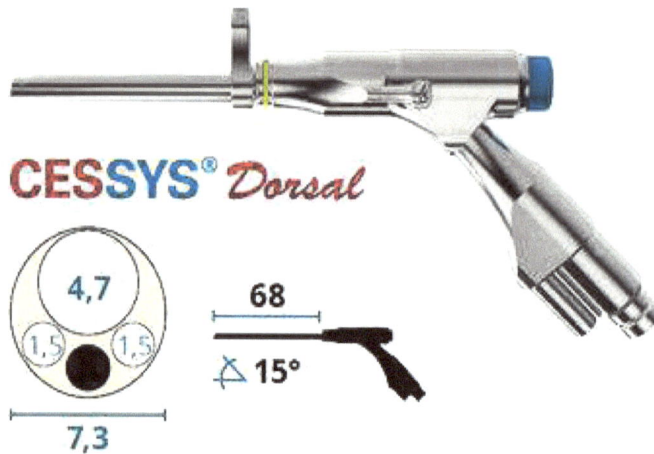

Fig. (1). Cervical endoscope CESSYS® Dorsal of Joimax™ with a 4.7 mm inner working channel.

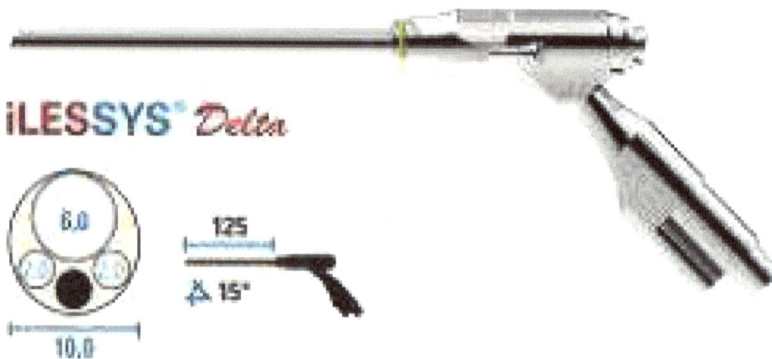

Fig. (2). The iLESSYS® Delta endoscope by Joimax™ with a 6.0 mm inner working channel is also suitable for the posterior cervical decompression.

Patient Positioning

Bleeding during the posterior microsurgical technique from epidural vessels may complicate the decompression of the cervical spinal cord. Therefore, the patient is often placed in a sitting position to reduce bleeding. In endoscopy, there is no need for this more complex and time-consuming setup. Positioning patients in the prone position is more straightforward. The head should be placed in what is known as the military position - slight capital flexion with the extension of the subaxial cervical spine (Fig. **3**) [36]. Approaching the upper levels of the subaxial cervical spine sometimes poses difficulties to establish enough inclination by the use of a head shell. In such cases, a clamp might be useful. In the lower levels of the cervical spine, sufficient kyphosis can usually be induced with a chest roll (without the additional need of a clamp). Since it still remains unclear if the rare event of a postoperative C5 palsy after cervical decompression is due to shoulder traction [37], extensive pulling/taping down of the shoulder should be avoided. Individually adapted traction necessity can be checked under fluoroscopy before draping.

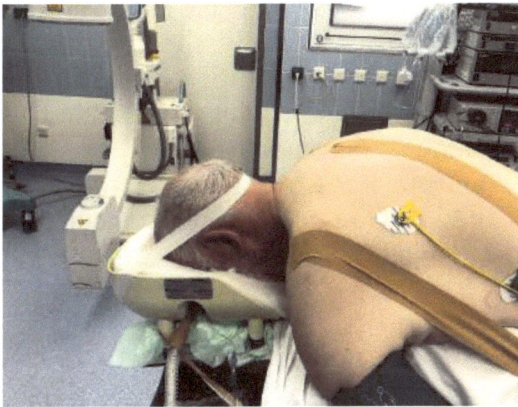

Fig. (3). Prone positioning of the patient in capital flexion and cervical extension over a chest roll.

The endoscopic procedure is done under continuous irrigation, which diminishes bleeding. At times, however, bipolar cautery may be used to control bleeding. It should be largely avoided, though, especially in the epidural space, as it may cause shrinkage of the dura and possibly contribute to a neurological deficit. Instead, hemostatic agents should be employed. If available, it is advisable to use intraoperative monitoring. This can bring forthcoming harm to the myelon to the surgeon's attention. Adaption of irrigation pressure all the way to interrupting the procedure are possible consequences.

Approach Planning

The anatomical landmarks relevant to this procedure include the posterior element, including the spinous process in the midline and the lateral masses bilaterally. They should be marked on the skin under fluoroscopic guidance in the posterior-anterior view (PA). The intended trajectory (line parallel to the target levels disc space) should be drawn in the lateral view of the patient's neck.

Incision Placement

The off-midline distance for the skin incision depends on whether there is ipsilateral foraminal stenosis and how extensive the contralateral decompression has to be. These scenarios dictate the usual medial-to-lateral distance between 0.5 and 1.5 cm (0.5 cm if an ipsilateral foraminotomy is necessary, 1.5 cm if a sufficient contralateral decompression has priority). After the skin incision is made, the rigid guiding rod is placed on the facet joint of the target level under fluoroscopic guidance. Usually, this is done in PA-view in order to have better control of placing the tip of the guiding rod on the posterior surface of the facet joint. It should also be placed rather towards the lateral aspect of the facet joint to have the least possible risk of accidentally slipping towards the spinal canal. Slipping off the lateral aspect contains little chance of injuring the vertebral artery, since it is protected by the facet joint. Since guide wires could sever the spinal cord, this team of authors does not use them. Serial soft tissue dilators are advanced over which the endoscopic beveled working sleeve is introduced. Initially, the bevel of the working cannula faces medially. After fluoroscopic verification of the working sleeves position, the cervical endoscope is inserted (Fig. **4**).

Irrigation Settings

Many surgeons still use gravity-assisted irrigation. Irrigation pumps, on the other hand, may allow for better control of irrigation. Yet, so far, there are no reliable guidelines on the settings of the irrigation pump, neither for lumbar endoscopic surgery nor for cervical endoscopic surgery. There are case reports where intra- and postoperative complications such as seizures and severe headaches occurred and have been attributed to excessive use of irrigation fluid at unreasonably high-pressure levels. The perioperative problems are presumably related to a high infusion rate, a prolonged operative time, a dural tear [38]. Since infusion rate is one possible risk factor, the settings should be as low as possible. When bleeding increases, it is advisable to adjust the pressure- and flow settings temporarily.

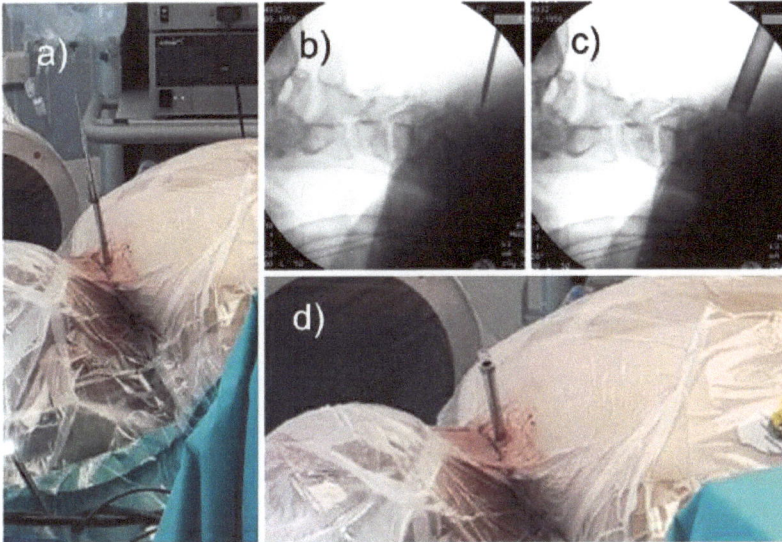

Fig. (4). Before serial dilators are advanced **(a)**, the guide rod is placed on the posterior surface of the facet joint C5/6 under fluoroscopic control **(b)**. The working sleeve is placed over the last dilator and its position is fluoroscopically verified **(c, d)**. Initially, the bevel should be oriented medially.

Apart from the infusion rate, a prolonged surgery time is a putative risk factor as well. Suppose the surgery cannot be accomplished within a satisfactory amount of time. In that case, one might even think of ending the procedure and having to perform a second surgery in the worst-case scenario. Another consideration is the position of the pump in relation to the patient. State-of-the-art irrigation pumps such as the Joimax Versicon® have a 'Level'-function to adjust for patient-position-related problems. Nevertheless, the absolute numbers for flow rate and irrigation pressures should be set at the surgeon's clinical judgement of appropriate settings considering intraoperative factors. In the future, studies and guidelines will have to establish recommendations of the settings. Until then, the authors' advice is simple: keep irrigation flow rates and pressure levels as high as necessary and as low as possible.

Anatomical Landmarks

After inserting the endoscope, the bone of the posterior cervical elements should be palpated. The target area is constituted by the cranial and caudal lamina, which defines the "V-point" (Fig. **5**). After that, the immediate layer of soft tissue is removed, exposing the facet joint, especially its medial border.

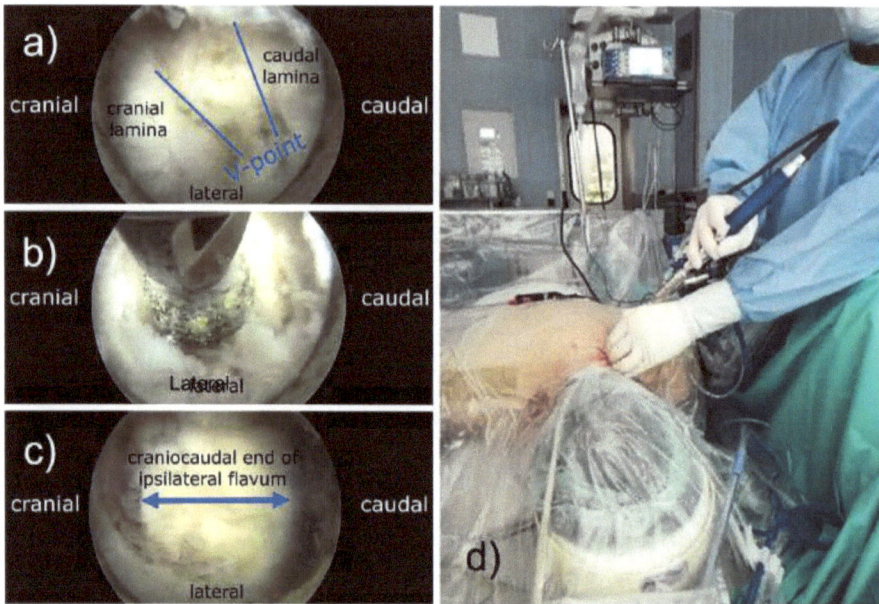

Fig. (5). Initially, the V-point is exposed (**a**). Then, the ipsilateral laminotomy is performed using a diamond drill (**b**) until the ipsilateral ligamentum flavum is exposed (**c**). If needed, a contralateral laminotomy is added (**d**).

Decompression

The most crucial goal of this procedure is not to harm the myelon. Accidentally compressing the spinal cord with the working sleeve or endoscope is one risk factor. It is, therefore, necessary to pay attention to the position of the working tube and endoscope throughout the whole procedure. Since this cannot be guaranteed by the surgeon itself, especially less experienced surgeons, a holding arm can help reduce this risk. The bony decompression is commenced by establishing the V-point as the significant starting point landmark (Fig. **6**). While it is legitimate to use bone resector blades performing a lumbar bony decompression, these blades should be avoided in cervical surgery. Not only the lamina but also the ligamentum flavum is much thinner than in the lumbar spine. Therefore, there is no need for this more efficient but also more dangerous blade. A diamond abrasor is sufficient (Fig. **3b**). The ligamentum flavum is left in place as long as possible to avoid irrigation fluid entering the spinal canal and compressing the dura. After completing the ipsilateral laminotomy, the contralateral laminotomy is performed before moving on to completing the bilateral flavectomy (Fig. **6**).

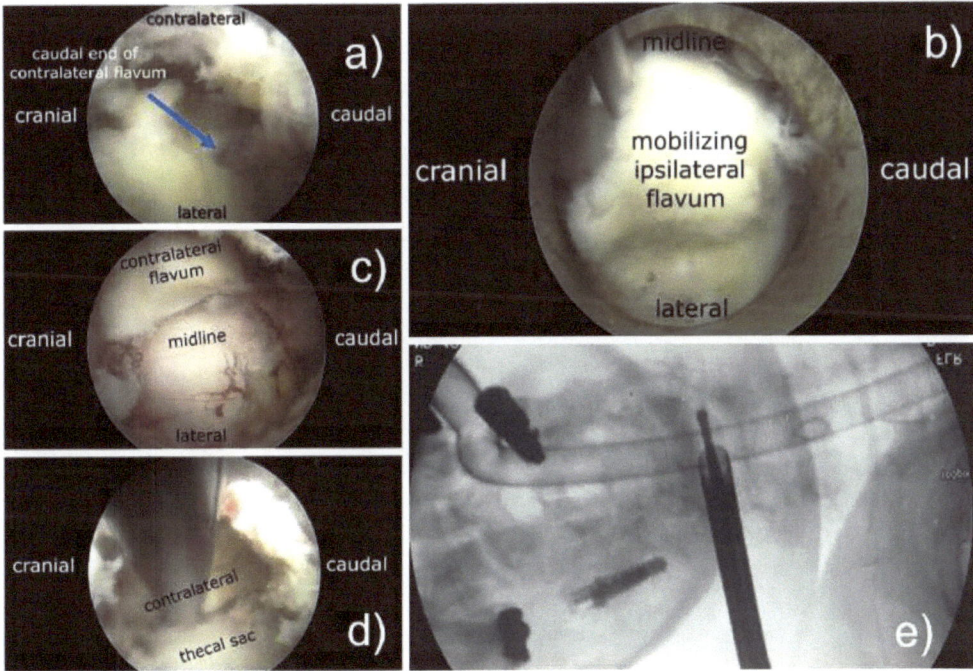

Fig. (6). The caudal end of the contralateral flavum is exposed after contralateral laminotomy **(a)**. The ipsilateral ligamentum flavum is mobilized **(b)** and removed to expose the ipsilateral dura **(c)**. After the contralateral flavectomy **(d)**, the extent of contralateral decompression is additionally assessed *via* fluoroscopy **(e)**.

If apart from a central stenosis there is also a foraminal stenosis, usually the myelopathy caused by the central stenosis outweighs the foraminal stenosis in importance to treat. Therefore, it should be the primary target of decompression. If needed, the foraminal decompression is done as the last step. Keep in mind, that the amount of partial facetectomy should not exceed 50% of the joint in order to preserve its function. A final inspection of the extent of decompression should be performed, including fluoroscopy (Figs. **6** and **7**).

POSTOPERATIVE CARE

After ventral approaches to the cervical spine, the patient is usually monitored on the intensive care unit (ICU) or at least the intermediate care unit (IMC). The authors adopted this management style because of the risk of developing dyspnea due to soft tissue swelling. Since this is not a risk with posterior approaches, there is no need for intensive postoperative monitoring after a CE-ULBD. Even more, patients can be mobilized few hours after the end of surgery. So far, several studies have shown very low-risk profiles for this procedure, allowing for a shorter hospital stay compared to other cervical spine decompression procedures

[5]. The authors recommend a soft cervical brace for comfort for the first three weeks. Perhaps this approach to postoperative management is ultra-conservative but has worked well for the authors. While patients usually do not return to work for two to three months after conventional c-spine surgery, the author's team observed a faster return to work after a posterior endoscopic bilateral decompression.

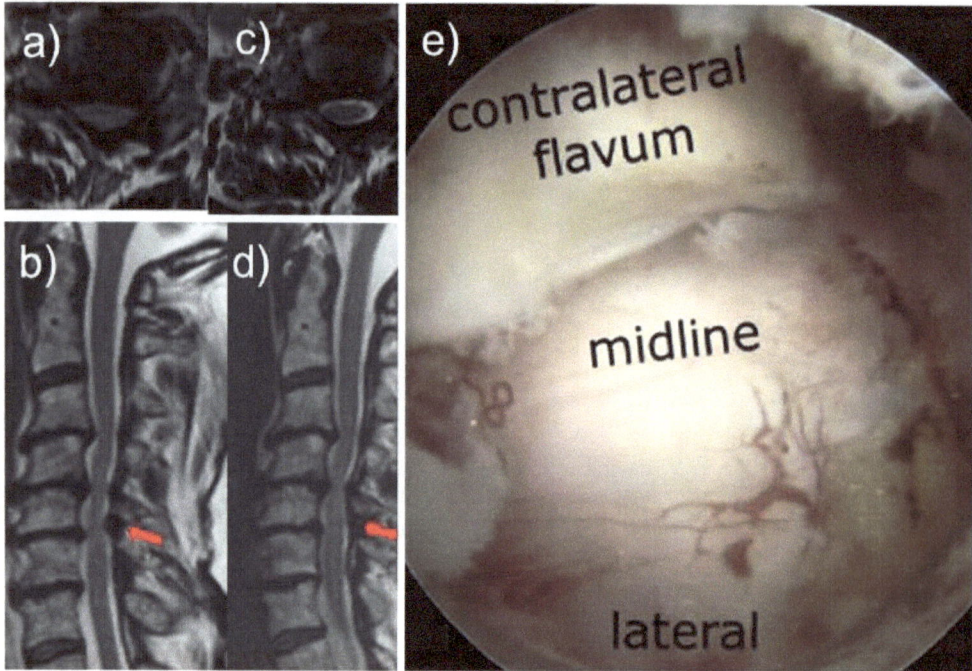

Fig. (7). Pre **(a, b)**- and postoperative **(c, d)** T2-weighted axial **(a, c)** and sagittal **(b, d)** MRI scans are shown. The direct video-endoscopic visualization shows excellent spinal cord decompression from the ipsilateral approach to the contralateral side, just as confirmed with the postoperative MRI scans two months after the procedure.

COMPLICATIONS

The clinical evidence on endoscopic surgery of the cervical spine is scarce. The few studies available suffer from low patient numbers. This team of authors is only aware of a few randomized controlled trials (RCTs) or comparative cohort studies addressing endoscopic *versus* open spine surgery [39 - 43]. Consequently, there are a few studies having analyzed the incidence of complications with the CE-ULBD decompression procedures but have found few [5, 31, 35, 42, 44 - 52]. This dynamic may change as more surgeons decide to treat their patients endoscopically. In our patient series, we did not encounter any significant complications or transient neurological deficits that did require any aftercare or additional surgery.

CLINICAL SERIES

Five patients with cervical myelopathy caused by central canal stenosis were treated in a single center between September 2020 and June 2021. Three patients were male, and two were female, with an average age of 57.4 (range 37 – 73) years. All patients received preoperative MRI scans. One patient had two-level stenosis, and the remaining four patients had single-level stenosis. In 4 patients, the leading site of compression was a hypertrophic ligamentum flavum. One patient had a mainly anterior compression (disc herniation/spondylophyte). All patients suffered from fine motor deficits as well as hypesthesia of the upper extremities. One patient had additional decreased sensory function of the lower extremities. Another patient showed walking impairment. Three out of 5 patients showed a myelomalacia on the preoperative MRI scan. Inclusion criteria were radiological or clinical signs of myelopathy, fine motor deficit, decreased sensory function, pathological upper motor neuron signs, and an abnormal JOA score. Patients with ≥ three-level stenosis were excluded. Compression caused by a central disc herniation or ossification of the posterior longitudinal ligament was an exclusion criterion. Patients with a preceding surgery (ACDF) on the target level were also excluded. Finally, instability and severe kyphosis are known contraindications for a posterior approach to the cervical spine. Macnab criteria and JOA scores were the primary outcome measures. Secondary outcome measures were operation time and duration of hospital stay. In the three-month follow-up, every patient improved in the JOA score, by average 2.4 points (range 1 to 4). Clinical outcomes (Macnab) in the follow-up were excellent in 3 patients (60%), good in 1 patient (20%) as well as fair in 1 patient (20%). Preoperative neck pain was present in 3 of the five patients. In 2 patients, neck pain was reduced (by 1 and 3 points on the VAS) in the three months follow-up. One patient described the neck pain as unchanged. None of the five patients mentioned new/increased neck pain postoperatively. Four patients complained of brachialgia preoperatively. Altogether, the brachialgia VAS was 5.2 by average (ranging from 0 to 7). Only one patient mentioned residual arm pain (VAS 2, preoperative VAS 7). The duration of surgery was 85.2 min by average (range 71-148 min). The average hospital stay was 2.4 days (range 2-3 days). No complication was observed, *i.e.*, no new neurological deficit, no infection, no hematoma, no dural tear.

DISCUSSION

To date, there are countless studies about endoscopic cervical spine decompression surgery. However, there are only two RCTs or comparative cohort studies. The over-the-top decompression integral to the CE-ULBD procedure is unique and novel. It relies on advanced and highly controllable decompression tools, including power burs, that can be handled with finesse and accuracy to get the job done safely. The risk of catastrophic neurological damage is much higher in the cervical spine with any iatrogenic injury to the cervical spinal cord or its exiting nerve roots. With that much at stake, the authors' techniques focused on performing the decompression safely, efficacious, and in a relatively short amount of time to minimize spinal cord irritation and migration of irrigation fluid past the boundaries of the surgical level into the spinal canal and beyond. Based on our clinical observations in our patients and the few existing articles, the authors of this chapter conclude that the CE-ULBD procedure in skilled hands is safe and effective.

While it seems intuitive that the perioperative and short-term clinical primary and secondary clinical outcome measures will likely be better than with open cervical decompression surgery by the pure nature of the minimally invasive endoscopic surgery that comes at a very low burden to the patient and can often be done in an outpatient setting, it remains to be seen whether or not there are any long-term benefits with lower rates of post decompression kyphosis, instability, and unrelenting axial neck pain when compared to open surgery. At a minimum, Minamide *et al*. showed that conventional cervical laminoplasty usually adds to a loss of lordosis. On the other hand, microendoscopic posterior cervical decompression adds to a gain of lordosis and has also been associated with significantly less postoperative axial neck pain. One would expect that this dynamic would also play out with the posterior cervical endoscopic decompression. The burden of proof rests with those surgeons who advocate breaking with the traditional dogma of avoiding posterior cervical approaches in patients with straightening or kyphosis of the cervical spine to avoid increased posterior axial neck pain.

Regardless of whether that is or is not the case, there are other less obvious advantages of endoscopic decompression - namely, the lower cost of outpatient spine care, faster recovery, and lower narcotic utilization in the immediate postoperative period. While these were not explicitly investigated in this chapter, the authors are currently conducting a clinical review of these peri- and postoperative primary and secondary outcome data to better position the overall value of the CE-ULBD within the framework of reimbursing cervical decompression surgeries.

CONCLUSION

The CE-ULBD procedure is made possible by recent technology advances in endoscopic instrumentation and decompression tools that fit down the single central working channel of a smaller diameter spinal endoscope. Being able to control the surgical corridor and the access area where the decompression takes place in terms of the hydrostatic pressure of the irrigation fluid to control bleeding and improve visualization without excessive pressures is at the heart of making the CE-ULBD procedure work. Performing the decompression quickly and effectively at low morbidity to the patient is the basis for a low complication rate [35, 48] and excellent and good clinical outcomes found in our patient series. The CE-ULBD requires a high-skill level and advanced understanding of the applied endoscopic cervical spine anatomy. It should be practiced only by those surgeons who have high confidence in their abilities and experience with endoscopic surgery in other areas of the spine. Further investigation should focus on how to master the learning curve and integrate this demanding operation into one's surgical portfolio.

CONSENT FOR PUBLICATION

Not applicable.

CONFLICT OF INTEREST

The authors declare no conflict of interest, financial or otherwise.

ACKNOWLEDGEMENT

Declared none.

REFERENCES

[1]   König SA, Spetzger U. Surgical management of cervical spondylotic myelopathy - indications for anterior, posterior or combined procedures for decompression and stabilisation. Acta Neurochir (Wien) 2014; 156(2): 253-8.
        [http://dx.doi.org/10.1007/s00701-013-1955-y] [PMID: 24292777]

[2]   Law MD Jr, Bernhardt M, White AA III. Cervical spondylotic myelopathy: a review of surgical indications and decision making. Yale J Biol Med 1993; 66(3): 165-77.
        [PMID: 8209553]

[3]   Law MD Jr, Bernhardt M, White AA III. Evaluation and management of cervical spondylotic myelopathy. Instr Course Lect 1995; 44: 99-110.
        [PMID: 7797896]

[4]   Levin KH, Maggiano HJ, Wilbourn AJ. Cervical radiculopathies: comparison of surgical and EMG localization of single-root lesions. Neurology 1996; 46(4): 1022-5.
        [http://dx.doi.org/10.1212/WNL.46.4.1022] [PMID: 8780083]

[5]   Lin Y, Rao S, Li Y, Zhao S, Chen B. Posterior percutaneous full-endoscopic cervical laminectomy and decompression for cervical stenosis with myelopathy: a technical note. World Neurosurg 2019; S1878-8750(19)30051-8.
        [http://dx.doi.org/10.1016/j.wneu.2018.12.180] [PMID: 30648610]

[6]   Matsunaga S, Kukita M, Hayashi K, *et al.* Pathogenesis of myelopathy in patients with ossification of the posterior longitudinal ligament. J Neurosurg 2002; 96(2) (Suppl.): 168-72.
        [PMID: 12450279]

[7]   Medow JE, Trost G, Sandin J. Surgical management of cervical myelopathy: indications and techniques for surgical corpectomy. Spine J 2006; 6(6) (Suppl.): 233S-41S.
[http://dx.doi.org/10.1016/j.spinee.2006.05.007] [PMID: 17097543]

[8]   Morishita Y, Naito M, Hymanson H, Miyazaki M, Wu G, Wang JC. The relationship between the cervical spinal canal diameter and the pathological changes in the cervical spine. Eur Spine J 2009; 18(6): 877-83.
[http://dx.doi.org/10.1007/s00586-009-0968-y] [PMID: 19357877]

[9]   Nakagawa H, Saito K, Mitsugi T, Yagi K, Kanno A. Microdiscectomy and foraminotomy in cervical spondylotic myelopathy and radiculopathy: anterior *versus* posterior, microendoscopic surgery *versus* mini-open microsurgery. World Neurosurg 2014; 81(2): 292-3.
[http://dx.doi.org/10.1016/j.wneu.2013.01.122] [PMID: 23376389]

[10]   Nouri A, Cheng JS, Davies B, Kotter M, Schaller K, Tessitore E. Degenerative cervical myelopathy: a brief review of past perspectives, present developments, and future directions. J Clin Med 2020; 9(2): E535.
[http://dx.doi.org/10.3390/jcm9020535] [PMID: 32079075]

[11]   Oshima Y, Seichi A, Takeshita K, *et al.* Natural course and prognostic factors in patients with mild cervical spondylotic myelopathy with increased signal intensity on T2-weighted magnetic resonance imaging. Spine 2012; 37(22): 1909-13.
[http://dx.doi.org/10.1097/BRS.0b013e318259a65b] [PMID: 22511231]

[12]   Epstein NE. Reperfusion injury (RPI)/White Cord Syndrome (WCS) due to cervical spine surgery: a diagnosis of exclusion. Surg Neurol Int 2020; 11: 320.
[http://dx.doi.org/10.25259/SNI_555_2020] [PMID: 33093997]

[13]   Goh GS, Liow MHL, Ling ZM, *et al.* Severity of preoperative myelopathy symptoms affects patient-reported outcomes, satisfaction, and return to work after anterior cervical discectomy and fusion for degenerative cervical myelopathy. Spine 2020; 45(10): 649-56.
[http://dx.doi.org/10.1097/BRS.0000000000003354] [PMID: 31809467]

[14]   Hattori T, Sakakibara R, Yasuda K, Murayama N, Hirayama K. Micturitional disturbance in cervical spondylotic myelopathy. J Spinal Disord 1990; 3(1): 16-8.
[http://dx.doi.org/10.1097/00002517-199003000-00003] [PMID: 2134406]

[15]   Tetreault L, Goldstein CL, Arnold P, *et al.* Degenerative cervical myelopathy: a spectrum of related disorders affecting the aging spine. Neurosurgery 2015; 77 (Suppl. 4): S51-67.
[http://dx.doi.org/10.1227/NEU.0000000000000951] [PMID: 26378358]

[16]   Abiola R, Rubery P, Mesfin A. Ossification of the posterior longitudinal ligament: etiology, diagnosis, and outcomes of nonoperative and operative management. Global Spine J 2016; 6(2): 195-204.
[http://dx.doi.org/10.1055/s-0035-1556580] [PMID: 26933622]

[17]   Nouri A, Tetreault L, Singh A, Karadimas SK, Fehlings MG. Degenerative cervical myelopathy: epidemiology, genetics, and pathogenesis. Spine 2015; 40(12): E675-93.
[http://dx.doi.org/10.1097/BRS.0000000000000913] [PMID: 25839387]

[18]   Young WF. Cervical spondylotic myelopathy: a common cause of spinal cord dysfunction in older persons. Am Fam Physician 2000; 62(5): 1064-70.

[19]   Karadimas SK, Gatzounis G, Fehlings MG. Pathobiology of cervical spondylotic myelopathy. Eur Spine J 2015; 24 (Suppl. 2): 132-8.
[http://dx.doi.org/10.1007/s00586-014-3264-4] [PMID: 24626958]

[20]   Deora H, Kim SH, Behari S, *et al.* Anterior Surgical Techniques for Cervical Spondylotic Myelopathy: WFNS Spine Committee Recommendations. Neurospine 2019; 16(3): 408-20.
[http://dx.doi.org/10.14245/ns.1938250.125] [PMID: 31607073]

[21]   Hussain I, Schmidt FA, Kirnaz S, Wipplinger C, Schwartz TH, Härtl R. MIS approaches in the cervical spine. J Spine Surg 2019; 5 (Suppl. 1): S74-83.

[http://dx.doi.org/10.21037/jss.2019.04.21] [PMID: 31380495]

[22]   Minamide A, Yoshida M, Simpson AK, *et al.* Microendoscopic laminotomy *versus* conventional laminoplasty for cervical spondylotic myelopathy: 5-year follow-up study. J Neurosurg Spine 2017; 27(4): 403-9.
[http://dx.doi.org/10.3171/2017.2.SPINE16939] [PMID: 28708041]

[23]   Oezdemir S, Komp M, Hahn P, Ruetten S. Decompression for cervical disc herniation using the full-endoscopic anterior technique. Oper Orthop Traumatol 2019; 31 (Suppl. 1): 1-10.
[http://dx.doi.org/10.1007/s00064-018-0531-2] [PMID: 29392340]

[24]   Ruetten S, Hahn P, Oezdemir S, Baraliakos X, Godolias G, Komp M. Full-endoscopic uniportal retropharyngeal odontoidectomy for anterior craniocervical infection. Minim Invasive Ther Allied Technol 2019; 28(3): 178-85.
[http://dx.doi.org/10.1080/13645706.2018.1498357] [PMID: 30179052]

[25]   Shen J, Telfeian AE, Shaaya E, Oyelese A, Fridley J, Gokaslan ZL. Full endoscopic cervical spine surgery. J Spine Surg 2020; 6(2): 383-90.
[http://dx.doi.org/10.21037/jss.2019.10.15] [PMID: 32656375]

[26]   Tan J, Zheng Y, Gong L, Liu X, Li J, Du W. Anterior cervical discectomy and interbody fusion by endoscopic approach: a preliminary report. J Neurosurg Spine 2008; 8(1): 17-21.
[http://dx.doi.org/10.3171/SPI-08/01/017] [PMID: 18173342]

[27]   Yadav YR, Parihar V, Ratre S, Kher Y, Bhatele PR. Endoscopic decompression of cervical spondylotic myelopathy using posterior approach. Neurol India 2014; 62(6): 640-5.
[http://dx.doi.org/10.4103/0028-3886.149388] [PMID: 25591677]

[28]   Yadav YR, Ratre S, Parihar V, Dubey A, Dubey MN. Endoscopic partial corpectomy using anterior decompression for cervical myelopathy. Neurol India 2018; 66(2): 444-51.
[http://dx.doi.org/10.4103/0028-3886.227270] [PMID: 29547169]

[29]   Zhang C, Li D, Wang C, Yan X. Cervical endoscopic laminoplasty for cervical myelopathy. Spine 2016; 41 (Suppl. 19): B44-51.
[http://dx.doi.org/10.1097/BRS.0000000000001816] [PMID: 27656783]

[30]   Park SM, Park J, Jang HS, *et al.* Biportal endoscopic *versus* microscopic lumbar decompressive laminectomy in patients with spinal stenosis: a randomized controlled trial. Spine J 2019; 20(2): 156-65.
[PMID: 31542473]

[31]   Platt A, Gerard CS, O'Toole JE. Comparison of outcomes following minimally invasive and open posterior cervical foraminotomy: description of minimally invasive technique and review of literature. J Spine Surg 2020; 6(1): 243-51.
[http://dx.doi.org/10.21037/jss.2020.01.08] [PMID: 32309662]

[32]   Herkowitz HN, Kurz LT, Overholt DP. Surgical management of cervical soft disc herniation. A comparison between the anterior and posterior approach. Spine 1990; 15(10): 1026-30.
[http://dx.doi.org/10.1097/00007632-199015100-00009] [PMID: 2263967]

[33]   Hukuda S, Mochizuki T, Ogata M, Shichikawa K, Shimomura Y. Operations for cervical spondylotic myelopathy. A comparison of the results of anterior and posterior procedures. J Bone Joint Surg Br 1985; 67(4): 609-15.
[http://dx.doi.org/10.1302/0301-620X.67B4.4030860] [PMID: 4030860]

[34]   Yuan H, Zhang X, Zhang LM, Yan YQ, Liu YK, Lewandrowski KU. Comparative study of curative effect of spinal endoscopic surgery and anterior cervical decompression for cervical spondylotic myelopathy. J Spine Surg 2020; 6 (Suppl. 1): S186-96.
[http://dx.doi.org/10.21037/jss.2019.11.15] [PMID: 32195427]

[35]   Park SM, Kim HJ, Kim GU, *et al.* Learning Curve for Lumbar Decompressive Laminectomy in Biportal Endoscopic Spinal Surgery Using the Cumulative Summation Test for Learning Curve.

World Neurosurg 2019; 122: e1007-13.
[http://dx.doi.org/10.1016/j.wneu.2018.10.197] [PMID: 30404053]

[36]   Manabe N, Shimizu T, Tanouchi T, *et al.* A novel skull clamp positioning system and technique for posterior cervical surgery: clinical impact on cervical sagittal alignment. Medicine (Baltimore) 2015; 94(17): e695.
[http://dx.doi.org/10.1097/MD.0000000000000695] [PMID: 25929898]

[37]   Park P, Lewandrowski KU, Ramnath S, Benzel EC. Brachial neuritis: an under-recognized cause of upper extremity paresis after cervical decompression surgery. Spine 2007; 32(22): E640-4.
[http://dx.doi.org/10.1097/BRS.0b013e3181573d1d] [PMID: 18090073]

[38]   Lin CY, Chang CC, Tseng C, *et al.* Seizure after percutaneous endoscopic surgery-incidence, risk factors, prevention, and management. World Neurosurg 2020; 138: 411-7.
[http://dx.doi.org/10.1016/j.wneu.2020.03.121] [PMID: 32251806]

[39]   Dunn C, Moore J, Sahai N, *et al.* Minimally invasive posterior cervical foraminotomy with tubes to prevent undesired fusion: a long-term follow-up study. J Neurosurg Spine 2018; 29(4): 358-64.
[http://dx.doi.org/10.3171/2018.2.SPINE171003] [PMID: 29957145]

[40]   Fang W, Huang L, Feng F, *et al.* Anterior cervical discectomy and fusion *versus* posterior cervical foraminotomy for the treatment of single-level unilateral cervical radiculopathy: a meta-analysis. J Orthop Surg Res 2020; 15(1): 202.
[http://dx.doi.org/10.1186/s13018-020-01723-5] [PMID: 32487109]

[41]   Foster MT, Carleton-Bland NP, Lee MK, Jackson R, Clark SR, Wilby MJ. Comparison of clinical outcomes in anterior cervical discectomy *versus* foraminotomy for brachialgia. Br J Neurosurg 2019; 33(1): 3-7.
[http://dx.doi.org/10.1080/02688697.2018.1527013] [PMID: 30450995]

[42]   Li XC, Zhong CF, Deng GB, Liang RW, Huang CM. Full-endoscopic procedures *versus* traditional discectomy surgery for discectomy: a systematic review and meta-analysis of current global clinical trials. Pain Physician 2016; 19(3): 103-18.
[PMID: 27008284]

[43]   McClelland S III, Goldstein JA. Minimally Invasive *versus* Open Spine Surgery: What Does the Best Evidence Tell Us? J Neurosci Rural Pract 2017; 8(2): 194-8.
[http://dx.doi.org/10.4103/jnrp.jnrp_472_16] [PMID: 28479791]

[44]   Chiu JC, Clifford TJ, Greenspan M, Richley RC, Lohman G, Sison RB. Percutaneous microdecompressive endoscopic cervical discectomy with laser thermodiskoplasty. Mt Sinai J Med 2000; 67(4): 278-82.
[PMID: 11021777]

[45]   Deng ZL, Chu L, Chen L, Yang JS. Anterior transcorporeal approach of percutaneous endoscopic cervical discectomy for disc herniation at the C4-C5 levels: a technical note. Spine J 2016; 16(5): 659-66.
[http://dx.doi.org/10.1016/j.spinee.2016.01.187] [PMID: 26850173]

[46]   Du Q, Lei LQ, Cao GR, *et al.* Percutaneous full-endoscopic anterior transcorporeal cervical discectomy and channel repair: a technique note report. BMC Musculoskelet Disord 2019; 20(1): 280.
[http://dx.doi.org/10.1186/s12891-019-2659-0] [PMID: 31182078]

[47]   Fessler RG, Khoo LT. Minimally invasive cervical microendoscopic foraminotomy: an initial clinical experience. Neurosurgery 2002; 51(5) (Suppl.): S37-45.
[http://dx.doi.org/10.1097/00006123-200211002-00006] [PMID: 12234428]

[48]   Haufe SM, Mork AR. Complications associated with cervical endoscopic discectomy with the holmium laser. J Clin Laser Med Surg 2004; 22(1): 57-8.
[http://dx.doi.org/10.1089/104454704773660985] [PMID: 15117488]

[49]   Komp M, Oezdemir S, Hahn P, Ruetten S. Full-endoscopic posterior foraminotomy surgery for

cervical disc herniations. Oper Orthop Traumatol 2018; 30(1): 13-24.
[http://dx.doi.org/10.1007/s00064-017-0529-1] [PMID: 29318337]

[50] Kong W, Xin Z, Du Q, Cao G, Liao W. Anterior percutaneous full-endoscopic transcorporeal decompression of the spinal cord for single-segment cervical spondylotic myelopathy: The technical interpretation and 2 years of clinical follow-up. J Orthop Surg Res 2019; 14(1): 461.
[http://dx.doi.org/10.1186/s13018-019-1474-5] [PMID: 31870395]

[51] Li C, Tang X, Chen S, Meng Y, Zhang W. Clinical application of large channel endoscopic decompression in posterior cervical spine disorders. BMC Musculoskelet Disord 2019; 20(1): 548.
[http://dx.doi.org/10.1186/s12891-019-2920-6] [PMID: 31739780]

[52] Liao C, Ren Q, Chu L, *et al.* Modified posterior percutaneous endoscopic cervical discectomy for lateral cervical disc herniation: the vertical anchoring technique. Eur Spine J 2018; 27(6): 1460-8.
[http://dx.doi.org/10.1007/s00586-018-5527-y] [PMID: 29478117]

SUBJECT INDEX

Kai-Uwe Lewandrowski, Jorge Felipe Ramírez León, Anthony Yeung, Gun Choi, Stefan Hellinger and Álvaro Dowling (Eds.)